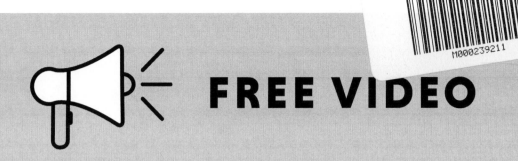

FREE VIDEO

Essential Test Tips Video from Trivium Test Prep!

Thank you for purchasing from Trivium Test Prep!
We're honored to help you prepare for your exam.
To show our appreciation, we're offering a

FREE *Essential Test Tips* Video

Our video includes 35 test preparation strategies that will make you successful
on your big exam. All we ask is that you email us your feedback and describe
your experience with our product. Amazing, awful, or just so-so:
we want to hear what you have to say!

> To receive your **FREE** *Essential Test Tips* **Video**, please email us at
> **5star@triviumtestprep.com.**

Include "Free 5 Star" in the subject line and the following information in your email:

1. The title of the product you purchased.

2. Your rating from 1 – 5 (with 5 being the best).

3. Your feedback about the product, including how our materials helped you meet
    your goals and ways in which we can improve our products.

4. Your full name and shipping address so we can send your
    FREE *Essential Test Tips* **Video**.

If you have any questions or concerns please feel free to contact us directly at:
5star@triviumtestprep.com.

Thank you!

– Trivium Test Prep Team

M000239211

CCRN Study Guide 2022-2023:

ADULT CRITICAL CARE REGISTERED NURSE EXAM
REVIEW BOOK WITH PRACTICE TEST QUESTIONS

E.M. FALGOUT

Copyright © 2022 by Ascencia Test Prep

ISBN-13: 9781637981917

ALL RIGHTS RESERVED. By purchase of this book, you have been licensed one copy for personal use only. No part of this work may be reproduced, redistributed, or used in any form or by any means without prior written permission of the publisher and copyright owner. Ascencia Test Prep, Trivium Test Prep, Accepted, and Cirrus Test Prep are all imprints of Trivium Test Prep, LLC.

The American Association of Critical-Care Nurses (AACN) was not involved in the creation or production of this product, is not in any way affiliated with Ascencia Test Prep, and does not sponsor or endorse this product.

Image(s) used under license from Shutterstock.com

TABLE OF CONTENTS

INTRODUCTION

Congratulations on choosing to take the CCRN Exam! Passing this exam is an important step forward in your nursing career, and we're here to help you feel prepared on exam day.

The CCRN Certification Process

The **CCRN Exam** is developed by the **American Association of Critical-Care Nurses (AACN)** as part of its certification program for critical care nurses. The CCRN measures the nursing skills necessary to excel as a nurse in critical care settings, including intensive care units, cardiac care units, trauma units, and critical care transport.

To qualify for the exam, you must have a current Registered Nurse license in the United States or its territories. You must also have completed a certain number of clinical hours. There are two paths for meeting these clinical requirements:

1. 11,750 hours in direct care of critically ill patients during the previous two years (875 of those hours accrued in the year before applying for certification)

2. at least five years of clinical experience with a minimum of 2,000 hours in direct care of critically ill patients (144 of those hours accrued in the year before applying for certification)

You can apply for the CCRN exam through the AACN website (www.aacn.org/certification/get-certified/ccrn-adult). You will need to provide proof of clinical hours when applying for the exam. Once you are approved, you will receive an email with directions for scheduling your exam.

The CCRN Exam

When taking the CCRN exam, you will have **three hours** to complete **150 multiple-choice questions**. Only 125 questions will be scored. The other twenty-five questions are pretest items included by the test makers to gauge their appropriateness for future exams. However, these pretest items will not be specified, so you must answer all questions on the exam.

There is no penalty for incorrect answers, so you should answer every question on the exam (even if you aren't sure of the answer).

The CCRN Adult test plan is broken into two sections: clinical judgement (80 percent) and professional caring and ethical practice (20 percent). The clinical judgement section is further broken down into five categories.

A summary of the test outline is given in the table below. The conditions included in each category are listed at the beginning of each chapter in this guide; you can also see the full test plan on the AACN website.

CCRN Exam Outline	
Category	Percent of Test
Cardiovascular	17%
Respiratory	15%
Endocrine, Hematology, Gastrointestinal, Renal, and Integumentary	20%
Musculoskeletal, Neurological, and Psychosocial	14%
Multisystem	14%
Professional Caring and Ethical Practice	20%

The questions on the exam will focus on patient care for the conditions listed in each category. You should be able to recognize the most common diagnostic criteria for each condition and understand how each condition is managed in the critical care setting.

CCRN Exam Scoring

If you are taking a computer-based exam, you will receive your score when the exam is over. If you take the pen-and-paper version of the test, you must wait six to eight weeks to receive your results.

To pass the CCRN Adult exam, you must answer **eighty-three questions correctly** out of the 125 scored questions. If you pass the exam, you will receive your certification in the mail. If you do not pass the exam, you may apply through AACN to retake the test.

You can retake the test four times within a year of your original application.

Using This Book

This book is divided into two sections. In the content review, you will find the pathophysiology, risk factors, signs and symptoms, diagnostic findings, and treatment protocols for the conditions included in the CCRN test plan. Throughout the chapters, you'll also see Quick Review Questions that will help reinforce important concepts and skills.

The book also includes two full-length practice tests with answer rationales. You can use these tests to gauge your readiness for the test and determine which content areas you may need to review more thoroughly.

Ascencia Test Prep

With health care fields such as nursing, pharmacy, emergency care, and physical therapy becoming the fastest-growing industries in the United States, individuals looking to enter the health care industry or rise in their field need high-quality, reliable resources. Ascencia Test Prep's study guides and test preparation materials are developed by credentialed industry professionals with years of experience in their respective fields. Ascencia recognizes that health care professionals nurture bodies and spirits, and save lives. Ascencia Test Prep's mission is to help health care workers grow.

1

CARDIOVASCULAR REVIEW

CCRN TEST PLAN: CARDIOVASCULAR

- Acute coronary syndrome (ACS)
- Acute peripheral vascular insufficiency
- Acute pulmonary edema
- Aortic aneurysm
- Aortic dissection
- Aortic rupture
- Cardiac surgery
- Cardiac tamponade
- Cardiac trauma
- Cardiac/vascular catheterization
- Cardiogenic shock
- Cardiomyopathies
- Dysrhythmias
- Heart failure
- Hypertensive crisis
- Myocardial conduction system abnormalities
- Papillary muscle rupture
- Structural heart defects (acquired and congenital, including valvular disease)
- Transcatheter aortic valve repair (TAVR)

Cardiovascular Physiology and Assessment

- During the **cardiac cycle**, the heart alternates between **diastole** (relaxation) and **systole** (contraction) to move blood.
  - When both chambers are in diastole, the atria passively fill the ventricles.
  - During atrial systole, the atria force blood into the ventricles.
  - During ventricular systole, the ventricles force blood into the arteries.

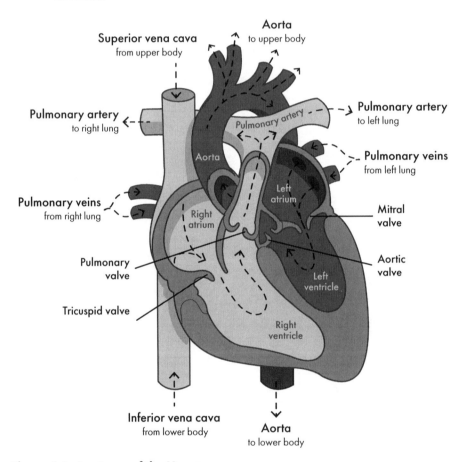

Figure 1.1. Anatomy of the Heart

- **Stroke volume (SV)** is the volume of blood pumped from the left ventricle during one contraction. Stroke volume is determined by:
  - **preload:** how much the ventricles stretch at the end of diastole (a measure of ventricular end-diastolic volume)
  - **afterload:** resistance the heart must overcome during systole to pump blood into circulation (a measure of aortic pressure and systemic vascular resistance [SVR])

□ **contractility:** the force of the heart independent of preload and afterload

Component of stroke volume	Preload	Afterload	Contractility
	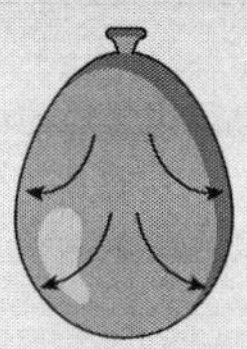	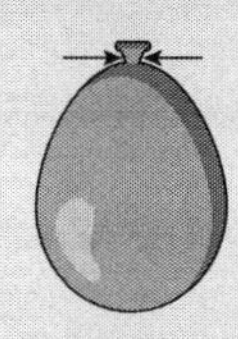	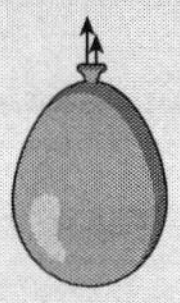
	How much the balloon stretches.	The resistance to air leaving the balloon.	The force of the air leaving the balloon.
Increase with	vasopressors IV fluids	vasopressors	positive inotropes (e.g., digoxin, dobutamine)
Decrease with	diuretics nitrates	antihypertensives nitrates	negative inotropes (e.g., beta blockers, non-dihydropyridine calcium channel blockers)

Figure 1.2. Management of Stroke Volume

TABLE 1.1. Hemodynamic Parameters

Parameter	Description	Normal Range
Blood pressure (BP)	vascular BP given as systolic blood pressure (SBP, top number) and diastolic blood pressure (DBP, bottom number)	90/60 – 120/80 mm Hg
Central venous pressure (CVP) or right atrial pressure (RAP)	pressure in the vena cava; used to estimate preload	2 – 6 mm Hg
Pulmonary artery pressure (PAP)	pressure in the pulmonary artery	8 – 20 mm Hg
Stroke volume (SV)	volume of blood forced from the left ventricle with each contraction	60 – 100 mL/beat
Cardiac output (CO)	volume of blood pumped in a unit of time (usually per minute) $CO = SV \times HR$	4 – 8 mL/min
Cardiac index (CI)	CO relative to patient size $CI = CO/BSA$	2.5 – 4 L/min/m^2
Mean arterial pressure (MAP)	average BP during a complete cardiac cycle $MAP = SBP + (2 \times DBP)/3$	70 – 100 mm Hg

continued on next page

TABLE 1.1. Hemodynamic Parameters (continued)

Parameter	Description	Normal Range
Systemic vascular resistance (SVR)	total peripheral vascular system resistance to blood flow SVR = 80 × (MAP − CVP)/CO	700 – 1200 dyne · sec/cm^5
Pulmonary artery occlusion pressure (PAOP) or pulmonary capillary wedge pressure (PCWP)	indirect measurement of left atrial pressure; uses Swan-Ganz catheter to "wedge" inflated balloon into a branch of the pulmonary artery	6 – 12 mm Hg
Pulmonary vascular resistance (PVR)	vascular resistance to blood flow in the lungs PVR = 80 × (MPAP − PAOP)/CI	255 – 285 dyne · sec/cm^5
Left ventricular end-diastolic pressure (LVEDP)	pressure in the left ventricle before systole	5 – 12 mm Hg
Arterial oxygen saturation (SaO$_2$)	fraction of oxygen-saturated hemoglobin in arteries	95% – 100%
Mixed venous saturation (SvO$_2$)	fraction of oxygen-saturated hemoglobin in veins (taken from pulmonary artery catheter [PAC])	60% – 80%
Central venous oxygen saturation (ScvO$_2$)	fraction of oxygen-saturated hemoglobin in veins; surrogate for SvO$_2$ (taken from central venous catheter)	>70%
Arterial oxygen content (CaO$_2$)	volume of oxygen delivered to tissue per unit of blood	16 – 22 mL/dL
Oxygen delivery (DO$_2$)	volume of blood oxygen being transported to tissues per unit of time	arterial = 1000 mL/min venous = 775 mL/min
Oxygen consumption (VO$_2$)	volume of oxygen used by the body per unit of time	200 – 250 mL/min

- **Heart sounds** are produced as blood moves through the heart.
  - **S1:** caused by the closure of the AV valves; indicates the end of diastole and the beginning of systole
  - **S2:** caused by the closure of the semilunar valves; indicates the end of systole and the beginning of diastole

- □ **S3 (ventricular gallop):** an extra heart sound heard after S2, caused by a rush of blood into a ventricle; a normal finding in children and young adults
- □ **S4 (atrial gallop):** an extra heart sound heard before S1, caused by the atrial contraction of blood into a noncompliant ventricle; can be a normal finding in older adults

S4 heart sound is associated with decreased ventricular compliance (e.g., hypertrophic cardiomyopathy, hypertension, or aortic stenosis).

- ▪ **Cardiac biomarkers** measure damage to heart tissue.

HELPFUL HINT:

S3 heart sound is associated with ventricular dysfunction or volume overload in the ventricles (e.g., MI, systolic heart failure [HF], dilated cardiomyopathy, or mitral valve regurgitation).

TABLE 1.2. Cardiac Biomarkers

Test	Description	Normal Range
Troponin I (cTnI) and troponin T (cTnT)	proteins released when the heart muscle is damaged; high levels can indicate an MI but may also be due to other conditions that stress the heart (e.g., renal failure, HF, pulmonary embolism [PE]); levels peak 24 hours post-MI and can remain elevated for up to 2 weeks	cTnI: <0.04 ng/mL cTnT: <0.01 ng/mL
Creatine kinase (CK)	responsible for muscle cell function; an increase indicates cardiac or skeletal muscle damage	22 – 198 U/L
Creatine kinase–muscle/brain (CK-MB)	cardiac marker for damaged heart muscle; often used to diagnose a second MI or ongoing cardiovascular conditions; a high ratio of CK-MB to CK (high CK-MB/CK) indicates damage to heart muscle (as opposed to skeletal muscle)	normal CK-MB: 5 – 25 IU/L CK-MB/CK suggesting possible MI: 2.5 – 3 IU/L

QUICK REVIEW QUESTION

1. The nurse is reassessing a patient with severe sepsis after a fluid bolus and administration of vasopressors. What hemodynamic value would indicate an improvement?

_____

Electrocardiogram

- A 12-lead **electrocardiogram (ECG)** includes 3 bipolar leads (I, II, and III), 3 unipolar leads (aVR, aVL, and aVF), and 6 precordial leads (V1 – V6).

- **Posterior leads** (V7, V8, and V9) are placed on the patient's back when a posterior infarction is suspected.

- **Right-side leads** (V3R, V4R, V5R, and V6R) are placed on the patient's right side in a mirror image of V3 – V6 when a right ventricular infarction is suspected.

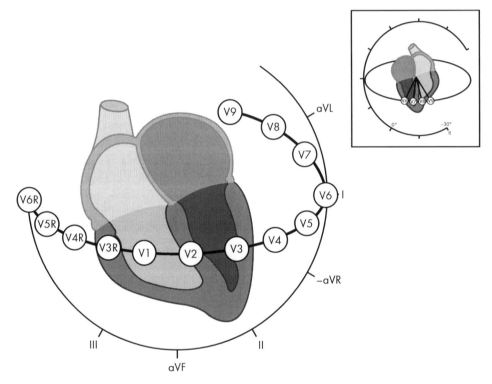

Figure 1.3. ECG Leads

- The waveforms and intervals on the ECG strip correspond to the cardiac cycle.
    - **P wave:** represents atrial depolarization and should measure 0.06 – 0.11 seconds
    - **PR interval:** represents the AV conduction time and should measure 0.12 – 0.20 seconds

- **QRS complex:** represents ventricular depolarization and should measure 0.08 – 0.10 seconds
- **T wave:** represents the repolarization of the ventricles
- **U wave:** theorized to represent late repolarization of the His-Purkinje system
- **QT interval:** represents the total time of ventricular activity (depolarization and repolarization) and should measure 0.36 – 0.44 seconds
- **ST segment:** shows the early part of ventricular repolarization

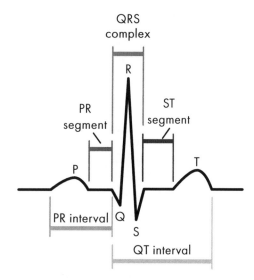

Figure 1.4. Waveforms and Intervals on an ECG

QUICK REVIEW QUESTION

2. A patient with chest pain and ST elevation undergoes a cardiac catheterization with PCI for a right ventricular infarction. The RCA was stented. After 3 hours, the patient starts having chest pain. Which leads of an ECG should the nurse focus on to identify early restenosis?

Cardiovascular Pharmacology

TABLE 1.3. Cardiovascular Medications

Category	Action	Therapeutic Uses
ACE inhibitors (ACE-Is): lisinopril, ramipril, enalapril, benazepril	lower SVR, resulting in decreased BP	• hypertension (first line) • CHF • medical management post-MI
Alpha1-adrenergic agonists: methoxamine, midodrine, phenylephrine	increase SVR, resulting in increased BP	• hypotension • shock

continued on next page

TABLE 1.3. Cardiovascular Medications (continued)

Category	Action	Therapeutic Uses
Beta-adrenergic antagonists (beta blockers): metoprolol, carvedilol, atenolol, propranolol, labetalol	lower BP and heart rate, decrease CO, and slow AV node conduction	• medical management post-MI (first line) • chronic angina • hypertension (second line) • cardiac dysrhythmias (A-fib, SVT)
Angiotensin II receptor blockers (ARBs): valsartan, losartan, irbesartan	use a mechanism of action similar to that of ACE inhibitors but cause fewer adverse effects	• hypertension (second line if intolerant to ACE inhibitors) • HF • medical management post-MI (second line if intolerant to ACE inhibitors)
Anticoagulants: warfarin, apixaban, rivaroxaban, enoxaparin, heparin	increase clotting time via various mechanisms that disrupt production of clotting factors	• known thrombosis (e.g., PE or DVT) • prophylaxis of thrombosis (e.g., after A-fib, cardiac post-op procedures) • adjunct therapy in mechanical valve replacements, MI, and stroke
Antidysrhythmics: amiodarone, flecainide, procainamide	suppress cardiac dysrhythmias and restore normal cardiac conduction	• dysrhythmias (hemodynamically stable)
Antiplatelets: clopidogrel, ticagrelor, prasugrel, aspirin	decrease platelet aggregation and inhibit thrombus production	• unstable angina • PCI/stent placement for ACS • treatment and prophylaxis for ischemic stroke
Calcium channel blockers: amlodipine, nicardipine, diltiazem, verapamil	cause coronary vasodilation, which slows cardiac conduction, decreases heart rate, and decreases myocardial contraction	• hypertension • variant (Prinzmetal) angina • artery vasospasm

Category	Action	Therapeutic Uses
Cardiac glycosides: digoxin	increase myocardial contraction, decrease heart rate, slow cardiac conduction, and increase CO	• atrial dysrhythmias (e.g., A-fib) • paroxysmal SVT conversion • HF
Diuretics: furosemide, bumetanide, mannitol	increase excretion of water and electrolytes	• hypertension • HF • edema • osmotic diuretics: ICP
Nitrates: nitroprusside, nitroglycerin	cause vasodilation, which decreases preload, afterload, and CO; reduces work effort of LV	• ACS • hypertension
Inotropic/vasodilator agents: milrinone	vasodilator; increase SV and CO	• emergent HF
Sympathomimetics: epinephrine, norepinephrine, dobutamine, dopamine	alpha- and beta-adrenergic agonists that cause vasoconstriction, increased force of cardiac contraction, or increased rate of cardiac conduction (depending on the affected receptors)	• hypotension • HF • cardiogenic shock • cardiac arrest, asystole, PEA • acute bronchospasm • anaphylaxis
Thrombolytics (fibrinolytics): tPA or alteplase, tenecteplase	promote destruction of fibrin clots	• MI when coronary angiography is unavailable • acute CVA • massive PE

QUICK REVIEW QUESTION

3. Why are beta blockers contraindicated for patients with second-degree AV blocks?

_____

Cardiac Interventions
Cardioversion, Defibrillation, and Pacing

- **Synchronized electrical cardioversion** uses electrical current supplied by external electrode pads placed on the anterior chest to reset the heart to a normal sinus rhythm.
  - Current is supplied during the R wave of the QRS complex.
  - Cardioversion is indicated for narrow-complex tachycardias, V-tach with a pulse, A-fib, and atrial flutter.
- During **defibrillation**, also known as **unsynchronized cardioversion**, electrical current is used to reset the heart to a normal sinus rhythm.
  - The electrical current is supplied randomly during the cardiac cycle, disrupting the heart's electrical rhythm and allowing the SA node's normal sinus rhythm to restart.
  - Defibrillation is an emergent treatment for patients with V-fib and unstable V-tach.
- An **implantable cardioverter-defibrillator (ICD)** can be programmed to provide cardioversion or defibrillation to prevent sudden cardiac death in patients at high risk for V-tach or V-fib.
- A **pacemaker** is a device that uses electrical stimulation to regulate the heart's electrical conduction system and maintain a normal heart rhythm.
  - **Temporary pacemakers** can include transvenous leads or transcutaneous adhesive pads attached to the chest (**transcutaneous pacing [TCP]**). Temporary pacemakers are controlled by an external pulse generator.
  - **Permanent pacemakers** are implanted subcutaneously, and the leads are then run through the subclavian vein into the heart. The device is battery operated and allows the physician to continuously monitor the patient's cardiac rhythm.

Cardiac Catheterization

- In **cardiac catheter procedures**, a catheter is inserted into a large blood vessel to diagnose and treat damage in the arteries, heart muscles, and valves.
- The most common sites for catheter procedures are the femoral, brachial, or radial arteries.
- Post-procedure complications include:
  - retroperitoneal bleeding
  - cardiac ischemic pain

- ☐ excessive bleeding
- ☐ dysrhythmia
- ☐ hematoma
- ☐ neurovascular insufficiency

ANGIOPLASTY

- During an **angioplasty**, a balloon is placed in the stenotic artery via a catheter and is inflated to open the artery. A **stent** may be placed to hold the artery open.

- **Percutaneous coronary intervention (PCI)** (also called coronary angioplasty) is used to revascularize the coronary arteries in patients with ACS.

- **Percutaneous transluminal angioplasty (PTA)** is used to widen the arteries in patients with peripheral artery disease or stenosis in the carotid, renal, or coronary arteries.

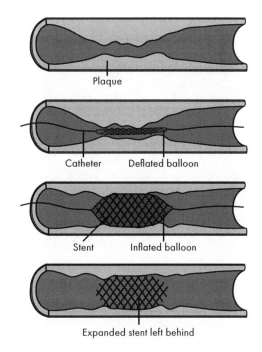

Figure 1.5. Angioplasty with Stent

CORONARY ARTERY BYPASS GRAFT (CABG)

- A **coronary artery bypass graft (CABG)** revascularizes ischemic heart tissue by diverting blood through the left internal thoracic artery or by grafting a section of the great saphenous vein to the aorta.

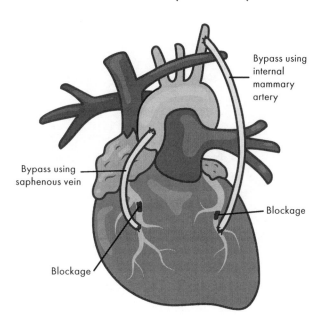

Figure 1.6. Coronary Artery Bypass Graft (CABG)

HELPFUL HINT:

Reperfusion pain—angina without the presence of restenosis—occurs in approximately 20% of patients after PCI. With reperfusion pain, the ECG should not show any significant changes, and the patient will respond to pharmacological treatment.

- CABG is performed in patients with cardiac ischemia who cannot be treated with PCI.
- Post-procedure complications include:
  - excessive bleeding or anemia (around 30% of patients will require a blood transfusion after CABG)
  - dysrhythmias (particularly A-fib): common postoperatively and may require medication or cardioversion; patient may be given prophylactic amiodarone
  - cardiac conditions, particularly perioperative MI and vasodilatory shock
  - post-pericardiotomy syndrome, due to pericardial injury; may cause pericarditis, pericardial effusion, or tamponade
  - neurological conditions, including stroke, post-cardiotomy delirium, and peripheral neuropathy

INTRA-AORTIC BALLOON PUMP (IABP)

- **Intra-aortic balloon pump (IABP) therapy** is used in patients with cardiogenic shock to increase coronary artery perfusion and raise blood pressure.
- The intra-aortic balloon is inserted into the ascending aortic arch via the femoral artery.
  - The balloon inflates during diastole and forces blood flow back into the coronary arteries.
  - During systole, the balloon deflates, which decreases afterload and increases cardiac output.
- The IABP should only be paused briefly, as thrombus formation can occur quickly.

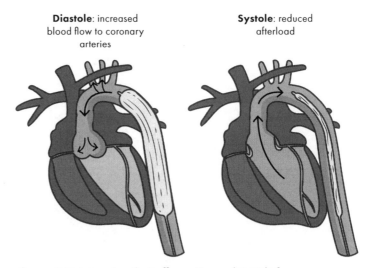

Diastole: increased blood flow to coronary arteries

Systole: reduced afterload

Figure 1.7. Intra-Aortic Balloon Pump (IABP) Therapy

- Contraindications for IABP include coagulopathies, aortic regurgitation, and dissecting/ruptured aortic aneurysm.

QUICK REVIEW QUESTION

4. A patient presents to the ED with chest pain and the ECG shown below. What priority intervention should the nurse expect?

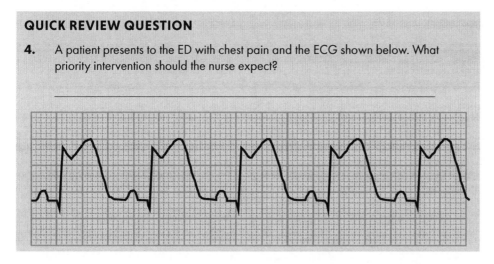

Acute Coronary Syndrome

Pathophysiology

Acute coronary syndrome (ACS) is an umbrella term for cardiac conditions in which thrombosis impairs blood flow in coronary arteries. **Angina pectoris** (commonly called just angina) is chest pain caused by narrowed coronary arteries and presents with negative troponin, an ST depression, and T wave changes.

- **Stable angina** usually resolves in about 5 minutes. It is resolved with medications or rest, and can be triggered by exertion, large meals, and extremely hot or cold temperatures.

- **Unstable angina** can occur at any time and typically lasts longer (>20 minutes). The pain is usually rated as more severe than stable angina and is not easily relieved with nitrates.

- **Variant angina** (also called Prinzmetal angina or vasospastic angina) is episodes of angina and temporary ST elevation caused by spasms in the coronary artery. Chest pain is easily relieved with nitrates.

A **myocardial infarction (MI)**, or ischemia of the heart muscle, occurs when the coronary arteries are partly or completely occluded. MI is diagnosed via positive troponin and ECG changes; it is classified by the behavior of the ST wave. A **non-ST-elevation myocardial infarction (NSTEMI)** includes an ST depression and a T wave inversion. An **ST-elevation myocardial infarction (STEMI)** includes an elevated ST (>1 mm), indicating a complete occlusion of a coronary artery.

HELPFUL HINT:

The starred topics are the ones most likely to appear on the exam.

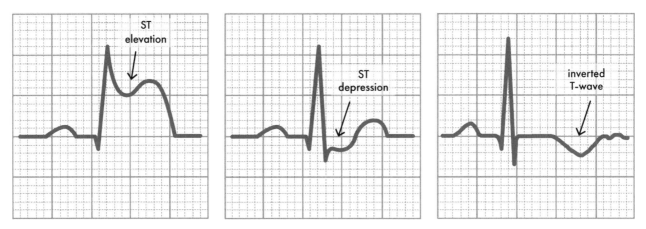

Figure 1.8. ECG Changes Associated with ACS

Signs, symptoms, and diagnostic findings for MI vary according to which coronary artery is occluded. The heart's blood supply comes from the aorta, which branches into the **left coronary artery (LCA)** and **right coronary artery (RCA)**. The LCA further divides into the **left anterior descending (LAD) artery** and **left circumflex artery**.

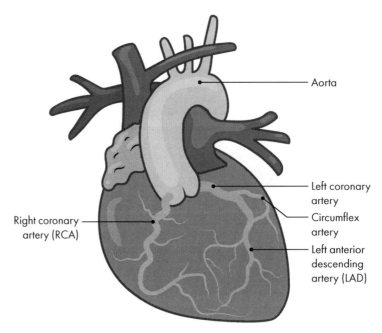

Figure 1.9. Coronary Arteries

- **Anterior-wall MI** is occlusion of the LAD artery, which supplies blood to the anterior of the left atrium and ventricle. **Septal MI** may occur alongside anterior-wall MI (but is rarely diagnosed in isolation).
  - ☐ ST changes in V1 – V4
  - ☐ increased risk of left ventricular failure (and subsequent cardiogenic shock)

□ increased risk of second-degree, type II heart block and BBB

□ increased risk of ventricular septal rupture (usually 2 – 7 days post-MI)

■ **Inferior-wall MI** is occlusion of the RCA, which supplies blood to the right atrium and ventricle, the SA node, and the AV node.

□ ST changes in II, III, aVF

□ presents with bradycardia and hypotension

□ increased risk of AV heart blocks (e.g., first-degree AV block)

□ increased risk for papillary muscle rupture

□ use beta blockers and nitrates cautiously to avoid reducing preload

HELPFUL HINT:

Papillary muscle rupture is a rare but serious complication that occurs 2 – 8 days post-MI. Patients will present with hemodynamic compromise; pulmonary edema; new, loud systolic murmur; and a large V wave in PAOP. Papillary muscle rupture usually requires immediate surgical repair.

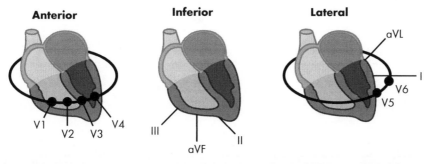

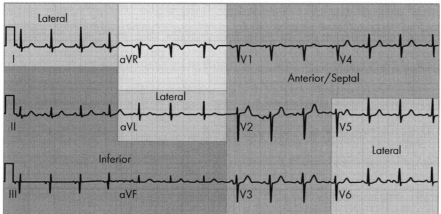

Figure 1.10. ECG Leads and Corresponding MI Location

■ **Right ventricular infarction** may occur with inferior-wall MI.

□ ST changes in V4R – V6R

□ presents with tachycardia, hypotension, and JVD

□ treat with positive inotropes

□ avoid preload-reducing medications (beta blockers, diuretics, morphine, nitrates)

■ **Lateral-wall MI** is occlusion of the left circumflex artery, which supplies blood to the left atrium and the posterior/lateral walls of the left ventricle. ST changes may be seen in I, aVL, V5, or V6.

HELPFUL HINT:

Contraindications for beta blocker use during STEMI include bradycardia, hypotension, cardiogenic shock, and heart block.

■ **Posterior-wall MI** is occlusion of the RCA or left circumflex artery, with ST elevation in V7 – V9 and ST depression in V1 – V4. Posterior-wall MI is rare but may be missed or read as an NSTEMI on a 12-lead ECG.

Signs and Symptoms

■ continuous chest pain that may radiate to the back, arm, or jaw (possible Levine's sign)

■ upper abdominal pain (more common in adults >65, people with diabetes, and women)

■ dyspnea

■ nausea or vomiting

■ dizziness or syncope

■ diaphoresis and pallor

■ palpitations

Diagnostic Tests

■ elevated troponin (>0.01 ng/mL)

■ elevated CK-MB (>2.5%)

Treatment and Management

■ pharmacological management
  □ nitroglycerin
  □ antiplatelets: aspirin and platelet P2Y12 inhibitors (e.g., clopidogrel or ticagrelor)
  □ anticoagulant (usually heparin)
  □ beta blocker
  □ morphine (only for severe pain not relieved by nitroglycerin)

■ isolated right ventricular infarction
  □ IV fluids
  □ antiplatelets and anticoagulants
  □ cautious use of nitrates, beta blockers, and morphine

■ NSTEMI: initially treated with medication (may require PCI)

■ STEMI: immediate fibrinolytics or PCI
  □ goal for door to balloon time: 90 minutes
  □ goal for door to fibrinolytics: 30 minutes
  □ post-procedure antithrombotic therapy (may include aspirin, clopidogrel, abciximab, eptifibatide, and/or heparin)

HELPFUL HINT:

Contraindications for beta blocker use during STEMI include bradycardia, hypotension, cardiogenic shock, and heart block.

QUICK REVIEW QUESTION

5. A 12-lead ECG on a patient with chest pain shows ST elevations in leads II, III, and aVF. Which medications are contraindicated for this patient?

Acute Peripheral Vascular Insufficiency

ARTERIAL OCCLUSION

Pathophysiology

Atherosclerosis, also called atherosclerotic cardiovascular disease (ASCVD), is a progressive condition in which **plaque** builds up in the tunica intima of arteries. Atherosclerosis that occurs in peripheral arteries leads to **peripheral vascular insufficiency** (also called **peripheral arterial disease [PAD]**).

Acute peripheral vascular insufficiency (also **acute arterial occlusion**) occurs when a thrombus or an embolus occludes a peripheral artery and causes ischemia and possibly the loss of a limb. This condition is a medical emergency requiring prompt treatment to prevent tissue necrosis.

Carotid artery occlusive disease (CAOD), or **stenosis**, is a narrowing or hardening of the carotid arteries, usually caused by atherosclerosis. The artery may be occluded, or plaque may break off and travel to the brain, causing a TIA, or an ischemic stroke. Carotid artery stenosis may be asymptomatic and is usually diagnosed after a CVA. It is the cause of most ischemic strokes.

Signs and Symptoms

- the 6 Ps (hallmark signs) of an arterial occlusion
    - pain (intermittent claudication)
    - pallor
    - pulselessness
    - paresthesia
    - paralysis
    - poikilothermia
- petechiae (visible with microemboli)
- ABPI <0.30 (indicating poor outcome of limb survivability)

→
CONTINUE

Diagnostic Tests

- duplex ultrasonography, CT angiography, or catheter-based arteriography
- elevated D-dimer

Treatment and Management

- medications: IV anticoagulants (usually heparin), thrombolytics, and/or antiplatelet agents
- surgical/catheter intervention: catheter-directed thrombolysis, bypass surgery, or embolectomy
  - ultrasound-enhanced thrombolysis: catheter-directed delivery of thrombolytic with ultrasound pressure
  - **carotid endarterectomy** indicated for patients with severe carotid artery stenosis
- nursing considerations
  - frequent pulse and neurovascular checks
  - do not elevate extremity
  - monitor for signs and symptoms of bleeding following use of anticoagulants or thrombolytics

---

QUICK REVIEW QUESTION

6. Catheter-directed thrombolysis is performed on a patient with an acute arterial occlusion in the lower right leg. What nursing interventions are the most important?

VENOUS OCCLUSION

Pathophysiology

A **deep vein thrombosis (DVT)** is the most common form of acute venous occlusion and occurs when a thrombus forms within a deep vein. DVT is most common in the lower extremities. Risk factors for acute venous occlusion include:

- Virchow's triad
  - hypercoagulability (e.g., due to estrogen, contraceptive use, or malignancy)
  - venous stasis (bed rest or any other activity that results in decreased physical movement)
  - endothelial damage (damage to the vessel wall from trauma, drug use, inflammatory processes, or other causes)

- pregnancy, hormone replacement therapy, or oral contraceptives
- recent surgery

Signs and Symptoms

- pain localized to a specific area (usually the foot, ankle, calf, or behind the knee)
- unilateral edema, erythema, and warmth
- positive Homans' sign

Diagnostic Tests

- elevated D-dimer
- venous duplex ultrasonography

Treatment and Management

- pharmacological management: anticoagulants (first line), thrombolytics (second line)
- surgical or endovascular thrombectomy (if medication is ineffective or contraindicated)
- inferior vena cava (IVC) filter may be placed to avoid a PE in patients who cannot tolerate anticoagulants

QUICK REVIEW QUESTION

7. A patient diagnosed with a DVT complains of dyspnea. What is the priority invention for this patient?

Acute Pulmonary Edema

Pathophysiology

Pulmonary edema (PE) is characterized by fluid accumulation in the lungs and is caused by extravasation of fluid from pulmonary vasculature into the interstitium and alveoli of the lungs. The fluid impairs respiration and may lead to acute respiratory failure.

Cardiogenic pulmonary edema develops secondary to a decrease in left ventricular function. The decrease in left-side function increases pulmonary venous pressure and capillary pressure in the lungs, forcing fluid from the vasculature into interstitial spaces. Common causes of **acute cardiogenic pulmonary edema (ACPE)** include acute decompensated HF, MI, severe dysrhythmias, hypertensive crises, valvular disease, or complications of cardiopulmonary bypass.

Signs and Symptoms

- severe, sudden onset of dyspnea
- blood-tinged sputum
- orthopnea (requiring high Fowler's positioning)
- anxiety, irritability, or restlessness
- tachycardia
- inspiratory fine crackles, rales, or wheezing
- other signs and symptoms of right-sided HF

Diagnostic Tests

- CXR shows intestinal edema
- PAOP >25 mm Hg

Treatment and Management

- immediate objective: to improve oxygenation and reduce pulmonary congestion
- noninvasive O_2 therapy (e.g., BiPAP) preferred; intubation may be required
- medications
  - □ morphine to reduce anxiety and afterload
  - □ diuretic to reduce fluid overload
  - □ vasodilator to reduce preload and afterload
  - □ medication to improve contractility
  - □ aminophylline to prevent bronchospasm (may increase risk of tachycardic dysrhythmias)

QUICK REVIEW QUESTION

8. A patient being treated for refractory V-tach develops severe orthopnea and dyspnea, and the lung sounds are coarse, with rales throughout. What is the probable cause of these signs and symptoms, and what testing is likely to be ordered to confirm the diagnosis?

Aortic Aneurysm

Pathophysiology

An **aortic rupture**, a complete tear in the wall of the aorta, rapidly leads to hemorrhagic shock and death. An **aortic dissection** is a tear in the aortic intima; the tear allows blood to enter the aortic media. Both aortic rupture and dissection will lead to hemorrhagic shock and death without immediate intervention.

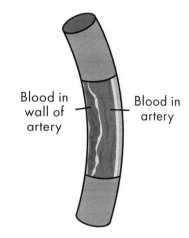

Blood in wall of artery

Blood in artery

Figure 1.11. Aortic Dissection

Signs and Symptoms

- sharp, severe pain in the chest, back, abdomen, or flank; often described as "tearing"
- rapid, weak, or absent pulse
- a blood pressure difference of ≥20 mm Hg between the left and right arms
- new-onset murmur
- diaphoresis
- nausea and vomiting
- pallor
- hypotension
- orthopnea

Diagnostic Tests

- CT scan, TEE, angiogram, or chest MRI

Treatment and Management

- pain management (usually morphine)
- beta blockers; nitroprusside may also be given
- hemodynamically unstable patients: immediate surgical repair usually required

HELPFUL HINT:

Positive inotropes are contraindicated in patients with aortic dissection because the medications increase stress on the aortic wall.

QUICK REVIEW QUESTION

9. A patient reports new-onset, sharp pain and describes it as tearing. The BP in the right arm is 85/62 mm Hg. What should the nurse do next?

Cardiac Tamponade

Cardiac tamponade is compression of the heart by excess fluid in the pericardium. The increased pressure reduces chamber compliance and filling. With enough pressure, venous return is reduced and cardiac output drops.

The onset of cardiac tamponade may be acute (usually due to trauma) or subacute. The most common etiology of subacute cardiac tamponade is idiopathic (likely viral). Other causes include malignancy, kidney dysfunction, MI, and infection (pericarditis).

HELPFUL HINT:

Constrictive pericarditis is fibrosis of the pericardial sac. It is usually chronic and is often caused by radiation therapy. Definitive treatment is pericardiectomy.

Symptoms and Physical Findings

- Beck's triad
  - low arterial BP
  - dilated neck veins
  - muffled heart sounds
- sudden and severe chest pain
  - increases with movement, lying flat, and inspiration
  - decreases by sitting up or leaning forward
- tachycardia (usually the earliest sign)
- hypotension
- pulsus paradoxus
- pericardial rub
- dyspnea

Diagnostic Tests

- ECG
  - ST elevation possible, usually in all leads except aVR and V1
  - tall, peaked T waves
- CXR showing "water bottle" silhouette in pericardial effusion
- echocardiogram may show pericardial effusion, thickening, or calcifications

HELPFUL HINT:

Positive pressure ventilation should be avoided in patients with cardiac tamponade because the pressure furthers limits venous return.

Management

- definitive treatment: pericardiocentesis or surgical drainage
- hemodynamically stable patients may be monitored while underlying condition is treated
  - maintain fluid volume
  - manage pain (positioning, analgesics)

QUICK REVIEW QUESTION

10. A patient who is 4 hours post-PCI presents with tachycardia, hypotension, dilated neck veins, and muffled heart sounds. What intervention should the nurse prepare for?

Cardiac Trauma

- **Cardiac trauma** occurs when an outside force causes injury to the heart. Cardiac trauma can cause rupture of heart chambers, dysrhythmias, damage to the heart valves, or cardiac arrest.

- **Blunt cardiac injury (BCI)** occurs when an object forcefully strikes the chest. Damage due to BCI may be caused by compression of the heart between the sternum and spine, pressure fluctuations in the thoracic cavity, or shearing forces. Because the right side of the heart is anteriorly positioned, it is typically the most affected.

  □ **Cardiac contusion** is a general term used to describe damage to the heart from blunt trauma.

  □ Common consequences of BCI include dysrhythmias; damage to chamber walls, septa, or valves; and decreased contractility and stroke volume.

  □ Management of BCI may include antidysrhythmic drugs, temporary pacemakers, medications to manage heart failure, and surgery to repair damaged heart tissues.

  □ Fluid and electrolytes should be monitored closely to preserve myocardial conduction and cardiac output.

  □ **Blunt aortic injury (BAI)** is a tear in the aorta resulting from compression of the aorta between the vertebrae and anterior chest wall. Patients with BAI are administered antihypertensives (sodium nitroprusside IV infusion) to maintain SBP <90 mm HG and usually require surgery.

- **Penetrating cardiac trauma** involves the puncture of the heart by a sharp object or a broken rib. The penetration causes blood to leak into the pericardial space or mediastinum.

  □ The most frequently affected area is the right ventricle (due to its anterior position).

  □ Blood leakage can result in cardiac tamponade, and blood loss from penetrating injuries can also result in shock.

  □ Penetrating objects should be stabilized and the patient prepped for surgery.

HELPFUL HINT:

The most common cause of blunt cardiac trauma is MVC. Any patient who experiences rapid deceleration forces during an MVC should be assessed for BCI.

HELPFUL HINT:

When assessing patients with suspected BCI, measure blood pressure in both arms; a tear in the aortic arch may create a pressure gradient between the upper extremities. An aortic disruption may also cause upper extremity hypertension and lower extremity relative hypotension.

QUICK REVIEW QUESTION

11. A patient arrives at the ED with a knife impaled in the chest. The patient is awake and alert but anxious and appears pale. What priority interventions should the nurse perform?

Cardiogenic Shock

Pathophysiology

Cardiogenic shock, a cyclical decline in cardiac function, results in decreased cardiac output in the presence of adequate fluid volume. A lack of coronary perfusion causes or escalates ischemia/infarction by decreasing the ability of the heart to pump effectively. The heart rate increases in an attempt to meet myocardial oxygen demands. However, the reduced pumping ability of the heart reduces cardiac output and the CI, and demands for coronary or tissue perfusion are not met. LVEDP increases, which leads to stress in the left ventricle and an increase in afterload. This distress results in lactic acidosis. Cardiogenic shock is most commonly seen after an MI but can be associated with trauma, infection, or metabolic disease.

HELPFUL HINT:

Left ventricular dysfunction caused by an anterior MI is the most common cause of cardiogenic shock.

Signs and Symptoms

- tachycardia and sustained hypotension (SBP <90 mm Hg)
- oliguria (<30 mL/hr or <0.5 mL/kg/hr output)
- crackles
- tachypnea and dyspnea
- pallor
- JVD
- altered LOC
- cool, clammy skin
- S3 heart sound possible

Diagnostic Tests

- CI <2.2 L/min/m^2
- PAOP >15 mm Hg

- elevated SVR, CVP
- decreased SvO_2, MAP
- elevated lactate
- ABG shows metabolic acidosis and hypoxia

Treatment and Management

- immediate goal: reduce cardiac workload and improve myocardial contractility
- immediate IV fluids
- medications given based on hemodynamic status
  - vasopressor (usually norepinephrine) for hypotensive patients
  - inotrope (usually dobutamine) and vasodilator for normotensive patients
- other interventions
  - IABP to reduce afterload and increase coronary perfusion
  - cardiac catheterization to improve myocardial perfusion and increase contractility
  - LVAD
- monitor patient for cardiac dysrhythmias

QUICK REVIEW QUESTION

12. A patient presents with tachycardia, pallor, JVD, and crackles after emergent PCI for anterior MI. What hemodynamic findings for this patient would indicate cardiogenic shock?

Cardiomyopathies

Pathophysiology

Cardiomyopathy is abnormal functioning of the heart muscles. Signs and symptoms of cardiomyopathy are similar to those of HF and vary with the location and degree of dysfunction. Types of cardiomyopathies include dilated, hypertrophic, and restrictive.

$\longrightarrow$
CONTINUE

TABLE 1.4. Pathophysiology and Management of Cardiomyopathy

Type of Cardiomyopathy	Management
Dilated congestive cardiomyopathy (DCCM) occurs when damage to the myofibrils causes dilation in the ventricles, causing enlargement and systolic impairment (<40% ejection fraction).	• beta blockers, ACE inhibitors (ARBs if patient is ACE intolerant), and diuretics • implantable defibrillator or cardiac resynchronization therapy
Hypertrophic cardiomyopathy (HCM) is an inherited disorder characterized by left ventricular hypertrophy and diastolic dysfunction. In **obstructive HCM**, cardiac output is decreased. The stiffening of the ventricle septum obstructs the left ventricle outflow tract and disrupts mitral valve function, resulting in a decreased preload and an increased afterload.	• beta blockers, calcium channel blockers, and antidysrhythmic agents • implantable defibrillator • alcohol septal ablation or surgical septal myectomy for severe symptoms • contraindicated: ACE inhibitors, digoxin, vasodilators, and diuretics
Restrictive cardiomyopathy (RCM) occurs when fibrous tissue builds up within the ventricles, resulting in diastolic dysfunction and decreased cardiac output. Systolic function is usually normal. Unlike other cardiomyopathies, in RCM the ventricles will not be enlarged or hypertrophic.	• diuretics; beta blockers and calcium channel blockers used cautiously • contraindicated: digoxin, nitrates
Ischemic cardiomyopathy is impaired left ventricular functioning caused by CAD and the resulting ischemia and ventricular remodeling.	• ACE inhibitors and beta blockers

QUICK REVIEW QUESTION

13. The nurse is completing a medication reconciliation on a patient admitted with HF symptoms and a history of HCM. Home medications include metoprolol, diltiazem, and digoxin. Which medication should the nurse be concerned about?

Dysrhythmias

A cardiac **dysrhythmia** is an abnormal heartbeat or rhythm. Dysrhythmias are typically caused by a malfunction in the heart's cardiac conduction system. Most dysrhythmias of clinical importance are caused by **reentry**: the re-excitation of the heart by an electrical impulse that did not die out. Reentry dysrhythmias include A-fib, atrial flutter, V-tach, and V-fib.

HELPFUL HINT:

When treating dysrhythmias, medical staff should always consider a hypotensive patient unstable.

TABLE 1.5. The Cardiac Conduction System

Component	Description
SA node	sets the heart's pace by sending out electrical signals that cause the atria to contract
AV node	relays the electrical impulse of the SA node to the ventricles; the impulse is delayed to allow the atria to fully contract and fill the ventricles
bundle of His	carries the electrical signal from the AV node to the right and left bundle branches
right and left bundle branches	carry the electrical signal from the bundle of His to Purkinje fibers
Purkinje fibers	endpoint of the conduction system; located in the endocardial layer; depolarize muscle cells, causing contraction of the ventricles

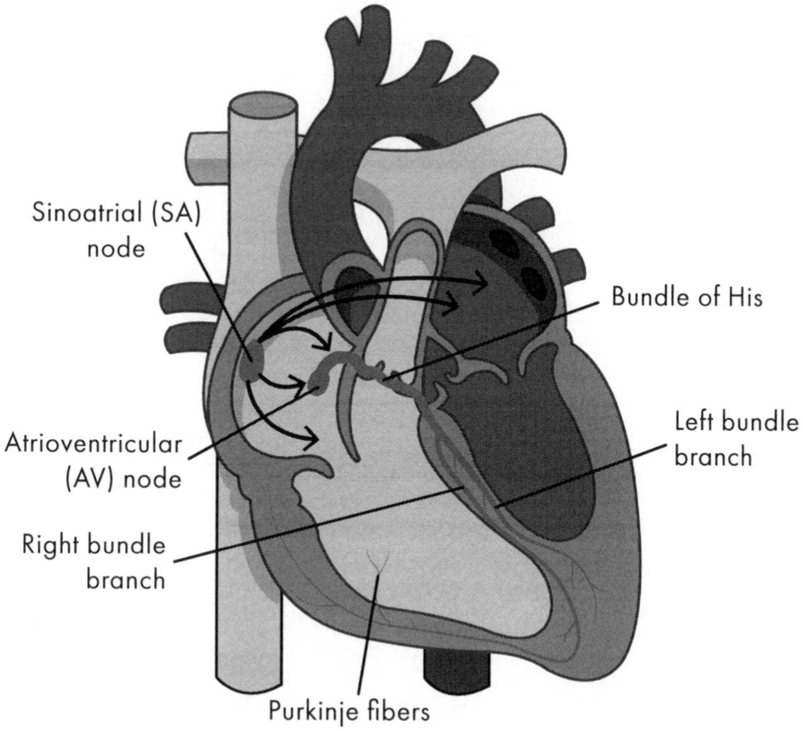

Figure 1.12. The Cardiac Conduction System

Treatment is based on whether the patient is deemed hemodynamically stable or unstable.

- Stable patients can receive noninvasive interventions or drugs as a priority intervention to correct an abnormal rhythm.

- Unstable patients should receive the appropriate electrical therapy.

BRADYCARDIA

Pathophysiology

Bradycardia is a heart rate of <60 bpm. It results from a decrease in the sinus node impulse formation (automaticity). Bradycardia is normal in certain individuals and does not require an intervention if the patient is stable. Symptomatic patients, however, need immediate treatment to address the cause of bradycardia and to correct the dysrhythmia. Symptoms of bradycardia may include hypotension, syncope, confusion, or dyspnea.

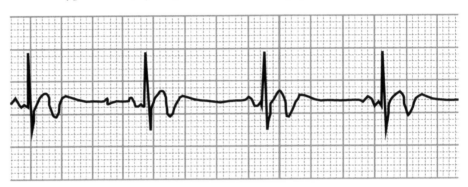

Figure 1.13. ECG: Bradycardia

Treatment and Management

- stable, asymptomatic patients: monitoring with no intervention required
- symptomatic, hemodynamically stable patients: monitor while determining underlying cause
- symptomatic, hemodynamically unstable patients: medication
  - first line: atropine 0.5 mg for first dose, with a maximum of 3 mg total
  - second line: dopamine or epinephrine if atropine is ineffective or if maximum dose of atropine already given and patient is still stable
  - patients with bradycardia and who have had a heart transplant: administer isoproterenol (atropine is ineffective in these patients)
- unstable patients who do not respond to medication: TCP

QUICK REVIEW QUESTION

14. A patient presents with complaints of confusion, dizziness, and dyspnea. The patient's blood pressure is 72/40 mm Hg, with a heart rate of 32 bpm and O_2 saturation of 92% on room air. What priority intervention should the nurse prepare for?

Narrow-Complex Tachycardias
Pathophysiology

Narrow-complex tachycardias (also called **supraventricular tachycardia [SVT]**) are dysrhythmias with >100 bpm and a narrow QRS complex (<0.12 seconds). The dysrhythmia originates at or above the bundle of His (supraventricular), resulting in rapid ventricular activation. Specific SBT rhythms include AV nodal reentrant tachycardia (AVNRT), AV reentrant tachycardia (AVRT), and atrial tachycardia (AT).

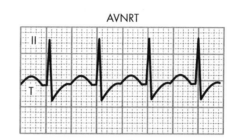

Figure 1.14. ECG: AV Nodal Reentrant Tachycardia (AVNRT)

Narrow-complex tachycardias are often asymptomatic. Symptomatic patients may have palpitations, chest pain, hypotension, and dyspnea.

Treatment and Management

- first line: vagal maneuvers
- second line: medication
  - rapid bolus dose of adenosine (6 mg)
  - second dose (this time 12 mg) if chemical cardioversion does not occur within 1 – 2 minutes
- refractory SVT
  - stable patients: calcium channel blockers, beta blockers, or digoxin
  - unstable patients and patients for whom medications are ineffective: synchronized cardioversion

QUICK REVIEW QUESTION

15. A patient in SVT is unresponsive to vagal maneuvers. What intervention is likely to be ordered next?

Atrial Fibrillation and Flutter
Pathophysiology

Atrial fibrillation (A-fib) is an irregular narrow-complex tachycardia. During A-fib, the heart cannot adequately empty, causing blood to pool and clots to form, increasing stroke risk. The irregular atrial contractions also decrease cardiac output. The ECG in A-fib will show an irregular rhythm with no P waves and an undeterminable atrial rate.

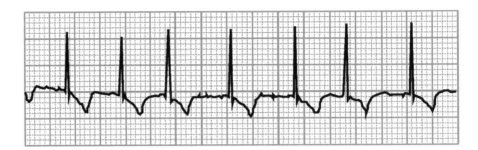

Figure 1.15. ECG: Atrial Fibrillation

During **atrial flutter**, the atria beat regularly but too fast (240 – 400 bpm), causing multiple atrial beats in between the ventricular beat. Atrial flutter can be regular or irregular. The ECG in atrial flutter will show a saw-toothed flutter and multiple P waves for each QRS complex.

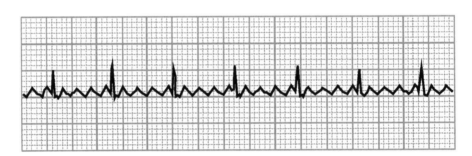

Figure 1.16. ECG: Atrial Flutter

Treatment and Management

- adenosine: slows the rhythm so that it may be identified, but will not convert dysrhythmia to a sinus rhythm
- hemodynamically stable patients: medication
  - □ calcium channel blockers, beta blockers, or cardiac glycoside to slow the rhythm
  - □ antidysrhythmics to convert to sinus rhythm
- hemodynamically unstable patients: cardioversion
- anticoagulants to lower risk of stroke
- cardiac ablation may be used to correct A-fib and atrial flutter

QUICK REVIEW QUESTION

16. A patient presents with A-fib. Vital signs are:

BP	125/80
HR	150
RR	23

What intervention should the nurse anticipate?

VENTRICULAR TACHYCARDIA AND FIBRILLATION
Pathophysiology

Ventricular tachycardia (V-tach) is tachycardia originating below the bundle of His, resulting in slowed ventricular activation. During V-tach, $\geq$3 consecutive ventricular beats occur at a rate >100 bpm. V-tach is often referred to as a **wide-complex tachycardia** because of the width of the QRS complex.

Because the ventricles cannot refill before contracting, patients in this rhythm may have reduced cardiac output, resulting in hypotension. V-tach may be short and asymptomatic, or it may precede V-fib and cardiac arrest.

HELPFUL HINT:

Torsades de pointes, a type of V-tach with irregular QRS complexes, occurs with a prolonged QT interval. It can be congenital or caused by antidysrhythmics, antipsychotics, hypokalemia, or hypomagnesemia.

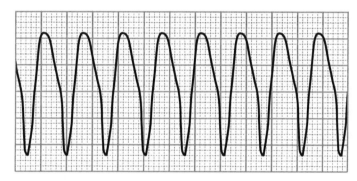

Figure 1.17. ECG: Ventricular Tachycardia

During **ventricular fibrillation (V-fib)** the ventricles contract rapidly (300 – 400 bpm) with no organized rhythm. There is no cardiac output. The ECG will initially show **coarse V-fib** with an amplitude >3 mm. As V-fib continues, the amplitude of the waveform decreases, progressing through **fine V-fib** (<3 mm) and eventually reaching asystole.

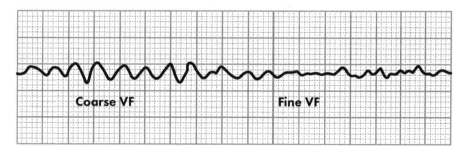

Figure 1.18. ECG: Ventricular Fibrillation

Treatment and Management

- V-fib: follow **advanced cardiac life support (ACLS)** protocols
  - □ immediately initiate high-quality CPR at 100 – 120 compressions per minute
  - □ defibrillation ASAP, before administration of any drugs
  - □ defibrillation doses: 200 J → 300 J → 360 J (biphasic)
  - □ ≥2 defibrillation attempts should be made for patients in V-fib before giving any medications
  - □ first line: epinephrine 1 mg every 3 – 5 minutes
  - □ shock-refractory V-fib: amiodarone (300 mg as first dose and 150 mg for second dose)
- priority intervention for V-tach: check for pulse
  - □ pulseless V-tach: follow ACLS protocols
  - □ V-tach with a pulse, patient stable: administer amiodarone
  - □ V-tach with a pulse, patient unstable: synchronized cardioversion
  - □ patients with recurrent V-tach: implantable defibrillator or radiofrequency ablation

---

QUICK REVIEW QUESTION

17. The nurse is participating in a cardiac resuscitation attempt of a patient found in V-fib. A total of 2 defibrillation attempts have been made, and 1 dose of epinephrine has been given 2 minutes earlier. What priority action should the nurse take next?

PULSELESS ELECTRICAL ACTIVITY/ASYSTOLE
Pathophysiology

Pulseless electrical activity (PEA) is an organized rhythm in which the heart does not contract with enough force to create a pulse. **Asystole**, also called a "flat line," occurs when there is no electrical or mechanical activity within the heart. Both PEA and asystole are nonshockable rhythms with a poor survival rate.

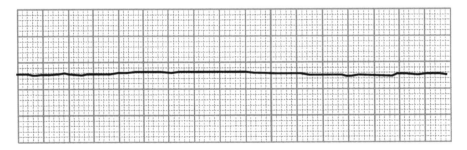

Figure 1.19. ECG: Asystole

Treatment and Management

- immediate CPR

- epinephrine 1 mg every 3 – 5 minutes until circulation returns or a shockable rhythm emerges

- immediate attempts to determine and treat underlying cause, particularly **Hs and Ts** (common causes of PEA and asystole)
    - hypovolemia
    - hypoxia
    - hydrogen ion (acidosis)
    - hyperkalemia/hypokalemia
    - hypothermia
    - toxins
    - tamponade
    - tension pneumothorax
    - thrombosis (coronary or pulmonary)

QUICK REVIEW QUESTION

18. A patient is found in bed unresponsive to commands. The patient appears cyanotic, and the nurse determines there is no pulse and no breathing present. What should the nurse do first?

Heart Failure

Pathophysiology

Heart failure (HF) occurs when either one or both of the ventricles in the heart cannot efficiently pump blood, resulting in decreased cardiac output. The condition is typically due to another disease or illness, most commonly CAD. **Acute decompensated heart failure** is the sudden onset or worsening of HF symptoms.

HF is classified according to the left ventricular ejection fraction. Impairment of systolic function results in **heart failure with reduced ejection fraction (HFrEF, or systolic HF)**, classified as an ejection fraction of <50%. **Heart failure with preserved ejection fraction (HFpEF, or diastolic HF)** is characterized by an ejection fraction of >50% and diastolic dysfunction.

→
CONTINUE

TABLE 1.6. Systolic Versus Diastolic Heart Failure (HF)

Systolic HF	Diastolic HF
• reduced ejection fraction (<50%)	• normal ejection fraction
• dilated left ventricle	• no enlargement of heart
• S3 heart sound	• S4 heart sound
• hypotension	• hypertension

HELPFUL HINT:

Cor pulmonale, or impaired functioning of the right ventricle, is caused by pulmonary disease or pulmonary hypertension.

HF can also be categorized as left-sided or right-sided, depending on which ventricle is affected. **Left-sided HF** is usually caused by cardiac disorders (e.g., MI, cardiomyopathy) and produces symptoms related to pulmonary function. **Right-sided HF** is caused by right ventricle infarction or pulmonary conditions (e.g., PE, COPD) and produces symptoms related to systemic circulation. Unmanaged left-sided HF can lead to right-sided HF.

Diagnostic Tests

- BNP >100 pg/mL
- echocardiogram to assess ejection fraction, ventricular hypertrophy, valve dysfunction
- CXR to show cardiomegaly or pulmonary congestion

Signs and Symptoms

TABLE 1.7. Signs and Symptoms of Right- and Left-Sided Heart Failure (HF)

Left-Sided HF	Right-Sided HF
increased LVEDP and left atrial pressures	increased right ventricular end-diastolic pressure (RVEDP) and right atrial pressures
increased PAP	increased CVP
dyspnea or orthopnea	increased PAP
pulmonary edema	dependent edema (usually in lower legs); ascites
tachycardia	JVD
bibasilar crackles	hepatomegaly
cough, frothy sputum, hemoptysis	right-sided S3 sound
left-sided S3 sound	weight gain
diaphoresis	nausea, vomiting, abdominal pain
pulsus alternans	nocturia
oliguria	

Treatment and Management

- goal of treatment: improve cardiac output and CI
- medications
    - first-line: loop diuretic, ACE inhibitor or ARB, and beta blocker
    - hydralazine and nitrate for patients who cannot tolerate ACE inhibitors or ARBs
    - calcium channel blockers used with caution (amlodipine or felodipine may be used to treat hypertension if first-line mediations are ineffective)
- other interventions: ICD, permanent pacemaker, IABP, VAD, or transplant

HELPFUL HINT:

Management of HF is complex. Patients will have varying needs for pharmacological and surgical interventions, depending on the type and degree of HF.

QUICK REVIEW QUESTION

19. A patient presents with sudden onset dyspnea, JVD, and peripheral edema. What laboratory test would confirm a diagnosis of acute decompensated heart failure?

Hypertensive Crisis

Pathophysiology

Hypertensive crises include hypertensive urgency and hypertensive emergencies. **Hypertensive urgency** occurs when blood pressure is >180/110 mm Hg without evidence of organ dysfunction. A **hypertensive emergency** occurs when systolic blood pressure is >180 mm Hg or when diastolic blood pressure is >120 mm Hg and when either of these is accompanied by evidence of impending or progressive organ dysfunction. Hypertensive crises increase the risk of cerebral infarction, and prolonged hypertension can lead to heart or renal failure.

Signs and Symptoms

- usually asymptomatic
- headache
- blurred vision
- dizziness
- dyspnea
- retinal hemorrhages
- epistaxis
- chest pain

Treatment and Management

- blood pressure reduction: limited to a decrease of ≤25% within the first 2 hours to maintain cerebral perfusion
- first-line medications: labetalol, hydralazine, clonidine, or metoprolol
- quiet, nonstimulating environment
- O₂ administration

QUICK REVIEW QUESTION

20. A patient is found to be alert and oriented with a blood pressure of 200/100 mm Hg and is asymptomatic. What priority intervention should the nurse take?

HELPFUL HINT:

If the R is far from P, then you have a *first degree.*

Longer, longer, longer, *drop,* this is how you know it's a *Wenckebach.*

If some Ps just don't go *through,* then you know it's a *type 2.*

If Ps and Qs don't *agree,* then you have a *third degree.*

Myocardial Conduction System Defects

Atrioventricular Blocks

Pathophysiology

An **atrioventricular (AV) block** is the disruption of electrical signals between the atria and ventricles. The electrical impulse may be delayed (first-degree block), intermittent (second-degree block), or completely blocked (third-degree block).

A **first-degree AV block** occurs when the conduction between the SA and the AV nodes is slowed, creating a prolonged PR interval. A first-degree AV block is a benign finding that is usually asymptomatic, but it can progress to a second-degree or third-degree block.

The ECG in a first-degree AV block will show a prolonged PR interval of >0.20 seconds.

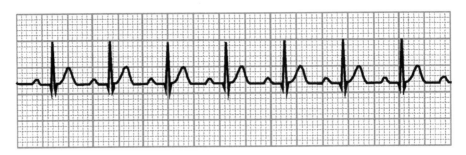

Figure 1.20. ECG: First-Degree Atrioventricular (AV) Block

A **second-degree AV block, type 1** (Wenckebach or Mobitz type 1), occurs when the PR interval progressively lengthens until the atrial impulse is completely blocked and does not produce a QRS impulse. This dysrhythmia occurs when the atrial conduction in the AV node or bundle of His is either being slowed or blocked. This type of block is cyclic; after the dropped QRS complex, the pattern will repeat itself.

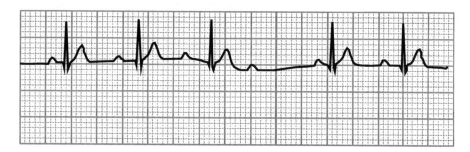

Figure 1.21. ECG: Second-Degree AV Block, Type 1

The ECG in second-degree AV block, type 1, will show progressively longer PR intervals until a QRS complex completely drops.

A **second-degree AV block, type 2** (Mobitz type 2), occurs when the PR interval is constant in length but not every P wave is followed by a QRS complex. This abnormal rhythm is the result of significant conduction dysfunction within the His-Purkinje system.

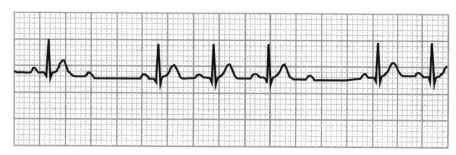

Figure 1.22. ECG: Second-Degree AV Block, Type 2

The ECG in second-degree AV block, type 2, will show constant PR intervals and extra P waves, with dropped QRS complexes.

A **third-degree AV block**, sometimes referred to as a complete heart block, is characterized by a complete dissociation between the atria and the ventricles. There are effectively 2 pacemakers within the heart, so there is no

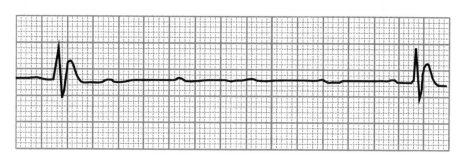

Figure 1.23. ECG: Third-Degree AV Block

correlation between the P waves and the QRS complexes. The most common origin of the block is below the bundle of His, but the block can also occur at the level of the bundle branches of the AV node.

The ECG for third-degree AV block will show regular P waves and QRS complexes that occur at different rates. There will be more P waves than QRS complexes, with P waves possibly buried within the QRS complex.

Signs and Symptoms

- first- and second-degree AV blocks usually asymptomatic
- may show symptoms of reduced cardiac output (e.g., hypotension, dyspnea, chest pain)
- bradycardia

Treatment and Management

- symptomatic patients: TCP possibly needed to manage symptoms
- implantable pacemaker if underlying cause cannot be resolved
- hypotensive patients: dopamine or epinephrine may be needed
- discontinue medications that slow electrical conduction in the heart (e.g., antidysrhythmics)

HELPFUL HINT:

Atropine is ineffective for Mobitz type 2 and third-degree AV blocks. It only increases the firing of the SA node, and the block prevents the SA node from influencing ventricular contraction.

> **QUICK REVIEW QUESTION**
>
> 21. A patient begins to complain of dizziness and weakness and appears diaphoretic. The nurse notes from the telemetry monitor that the patient has a third-degree AV block. BP is 71/55 mm Hg, and HR is 30 bpm. What interventions does the nurse expect?

SINUS NODE DYSFUNCTION
Pathophysiology

Sinus node dysfunction (SND), also known as sick sinus syndrome (SSS), refers to dysrhythmias caused by a dysfunction in the SA node. An individual with SND can have bouts of bradycardia or tachycardia or can alternate between the two. SND can also arise from an SA block or sinus arrest. Because of these irregular and usually unpredictable signals, most people with SND will need a permanent pacemaker.

- The ECG for SND will show alternating bradycardia and tachycardia and sinus arrest.

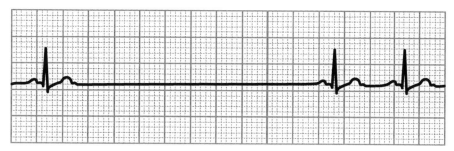

Figure 1.24. ECG: Sinus Arrest

Signs and Symptoms

- syncope
- fatigue
- dyspnea
- palpitations
- confusion

Treatment and Management

- stable, asymptomatic patients: monitoring only
- hemodynamically unstable patients: atropine and temporary pacing to correct bradycardia
- symptomatic patients with recurrent episodes of bradycardia: implantable pacemaker required

QUICK REVIEW QUESTION

22. A patient with recurring episodes of bradycardia due to SND tells the nurse that they do not want to have surgery for a pacemaker, since they currently have no symptoms. What is the nurse's best response?

BUNDLE BRANCH BLOCK
Pathophysiology

Right bundle branch block (RBBB) and **left bundle branch block (LBBB)** are interruptions in conduction through a bundle branch. Bundle branch blocks (BBB) usually occur secondary to underlying cardiac conditions, including MI, hypertension, and cardiomyopathies. LBBB in particular is associated with progressive underlying structural heart disease and is associated with poor outcomes post-MI. However, both RBBB and LBBB may occur in the absence of heart disease.

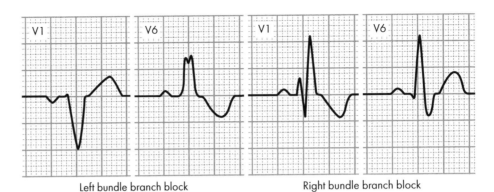

Left bundle branch block   Right bundle branch block

Figure 1.25. ECG: Bundle Branch Blocks

HELPFUL HINT:

LBBB may mask the characteristic signs of MI on an ECG.

Ischemic heart disease is the most common cause of both RBBB and LBBB. LBBB can also arise from other heart diseases, hyperkalemia, or digoxin toxicity. Other causes of RBBB include cor pulmonale, pulmonary edema, and myocarditis.

If the patient with a BBB is asymptomatic, no treatment is necessary. Patients with syncopal episodes may need to have a pacemaker inserted.

QUICK REVIEW QUESTION

23. A patient with HF develops a new-onset LBBB. What medication would be important to consider as a possible cause of the LBBB?

CONGENITAL CONDUCTION DEFECTS

- **Wolff-Parkinson-White syndrome**, caused by an early excitation of an extranodal accessary pathway, results in tachycardia.
  - □ May be asymptomatic or present as sudden A-fib or paroxysmal tachycardia with HR >150.
  - □ ECG shows short PR interval (<0.12 seconds) with a slurred QRS upstroke and a wide QRS (>0.12 seconds).
  - □ Treatment is synchronized cardioversion. Unstable patients may require catheter ablation.
  - □ Contraindicated medications include adenosine, digoxin, amiodarone, beta blockers, and calcium channel blockers.
- **Long QT syndrome** is a cardiac electrical disturbance that causes a prolonged ventricular repolarization (seen as a QT interval >0.44 seconds on ECG).
  - □ may be asymptomatic or present with dysrhythmias (especially torsades de pointes), syncope, seizure, or sudden cardiac death
  - □ management: beta blockers and placement of an ICD

□ medications likely to prolong the QT interval contraindicated

■ **Brugada syndrome** is a genetically inherited cardiac electrical pathway syndrome that is linked to 4% – 12% of all sudden cardiac deaths.

□ Diagnosed by characteristic ECG findings with sudden cardiac arrest, ventricular tachydysrhythmias, or syncopal episodes.

□ ECG shows pseudo-RBBB and persistent ST-segment elevation.

□ ECG abnormalities may be unmasked by sodium channel blockers.

□ Treated with medication (quinidine or flecainide) or ICD placement.

□ Medications likely to prolong the QT interval are contraindicated.

HELPFUL HINT:

Caution should be exercised when administering antipsychotics, antidepressants, and anticonvulsants if the QT is >0.45 seconds.

QUICK REVIEW QUESTION

24. A combative patient with schizophrenia develops torsades de pointes in the ICU. What medications may have caused this dysrhythmia?

Structural Heart Defects

■ In **aortic stenosis (AS)**, blood flow from the left ventricle to the aorta is impeded.

□ The pressure load on the left ventricle is increased, eventually leading to left ventricular hypertrophy, decreased cardiac output, and HF.

■ **Aortic regurgitation (AR)** occurs when blood flows backward from the aorta to the left ventricle.

□ Volume overload in the left ventricle leads to left ventricular hypertrophy and systolic dysfunction with a lowered ejection fraction.

■ In **mitral stenosis (MS)**, blood flow from the left atrium to the left ventricle is impeded, resulting in an enlarged atrium.

□ Almost all cases of mitral stenosis are caused by rheumatic heart disease, with most patients showing symptoms ≥15 years after the initial infection.

■ **Mitral regurgitation (MR)** occurs when the blood flows backward from the left ventricle to the left atrium.

□ This backward flow increases the preload and decreases the afterload.

■ Aortic and mitral valve disease presents with signs and symptoms similar to HF; they include dyspnea, exercise intolerance, angina, and dizziness or syncope.

- Symptomatic patients will require surgical valve repair or replacement.
- **Transcatheter aortic valve repair (TAVR)** is the replacement of the aortic valve via catheter. Common postoperative complications include bleeding, thrombosis, and endocarditis.

QUICK REVIEW QUESTION

25. What heart sound is associated with aortic stenosis?

ANSWER KEY

1. The nurse should focus on CVP as CVP is an indirect measure of right ventricular pressure and is highly influenced by fluid status. In sepsis, CVP is <2 mmHg, because of profound systemic vasodilation. Both treatments would be expected to increase preload, thereby increasing CVP.

2. As the initial MI involved the right ventricle, ST elevation changes will be enhanced with placement of leads V3 through V6 on the right side. Restenosis of the stent will present as an acute MI, whereas reperfusion pain will have little to no ECG changes and will respond to medical treatment.

3. Beta blockers depress conduction through the AV node; the reduced conduction may exacerbate an underlying AV block, resulting in severe bradycardia.

4. The patient is experiencing a STEMI and needs immediate transport to the catheterization lab for PCI for reperfusion.

5. The symptoms indicate inferior-wall MI, which puts the patient at risk for right ventricular infarctions. For patients with right ventricular infarction, medications that reduce preload (e.g., nitrates, diuretics, morphine) should be avoided.

6. The nurse should ensure strict bedrest and make sure that the affected extremity is kept straight. The nurse should also assess the site frequently and notify the physician for bleeding, coldness, increased pain, or decreased pulse. NPO status should be initiated 8 hours before reevaluation.

7. Patients with DVT and dyspnea should immediately have a CT scan ordered to rule out a PE. A PE is an emergent condition that needs immediate treatment.

8. Because of the patient's dysrhythmia and the presented symptoms, pulmonary edema should be suspected. Confirmation through a chest X-ray will reveal anomalies, especially pleural effusions and basal congestion due to accumulation of fluid within the alveolar space.

9. Since the patient describes the pain as tearing, the nurse should take the blood pressure in the other arm. A difference of $\geq$20 mm Hg can be a strong indicator that the patient is experiencing an aortic rupture or dissection.

10. The patient has signs and symptoms of cardiac tamponade, which is a possible complication following percutaneous cardiac interventions. The nurse should prepare for pericardiocentesis to drain the fluid.

11. The object should be stabilized and bleeding controlled. Two large-bore IVs should be placed for the administration of IV fluids and blood if needed. The patient should be prepped for surgery to have the object removed and to be assessed for underlying damage to organs and surrounding areas.

12. Cardiogenic shock is characterized by signs and symptoms of hypoperfusion combined with a systolic BP of <90 mm Hg, a CI of <2.2 L/min/m², and a normal or elevated PAOP (>15 mm Hg).

13. Digoxin is contradicted with this type of cardiomyopathy, as the medication is a positive inotropic and can reduce LV filling and increase obstruction of the left ventricular outflow tract. The medication should be verified with the patient, and the admitting physician should be notified immediately.

14. This patient is hemodynamically unstable because of bradycardia. The nurse should prepare to push IV atropine.

15. If the patient in SVT does not respond to vagal maneuvers, the patient will likely be administered 6 mg of adenosine to terminate the dysrhythmia.

16. The nurse should expect a hemodynamically stable patient with A-fib to receive calcium channel blockers, beta blockers, or cardiac glycosides to decrease the heart rate.

17. After 2 defibrillation attempts and the first dose of epinephrine has been given, the nurse should prepare the first dose of amiodarone (300 mg) to be given next.

18. The nurse should activate the code team and begin high-quality compressions immediately. CPR should not be delayed to administer epinephrine.

19. A BNP lab value of >100 pg/mL indicates HF.

20. After confirming that the BP reflects a hypertensive crisis, the nurse should administer an antihypertensive medication but should aim for a reduction of no more than 25% within the first 2 hours.

21. The nurse should prepare the patient for TCP. Dopamine and epinephrine may be appropriate medications to administer for a third-degree block as they will increase the overall heart rate.

22. The nurse should explain that the absence of symptoms does not mean that underlying conditions are gone. Without the pacemaker, the patient risks developing additional dysrhythmias or could go into sudden cardiac arrest without warning.

23. Digoxin, often administered for treatment of HF, has a narrow therapeutic index. Digoxin toxicity may manifest itself as an LBBB. Labs would need to be drawn to assess for digoxin toxicity.

24. There is a strong association between antipsychotic medication use and torsades de pointes in patients with prolonged QT. The patient may have been administered haloperidol, which is one of the most commonly used medications in the ICU associated with torsades de pointes.

25. In aortic stenosis, an S4 heart sound may be heard. This extra heart sound, heard before S1, is caused by the atrial contraction of blood into a noncompliant ventricle.

2 RESPIRATORY REVIEW

Respiratory Physiology

- The primary functions of the respiratory system are ventilation and respiration. The CCRN exam will focus on trauma- or disease-induced changes in these physiological functions.

- □ **Ventilation** is the inhalation and exhalation of air by the lungs.
- □ **Respiration** is the exchange of gas within the lungs.
- ■ **Lung compliance** is a measure of how easily the lungs inflate (distensibility or elasticity).
  - □ **Static compliance** is measured under no-flow conditions so that only lung compliance (not airway resistance) is being measured. Normal range is 57 – 85 mL/cm H_2O.
  - □ **Dynamic compliance** is measured during the patient's breathing cycle to measure both lung and airway elasticity. Normal range is 46 – 66 mL/cm H_2O.
- ■ **Lung volumes and capacities** are measured by spirometry at bedside in a critical care unit for clinical application in pulmonary management.
  - □ **Tidal volume (V_T)** is the volume of air exhaled after a normal resting inhalation. Normal value is 7 mL/kg.
  - □ **Vital capacity (VC)** is the maximal volume of air that can be exhaled after a maximal inhalation. It increases with height and decreases with age; the normal value is 60 – 70 mL/kg.
  - □ **Inspiratory capacity (IC)** is the maximal volume of gas that can be inspired from the resting expiratory level.
  - □ **Functional residual capacity (FRC)** is the volume of gas retained in the lungs when the patient is at rest and at the end of expiration.
  - □ **Total lung capacity (TLC)** is the volume of gas contained in the lungs at the end of a maximal inspiration.
  - □ **Normal resting minute ventilation** is the volume of air inhaled or exhaled per minute. Normal is 5 – 8 L/min.
- ■ **Ventilation/perfusion (V/Q) ratio** is the amount of air that reaches the alveoli (ventilation, V) divided by the amount of blood flow in lung capillaries (perfusion, Q).
  - □ Normal V/Q ratio is 0.8.
  - □ A **V/Q mismatch** occurs when either perfusion or ventilation is inadequate.
  - □ A low V/Q ratio (perfusion with low ventilation) causes intrapulmonary shunting (e.g., ARDS).
  - □ A high V/Q ratio (ventilation with low perfusion) causes increased dead space (e.g., PE).
- ■ **Intrapulmonary shunting (right-to-left shunting)** occurs under normal perfusion but with decreased ventilation, causing blood to enter the arterial system without being oxygenated.
  - □ PaO_2 decreases as shunting increases; $PaCO_2$ is essentially unchanged.

HELPFUL HINT:

A VC of 10 – 15 mL/kg (accompanied by a spontaneous RR of <24 breaths/min) is the minimal accepted value for weaning from mechanical ventilation.

- ☐ If left untreated, tissue demand for oxygen is unmet, leading to cellular hypoxia, lactic acidosis, and multiple organ dysfunction syndrome (MODS).
- ☐ Intrapulmonary shunting may occur because of fluid in alveoli (e.g., pulmonary edema), constriction of airways (e.g., asthma), or collapse of alveoli (e.g., atelectasis).
- ■ **Dead space** in the lungs is the volume of air that does not participate in gas exchange and is expired unchanged.
  - ☐ **Anatomical dead space** is the volume of inspired air that never reaches the alveoli. It includes the volume of air in the upper and lower respiratory tracts down to the terminal bronchioles.
  - ☐ **Alveolar dead space** is the volume of inspired air that reaches the alveoli but never participates in gas exchange. It is negligible in healthy lungs and increases because of alveoli hypoperfusion (e.g., PE).
  - ☐ **Physiologic dead space** is the sum of anatomical and alveolar dead space.

HELPFUL HINT:

Administering O_2 to patients with severe intrapulmonary shunting (very low V/Q) will have little effect on PaO_2 because air is not reaching the area where perfusion occurs.

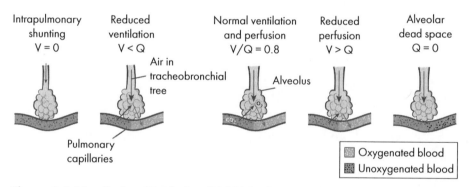

Figure 2.1. Ventilation/Perfusion (V/Q) Ratio

- ■ **Hypoxemia** is a decreased level of oxygen (O_2) in the blood (as measured by SaO_2, PaO_2, or A-a gradient). It can be caused by several different underlying pathophysiological processes.
  - ☐ V/Q mismatch (e.g., PE)
  - ☐ shunting (e.g., pneumonia, ARDS)
  - ☐ hypoventilation (e.g., sedation, brain injury)
  - ☐ impaired diffusion (e.g., pulmonary fibrosis)
- ■ **Hypoxia** is a deficiency in oxygenation at the tissue or cellular level. It may be caused by hypoxemia or other processes, including hypoperfusion (e.g., MI) or the inability of tissues to metabolize O_2 (e.g., cyanide poisoning).

QUICK REVIEW QUESTION

1. A SICU patient is now 5 hours post-extubation after a successful open-abdominal complete hysterectomy. When the nurse auscultates the patient's lungs, there are bronchial breath sounds over the lung fields, indicating consolidation, and the patient's SaO_2 is low. The surgical resident orders a mixed venous blood gas analysis after the patient is placed on an initial CPAP mask at 35% FiO_2. The nurse knows that a specific lung disease process has initiated. What physiological pulmonary process will the venous blood gas results indicate?

Respiratory Assessment Tools

- **Pulse oximetry** (peripheral capillary oxygen saturation, or **SpO$_2$**) is the noninvasive, continuous monitoring of patient's oxygen saturation.

- **Capnography** (patient end-tidal CO_2 measurement, or **PETCO$_2$**) is the noninvasive, continuous monitoring of patient's exhaled carbon dioxide (CO_2) gas. **PETCO$_2$** is used to assess:
  - ventilation status during procedural sedation
  - proper ET placement
  - effectiveness of CPR
  - physiologic dead space changes (increased gradient between $PaCO_2$ and $PETCO_2$ means worsening pulmonary impairment)

- An **arterial blood gas (ABG) test** measures the pH (acidity) and amount of dissolved CO_2 and O_2 in the blood. ABG tests provide information on acid-base balance and pulmonary gas exchange.

TABLE 2.1. Normal Values for ABG	
Elements of an ABG	**Normal Value**
pH	7.35 – 7.45
Partial pressure of oxygen (PaO_2)	75 – 100 mm Hg
Partial pressure of carbon dioxide ($PaCO_2$)	35 – 45 mm Hg
Bicarbonate (HCO_3-)	22 – 26 mEq/L
Oxygen saturation (SaO_2)	94% – 100%

  - The following tic-tac-toe method is one of many tools available for understanding the pathophysiology behind the ABG result in critically ill patients.

1. Identify the normal, acidic, and basic values.

Lower	Normal	Higher
	pH	
Acidic ←	7.35–7.45	→ Basic
	$PaCO_2$	
Basic ←	35–45 mm Hg	→ Acidic
	HCO_3^-	
Acidic ←	22–26 mEq/L	→ Basic

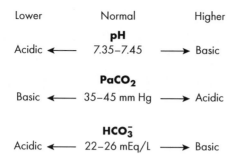

Figure 2.2. Normal ABG Values

2. Draw tic-tac-toe grid.

Acid	Normal	Base

Figure 2.3 ABG Tic-Tac-Toe Grid

3. Plug in the given values in the appropriate column.

Acid	Normal	Base
HCO_3^- 19		pH 7.5
		$PaCO_2$ 26

Figure 2.4 Example of a Completed ABG Tic-Tac-Toe Grid

4. Name the acid-base result by finding the "tic-tac-toe/3-in-a-row."

Tic-tac-toe: respiratory alkalosis

Abnormal: compensated

Acid	Normal	Base
HCO_3^- 19		pH 7.5
		$PaCO_2$ 26

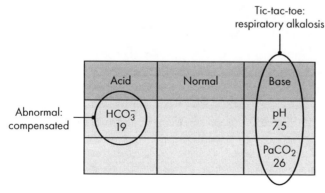

Figure 2.5 Analysis of an ABG Tic-Tac-Toe Grid

5. Determine if uncompensated, partially compensated, or fully compensated.

6. Consider possible causes of acid-base imbalance to implement plan of care.

TABLE 2.2. Common Causes of Changes in ABG Values

Abnormality	pH	ABG	Etiology
Respiratory acidosis	decreased	$PaCO_2$ increased	• asthma (late stage) • cardiac arrest • COPD • Guillain-Barre syndrome, ALS, myasthenia gravis • respiratory depressant drugs
Respiratory alkalosis	increased	$PaCO_2$ decreased	• asthma (early stage) • cirrhosis • CNS disorders • hypoxemia • salicylate overdose • sepsis
Metabolic alkalosis	increased	HCO_3- increased	• blood transfusions • GI: vomiting • hypokalemia
Metabolic acidosis	decreased	HCO_3- decreased	• DKA • GI: diarrhea • lactic acidosis • renal failure • rhabdomyolysis

■ The **alveolar-arterial (A-a) gradient** is the difference between oxygen concentration in the alveoli and the arterial oxygen concentration (A-a gradient = $PAO_2 - PaO_2$).
  □ assesses shunting and level of V/Q mismatch
  □ normal gradient is 5 – 10 mm Hg (in young adult, nonsmoker, breathing room air)

■ **P/F ratio** is PaO_2 divided by patient's fraction of inspired oxygen (FiO_2).
  □ A low P/F ratio indicates poor respiration; oxygen is entering the lungs but is not diffusing to the capillaries.

■ There are a variety of normal breath sounds.

- □ **bronchial:** high pitch, loud, auscultated over trachea
- □ **bronchovesicular:** moderate pitch, moderate intensity, upper sternum/between scapulae
- □ **vesicular:** low pitch, soft, peripheral, and basilar lung fields

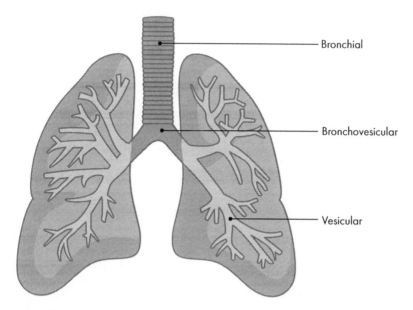

Figure 2.6. Three Types of Breath Sounds

TABLE 2.3. Abnormal and Adventitious Breath Sounds	
Sound	**Etiology**
Abnormal Breath Sounds	
Absent	• complete airway obstruction • pleural effusion • pneumothorax
Diminished	• atelectasis • pleural effusion
Bronchial sounds heard in lung fields	• pleural effusion • pneumonia • pulmonary edema
Adventitious breath sounds	
Crackles (rales)	• atelectasis • pulmonary edema • pneumonia

continued on next page

TABLE 2.3. Abnormal and Adventitious Breath Sounds (continued)

Sound	Etiology
Abnormal Breath Sounds	
Rhonchi	• asthma • bronchospasm • pneumonia
Wheeze	• asthma • bronchospasm
Friction rub	• pleural effusion • pleurisy

QUICK REVIEW QUESTION

2. A patient is in the critical care unit post-cardiac arrest with the following ABG values:

   pH: 7.30

   PaO_2: 95

   $PaCO_2$: 48

   HCO_3-: 28

   How should the nurse interpret these results?

Respiratory Gases

- **Oxygen (O_2)** is a vasodilator in lungs and a vasoconstrictor in all other vascular beds.
  - □ Room air = 21% oxygen
  - □ over-oxygenation can result in **oxygen toxicity**
    - ❑ may occur in any patient breathing >50% FiO_2 over 24 hours
    - ❑ a risk factor for ARDS
    - ❑ reduces hypoxic drive (especially with COPD)
    - ❑ clinical signs include substernal chest pain exacerbated by deep breathing, dry cough, tracheal irritation, dyspnea, absorption atelectasis, negative inotropic effects on the heart, and ocular toxicity
- **Nitric oxide (NO)** is a pulmonary selective vasodilator.
  - □ used with mechanically ventilated patients
  - □ may be an effective therapy in some respiratory diseases of critically ill adults (e.g., PH, COPD)

□ adverse effects include pulmonary edema, bronchospasm, and acidosis

■ **Heliox** is a mixture of room air (21% FiO_2) and helium (He).

□ has same viscosity as room air but is less dense, allowing it to move more easily to distal areas of lung

□ generates less airway resistance than room air

□ reduces work of breathing and assists in liberation from mechanical ventilation

---

QUICK REVIEW QUESTION

3. A critical care patient has been on >60% FiO_2 via a partial rebreathing mask for 36 hours. The patient tells the nurse about a sharp substernal pain on inhalation that worsens with deep breaths. The nurse notes the patient's RR is 22 – 24, with a frequent dry cough. The bedside monitor shows bradycardia in the 50 – 60 bpm range. What disease process does the nurse suspect has been initiated, and what serious respiratory disease process is a potential sequela?

Respiratory Procedures

FIBER-OPTIC BRONCHOSCOPY

■ **Fiber-optic bronchoscopy** is a common diagnostic and therapeutic bedside procedure in critical care units.

■ Pre- and intra-procedure medications include:

□ IV sedation

□ IV analgesia

□ pre-procedure atropine (decreases secretions, reduces vasovagal response)

□ pre-procedure IM codeine (decreases cough reflex)

■ Complications include laryngospasm and bronchospasm, vomiting, infection, anaphylaxis, and respiratory or cardiac impairment.

THORACENTESIS

■ In **thoracentesis**, a needle is inserted with local anesthetic as a diagnostic or therapeutic procedure to remove air or fluid from the pleural space.

■ Removal of greater than 1000 mL effusion fluid will increase negative intrapleural pressure and lead to **re-expansion pulmonary edema** if lung does not re-expand to fill the now-available pleural space.

- Signs and symptoms of re-expansion pulmonary edema include severe cough and dyspnea.
- If re-expansion pulmonary edema is suspected:
  - Stop procedure immediately.
  - Administer supplemental oxygen.
  - Consider positive pressure mechanical ventilation.
  - If pneumothorax develops, immediate chest tube insertion is needed.

CHEST TUBE

- **Chest tubes** (also tube thoracotomy) use suction to reestablish negative pleural pressure and re-expand the lung field; they may also be used to remove fluids from compromised thoracic spaces.
- Serial CXR is used to monitor lung improvement.
- Position patient with "good side" down so that air travels up and is evacuated by chest tube system.
- If chest tube is dislodged, immediately cover surgical insertion site with occlusive dressing and manual pressure.
- The water-seal system has a water-seal chamber, suction-control chamber, and collection chamber.
  - The **water-seal chamber** acts like a one-way valve: air escapes but can't reenter the pleural space.
  - Suction-control chamber is set to 10 – 20 cm H_2O suction on regulator.
  - Collect and measure fluid from collection chamber, per facility policy.
  - Heimlich valve is a one-way valve: air escapes but can't reenter the pleural space.

HELPFUL HINT:

Bubbling in water-seal column is normal only when used for pneumothorax. New bubbling may indicate an air leak in the system or a new pneumothorax.

EXTRACORPOREAL MEMBRANE OXYGENATION (ECMO)

- During **extracorporeal CO_2** removal, a venous catheter circuit pumps through a modified extracorporeal membrane oxygenation (ECMO) device to extract CO_2 from blood.
- ECMO is used for ARDS and COPD exacerbation.
- Contraindicated for cardiac failure.

SURGICAL PROCEDURES

Medical and postoperative nursing management of common complications of thoracic surgery may be a brief focus of the CCRN exam.

TABLE 2.4. Respiratory Surgical Procedures		
Procedure	**Description**	**Indications**
Pneumonectomy	removal of entire lung, with or without resection of mediastinal lymph nodes	• one-sided tuberculosis • unilateral bronchiectasis • malignant tumors • overwhelming hemoptysis • bronchopleural fistula
Lobectomy	resection of one or multiple lung lobes	• tuberculosis in single lobe • tumor in single lobe • cysts or abscesses in single lobe • bronchiectasis • traumatic injury
Segmental resection	resection of bronchovascular section of lung lobe	• bronchiectasis • cysts or blebs • small localized peripheral lesions
Wedge resection	removal of wedge-shaped section(s) of lung	• peripheral granulomas • blebs • small localized peripheral lesions without lymph involvement • empyema drainage • infection
Partial rib resection	removal of one or more ribs	• healing of chronic empyema
Video-assisted thoracoscopic surgery (VATS)	minimally invasive chest wall incisions with small videoscope insertion	• biopsy of lung lesions • recurrent spontaneous pneumothorax incidents • sympathectomy • adhesion lysis

■ Common complications of thoracic surgeries
  □ acute respiratory failure
  □ hemorrhage

HELPFUL HINT:

Lobectomy: position
patient with good
side down

Pneumonectomy:
position patient supine
with operative side
down.

□ bronchopleural fistula (opening into pleural space from suture line failure)

□ pulmonary edema

□ dysrhythmias

□ atelectasis (prevent through deep breathing/incentive spirometry and stabilization of V/Q mismatch)

QUICK REVIEW QUESTION

4. A bedside thoracentesis is ordered for drainage of a pleural effusion for a critical care patient. The ICU resident has determined the needle insertion site by reviewing the previously obtained chest CT scan and has appropriately administered local anesthetic prior to needle insertion. After 1400 mL of effusion fluid has been slowly removed, the patient suddenly demonstrates severe dyspnea and severe coughing. What has occurred, and what is the nursing response to this complication?

Mechanical Ventilation
OVERVIEW OF MECHANICAL VENTILATION

■ **Invasive mechanical ventilation** uses an advanced invasive airway.

■ **Endotracheal tube (ETT)** placement (oral or nasal) should be checked after intubation.

□ CXR remains gold standard for placement verification; tip of ETT should be 2 – 3 cm above carina.

□ Waveform capnography is an excellent tool to confirm ETT placement at bedside.

□ Chest auscultation simply identifies that bilateral breath sounds are present and equal, and not in stomach or right main-stem bronchus.

□ Cuff pressure should be 20 – 30 cm H_2O.

■ **Tracheostomy tubes** are placed emergently for obstruction and used for long-term ventilator support.

□ Deflate cuff and place one-way valve for patient to talk.

□ Always keep an extra trach tube at bedside (document every shift).

■ **Volume-limited ventilation** delivers a set volume.

□ **Assist-control (AC) ventilation** always delivers a set V_T and set respiratory rate (RR).

❏ Spontaneous patient breath receives full-delivery V_T.

❏ RR maintained even with spontaneous breaths.

❏ Requires neuromuscular blockade to not "fight vent."

- **Synchronized intermittent mandatory ventilation (SIMV)** always delivers a set V_T and a set RR.
  - Spontaneous patient breath receives only patient's own V_T.
  - Each ventilator breath is synchronized with patient's own RR.
  - Use sedation or neuromuscular blockade, per patient's needs.
- During **pressure-support ventilation (PSV)**, patient-initiated breaths receive positive pressure support on inspiration.
  - decreases work of breathing
  - very effective during weaning from ventilator
  - need backup apnea mode
- Ventilator settings
  - RR: 8 – 20 breaths/min
  - V_T: customized to the patient's predicted body weight (as part of lung-protective ventilation [LPV] bundles) to prevent volutrauma (6 – 8 mL/kg of patient's body weight)
  - The lowest tolerated FiO_2 should be used to maintain SaO_2 without oxygen toxicity.
  - **Positive end-expiratory pressure (PEEP)** is positive pressure applied at the end of exhalation to prevent the passive emptying of the lung, which causes end-expiratory alveolar collapse.
    - PEEP increases alveolar recruitment and allows for more gas exchange.
    - Complications of PEEP include barotrauma, decreased blood pressure and cardiac output, and air-leak disorders.
    - For most patients, extrinsic PEEP is set at 5 cm H_2O.
  - The normal **inspiratory-expiratory (I:E) ratio** is 1:2.
  - The **inspiratory flow rate** is usually set with a peak rate of 60 L/min.
- **Noninvasive ventilation (NIV)** uses a noninvasive interface such as a face mask or mouthpiece.
  - **Continuous positive airway pressure (CPAP)** delivers a single level of pressure for both inspiration and expiration. It is primarily used for obstructive sleep apnea and cardiogenic pulmonary edema.
  - **Bilevel positive airway pressure (BiPAP or BPAP)** delivers two levels of positive airway pressure, IPAP and EPAP.
    - **Inspiratory positive airway pressure (IPAP)** enhances airflow and augments patient's V_T; corresponds to pressure support.
    - **Expiratory positive airway pressure (EPAP)** reduces amount of pressure to ease expiratory effort; corresponds to PEEP.

HELPFUL HINT:

Asynchrony occurs when ventilator gas-flow delivery is not efficiently matched to the patient's needs. Machine-delivered breaths may be early or late, or the flow rate may not meet the patient's needs.with operative side down.

HELPFUL HINT:

Volutrauma is injury due to mechanical settings that deliver excessive volume to the alveoli. Ventilated patients with ARDS are at high risk for volutrauma and should receive a lower V_T.

- NIV may be used as an alternative to mechanical ventilation, with fewer risks; it reduces airway injuries, ventilator-associated pneumonia (VAP), and length of stay.
- Contraindications for NIV include:
  - life-threatening conditions, including hypoxemia and dysrhythmias
  - high risk of airway obstruction

QUICK REVIEW QUESTION

5. What is PEEP, and what are the complications of this therapy?

LIBERATION FROM MECHANICAL VENTILATION

- Critical care facilities have specific parameters for liberating patients from mechanical ventilation. Some general parameters are:
  - The patient must be awake and be able to follow commands, perform chin-to-chest movement, lift their head from the pillow, and protect their airway by coughing and deep breathing.
  - ABGs must reflect stabilization of underlying respiratory disease pathology.
  - The Richmond Agitation-Sedation Scale (RASS) must provide evidence of patient tolerance to lightened sedation and analgesia and daily "sedation holidays" that are part of facility-specific protocols.
  - Most patients are off vasopressors.
  - Nutrition status, especially phosphate and albumin levels, has been optimized.
- If all the above criteria are satisfactory, the following are generally accepted parameters for successful liberation from mechanical ventilation:
  - positive expiratory pressure >30 cm H_2O
  - vital capacity >10 mL/kg
  - spontaneous V_T >5 mL/kg
  - FiO_2 <50%
  - minute volume <10 L/min
  - rapid shallow breathing index (RSBI) <105 breaths/min/L
  - negative inspiratory force (NIF) <−20 cm H_2O
- The US Agency for Healthcare Research and Quality (AHRQ) has recommended specific protocols that coordinate the use of **spontaneous**

awakening trials (SAT) and **spontaneous breathing trials (SBT)** to evaluate patients' tolerance for removal from mechanical ventilation.

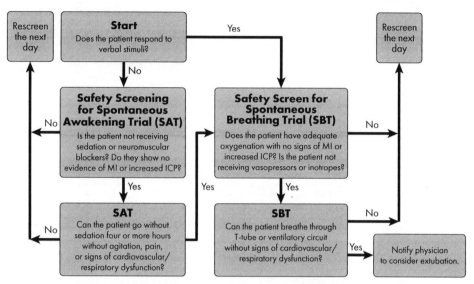

Figure 2.7. Summary of AHRQ Protocols for SAT and SBT

- Post-extubation adverse events include:
  - stridor: treated with heliox and steroids to reduce subglottal inflammation
  - post-extubation laryngeal edema: airway obstruction from ETT-generated mucosal damage that may require emergent re-intubation

QUICK REVIEW QUESTION

6. A patient has been successfully liberated from mechanical ventilation after 6 days of intubation, where the oral ETT soft cuff pressure was monitored at every shift and maintained at 20 – 25 cm H_2O, and ETT was repositioned in the mouth, per facility protocol. Then, 5 hours post-extubation, the patient's voice is raspy and they say their throat "feels tight." What does the nurse suspect is occurring?

_____

VENTILATOR-ASSOCIATED EVENTS

- Patients on mechanical ventilation are at high risk for ventilator-associated events (VAE).
  - **ventilator-associated conditions (VAC)**, which include atelectasis, fluid overload, and ARDS
  - **infection-related ventilator-associated conditions (IVAC)**, which include VAP

- The Society of Critical Care Medicine (SCCM) recommends the implementation of an LPV bundle and the ABCDEF bundle to reduce VAP.
  - LPV bundle
    - If $PaCO_2$ is in the tic-tac-toe, the imbalance is respiratory.
    - If HCO_3 is in the tic-tac-toe, the imbalance is metabolic.
    - If pH is normal, ABG is fully compensated; the body has done its job.
    - If pH is abnormal and the remaining value (not the tic-tac-toe/3-in-a-row) is abnormal, then the ABG is partially compensated: the body is trying but is not able to maintain acid-base balance.
    - If pH is abnormal and the remaining value is normal, then the ABG is uncompensated: the body isn't doing anything to fix the problem.
    - chest tube blood loss >100 mL
    - sudden increase in blood loss
    - place patient operative side down
    - emergent return to OR necessary for repair
    - emergent chest tube placement may be done at bedside to drain fluid
    - head of bed raised 30 – 45 degrees (to prevent aspiration)
    - oral care (chlorhexidine every 2 hours)
    - subglottic suction protocol
    - low VT settings
    - Choice of analgesia and sedation: treat pain before sedation, and routinely assess for agitation and depth of sedation
    - Delirium assessment and management
    - Early mobility and exercise
    - Family engagement and empowerment
  - ABCDEF bundle
    - Assess, prevent, and manage pain
    - Both SAT and SBT (see "Liberation from Mechanical Ventilation" section on page 58)
- Additional interventions to prevent VAE include:
  - GI prophylaxis
  - DVT prophylaxis
  - IV fluid administration (prevent fluid overload or dehydration)
  - vigilant monitoring for sepsis, per facility protocol (with targeted antibiotic therapy as needed)

QUICK REVIEW QUESTION

7.   What components of the LPV bundle help prevent VAP in the critical care setting?

Acute Pulmonary Embolus

Pathophysiology

A **pulmonary embolus (PE)** is a thromboembolus that occludes a pulmonary artery. The most common embolus is a blood clot caused by deep vein thrombosis (DVT), but fat emboli, tumor emboli, and amniotic fluid emboli can also reach the lungs.

Damage to the lungs during PE follows several pathways. The occlusion increases pulmonary dead space and causes V/Q mismatch, resulting in pulmonary shunting and hypoxemia. PE may also trigger bronchoconstriction and disrupt surfactant functioning, resulting in atelectasis and worsening hypoxemia.

Pulmonary hypertension develops from both the mechanical obstruction (clot) and the release of an injury-site mediator that causes pulmonary vasoconstriction. These processes elevate pulmonary vascular resistance (PVR), which in turn increases right ventricular workload and eventually results in right ventricular failure. Left ventricular preload decreases, cardiac output drops, hypotension follows, and shock occurs.

Etiology

- trauma (high risk with fracture)
- surgery
- A-fib
- immobility
- hypercoagulability states

Signs and Symptoms

- pleuritic chest pain
- tachycardia
- tachypnea and dyspnea
- hemoptysis

- increased pulmonary S2
- sudden onset
  - increased PA pressures
  - right-sided HF

Diagnostic Findings

- ABG showing low PaO_2
- increased A-a gradient
- V/Q scan (25% – 30% accuracy)
- spiral CT scan: a 30-second study with >90% sensitivity/specificity
- pulmonary angiogram: definitive diagnosis but with long study time
- ultrasound for DVT in lower extremities
- 12-lead ECG
  - tall, peaked T waves in II, III, aVF
  - transient RBBB
  - right-axis deviation
- D-dimer positive
- $ETCO_2$ value ≥ 36 rules out PE with high reliability

Treatment and Management

- IV fluid resuscitation
- IV anticoagulants once diagnosis is confirmed
- thrombolytics for unstable patients with no contraindications
- supportive treatment for symptoms
  - O_2 therapy
  - analgesics
  - vasopressors to manage blood pressure

QUICK REVIEW QUESTION

8. A 52-year-old patient is admitted to the critical care unit with tachycardia, tachypnea, hemoptysis, and chest pain. The patient is currently hemodynamically stable, and a diagnosis of a PE is suspected. What diagnostic study should the nurse expect to be ordered to confirm the diagnosis?

Acute Respiratory Distress Syndrome

Pathophysiology

Acute respiratory distress syndrome (ARDS) is a sudden and progressive form of **noncardiogenic pulmonary edema (NPE)** in which the alveoli fill with fluid following damage to the pulmonary endothelium. ARDS is the systemic response to lung injury and is initiated by the inflammatory-immune system, which releases inflammatory mediators from the site of injury within 24 – 48 hours.

There are three phases of ARDS, but the CCRN exam focuses on phase 1, the exudative phase. When inflammatory mediators injure pulmonary capillaries, the resultant permeability allows blood, proteins, fibrin, and other mediators to leak into the pulmonary interstitium, causing interstitial edema. This fluid is then forced back into the alveoli, causing alveolar edema. The combination of edema and protein in the alveolar fluid disrupts surfactant production, causing the alveoli to stiffen and collapse.

NPE with refractory hypoxemia ensues because of intrapulmonary shunting and V/Q mismatch. Compression also increases the work of breathing, decreases lung compliance, and reduces the functional residual capacity of the lungs. Hypoxic vasoconstriction, microthrombi, and patient fatigue all lead to increased alveolar dead space and pulmonary hypertension, which increases the right ventricular afterload. As increased right ventricular dysfunction continues, cardiac output is reduced.

Etiology

- gastric aspiration, pneumonia
- chemotherapy, transthoracic radiation
- toxic inhalation
- pulmonary contusion
- sepsis
- DIC
- pancreatitis
- TRALI

Signs and Symptoms

- restlessness, anxiety
- tachypnea with increased accessory-muscle usage for work of breathing

---

HELPFUL HINT:

Historically, respiratory distress with a P/F ratio between 200 and 300 was referred to as acute lung injury (ALI). That term is generally no longer used; instead, ARDS has been divided into mild, moderate, and severe, based on the P/F ratio.

HELPFUL HINT:

Hypermetabolism is an increase in resting energy expenditure often seen in critically ill patients. It is a complex stress response that impairs glucose metabolism, increases risk of infection, and impairs tissue healing. Adequate and early parenteral nutrition is vital to manage hypermetabolism in trauma, SIRS, and ARDS patients.

- elevated PAP
- PAOP normal or low
- progressive hypoxemia
- lungs clear initially; fine crackles as ARDS progresses
- decreased urine output
- tachycardia and hypotension

Diagnostic Findings

- CXR showing pulmonary infiltrates, ground-glass opacity, and an elevated diaphragm
- ABG findings
  - decreasing P/F ratio
    - <300 = mild ARDS
    - <200 = moderate ARDS
    - <100 = severe ARDS
  - refractory hypoxemia
  - increasing hypercapnia
- bronchoscopy showing increase in neutrophils and protein in aspirate
- lab results
  - lactic acidosis
  - elevated SGOT, ALP, bilirubin
  - increased PT/aPTT
  - decreased albumin

Treatment and Management

- use LPV methods
  - goal for reversing hypoxemia and preventing oxygen toxicity: PaO_2 = 55 – 65 mm Hg
  - PEEP: set at lowest possible amount (10 – 15 cm H_2O) to decrease intrapulmonary shunting while improving P/F ratio
  - low V_T (4 – 6 mL/kg) to reduce barotrauma and volutrauma
  - increased mechanical respiratory rate (20 – 30 breaths/min) for sufficient CO_2 elimination in low V_T settings
  - end-inspiratory plateau pressure goal: <30 cm H_2O
  - permissive hypercapnia with arterial pH ≥7.20 to avoid cardiopulmonary effects of acidosis
    - administer IV $NaHCO_3$

HELPFUL HINT:

Low PEEP can cause decreased cardiac output and hypotension.

- ❑ increase RR ventilator settings
  - ❑ increase V_T ventilator settings
- ▪ neuromuscular blockade agent; peripheral nerve stimulator (train of four) to titrate paralytic doses, with goal of $1 - 2$ twitches
- ▪ prone positioning to reduce damage to dependent areas of lungs
  - ☐ initiated early in treatment
  - ☐ maintained >16 hr/day
- ▪ improve tissue perfusion
  - ☐ low PAOP (intravascular volume) at $5 - 8$ mm Hg through fluid restriction and diuretics
  - ☐ positive inotropic therapy and other vasoactive medications to maintain cardiac output

QUICK REVIEW QUESTION

9. A 68-year-old patient was admitted from the ED to the critical care unit for aspiration pneumonitis after being found in bed, lethargic, weak, and confused, with dried vomit on their clothing and gurgling respirations. CXR shows bilateral lung infiltrates. Vital signs: temperature 38.4°C (101.2°F) oral, HR 118 bpm, RR labored at 26 breaths/min, BP 86/50 mm Hg. Fine bibasilar crackles are auscultated, and pulse oximetry reads 83%. ABG on 3 L nasal cannula shows a pH = 7.29, $PaCO_2$ = 62 mm Hg, PaO_2 = 55 mm Hg, and HCO_3^- = 24 mEq/L. The patient is intubated to correct uncompensated respiratory acidosis with hypoxemia secondary to aspiration pneumonitis and ARDS. What components of LPV would be included for this patient?

Acute Respiratory Failure

Pathophysiology

Acute respiratory failure is a critical condition of the respiratory system marked by insufficient gas exchange and pulmonary inflammation caused by direct or indirect injury to the lungs. Acute respiratory failure may be characterized by hypoxemia (acute hypoxemic respiratory failure), hypercapnia (acute hypercapnic respiratory failure), or both. Hypoxemia symptoms are related to impaired oxygen exchange in lung fields; hypercapnia symptoms are related to the retention and inability to clear carbon dioxide, even in the presence of increased FiO_2 delivery.

HELPFUL HINT:

Contraindications for permissive hypercapnia include pulmonary hypertension, increased ICP, heart failure, and seizures.

HELPFUL HINT:

Refractory hypoxemia—low oxygen levels that do not respond to increased FiO_2—is a hallmark of respiratory failure.

$\longrightarrow$
CONTINUE

TABLE 2.5. Types of Acute Respiratory Failure

Type	Description	Etiology
Type 1	hypoxemic: failure of O_2 exchange, with PaO_2 <60 mm Hg	• ARDS • atelectasis • PE • pneumonia
Type 2	hypercapnic: failure of CO_2 exchange, with $PaCO_2$ >45 mm Hg	• airway obstruction • blunt or penetrating trauma • COPD • drug overdose (e.g., opioids) • postoperative state • neuromuscular disease • spinal injury
Type 3	combined: failure of O_2 and CO_2 exchange, with PaO_2 <60 mm Hg and $PaCO_2$ >45 mm Hg	• ARDS • asthma • COPD

Signs and Symptoms

- hypoxemic
  - increased work of breathing
  - increased minute ventilation
  - tachypnea
  - dysrhythmias
- hypercapnic
  - reduced RR
  - altered mental status (including delirium and paranoia)
  - decreased LOC

Diagnostic Findings

- hypoxemia
  - PaO_2 <60 mm Hg
- hypercapnia
  - $PaCO_2$ >45 mm Hg
  - increased A-a gradient (>20 mm Hg)
  - pH <7.35 (in patients with acute hypercapnia)

Treatment and Management

- primary goals: improve ventilation and treat underlying etiology
- airway support (e.g., suctioning) as needed
- high FiO_2 likely needed, but should be reduced as quickly as possible
- noninvasive or invasive mechanical ventilation as needed
  - □ BiPAP for hypercapnic failure
  - □ CPAP for hypoxic failure
- ECMO for hypercapnia
- monitor and manage cardiac complications

QUICK REVIEW QUESTION

10. A patient with COPD develops acute-on-chronic hypercapnia ($PaCO_2$ 55 mm Hg and pH 7.30) that is unresponsive to bronchodilators and administration of oxygen via nasal cannula. The patient is hemodynamically stable. What intervention should the nurse anticipate?

Acute Respiratory Infection

Pathophysiology

Pneumonia is a lower respiratory tract infection that causes inflammation and consolidation in the alveoli. It is classified according to how it was acquired. **Community-acquired pneumonia (CAP)** is contracted in the community. **Hospital-acquired pneumonia (HAP)**, also called **nosocomial pneumonia**, is contracted in a medical care setting. Patients with gastric feeding tubes are at a higher risk of **aspiration pneumonia** caused by inhalation of oropharyngeal secretions. Patients who have been intubated are at risk for VAP. Signs, symptoms, and treatment of CAP, HAP, aspiration pneumonia, and VAP are similar.

Signs and Symptoms

- productive cough
- pleuritic chest pain
- fever
- dyspnea
- hemoptysis
- abnormalities in affected lung/lobe
  - □ decreased lung sounds
  - □ inspiratory crackles
  - □ dull percussion

Diagnostic Tests and Findings

- elevated WBC count
- CXR showing infiltrates
- positive blood cultures or sputum cultures

Treatment and Management

- oxygen adjuncts or mechanical ventilation where necessary
- broad-spectrum antibiotics until cultures determine sensitivity
- adequate hydration
- good pulmonary hygiene and chest physiotherapy

HELPFUL HINT:

In patients with unilateral lung disease (e.g., right lung pneumonia), the patient should be positioned with the "good" lung down to promote blood flow and perfusion in the healthy lung.

QUICK REVIEW QUESTION

11. A 70-year-old patient is transported from a nursing home with complaints of dyspnea, fever, chills, and a productive cough with thick brown sputum. The patient's pulse oximetry reading is 86% on room air. What are the first actions the nurse should take?

Aspiration

Pathophysiology

Pulmonary aspiration is the entry of foreign bodies or material from the mouth or GI tract into the upper and/or lower respiratory tract. The acidity of the ingested material damages alveoli and capillaries, resulting in inflammation, decreased lung compliance, and possible pulmonary edema.

Etiology

- mechanical ventilation
- NG tube, tracheostomy, or bronchoscopy
- sedation or other altered LOC
- dysphagia
- stroke
- seizures

Signs and Symptoms

- coughing
- dyspnea

- choking
- diminished breath sounds in affected lobe
- crackles
- reduced SaO_2 or SpO_2

Diagnostic Tests and Findings

- CXR, spiral CT scan showing pulmonary infiltrates
- elevated WBC, increasing lactic acid, and positive blood cultures

Treatment and Management

- preventative measures to decrease risk
  - HOB elevated $\geq 30°$, if not contraindicated
  - minimal amount of sedation for patient comfort
  - airway clearing and suctioning, where appropriate
  - maintain endotracheal cuff pressure <30 cm H_2O
  - assess placement of gastric tubes per sepsis protocols
  - continuous feedings instead of bolus; feeding tolerance assessed by monitoring residual formula
  - swallow assessment on extubated patients before PO delivery
- sepsis protocol

QUICK REVIEW QUESTION

12. An 84-year-old nursing home patient with dementia, a right-side CVA 10 years ago, residual lower extremity weakness, bilateral knee contractures, mild dysphagia, and a history of GERD is transferred to the MICU after 2 – 3 days of increasing lethargy. On arrival, the nurse notes a temperature of 38.5°C (101.3°F) oral, tachycardia, dyspnea, and SpO_2 of 88% on 4 L nasal cannula. Lung sounds are diminished in the RLL, with fine, scattered crackles. CXR on admission shows right-sided pulmonary infiltrates. Which diagnosis would the nurse expect, and which actions should be prioritized?

Chronic Conditions

- The conditions in this section are included in the CCRN text framework but are usually not covered in depth on the exam. Test takers should be familiar with the basic pathophysiology of the conditions and management of acute exacerbations in critical care settings.

- **Chronic obstructive pulmonary disease (COPD)** is characterized by a breakdown in alveolar tissue (emphysema), chronic productive cough (chronic bronchitis), and long-term obstruction of the airways; the condition worsens over time.
  - The most common cause of COPD is smoking, although the disease can be caused by other inhaled irritants (e.g., smoke, industrial chemicals, other air pollution).
  - COPD is characterized by low expiratory flow rates.
  - Acute exacerbations of COPD are characterized by increased sputum production and hypoxia or hypercapnia, which may require emergent treatment.
  - Dysrhythmias are a common complication of acute exacerbations.
  - First-line management of COPD is bronchodilators (not inhaled corticosteroids) such as short-acting beta agonists and anticholinergics with cautious use of oxygen (titrated to SaO_2 88% – 92% or PaO_2 of 60 mm Hg).
  - When administering oxygen, vigilantly monitor for hypercapnia.
  - Intubation is required if respiratory distress is accompanied by progressive deterioration of hemodynamic stability.
- **Pulmonary fibrosis** is a chronic, progressive lung disease in which the tissue surrounding the alveoli is damaged, leading to thickening, scarring, and impaired lung function.
  - Most cases of pulmonary fibrosis are idiopathic, but the condition has been linked to smoking and exposure to some environmental pollutants.
  - Secondary complications include pulmonary hypertension and right-sided HF.
  - Acute exacerbations of pulmonary fibrosis may present with signs and symptoms similar to respiratory infection, PE, or pneumothorax.
  - Management of acute exacerbations of pulmonary fibrosis is supportive and includes O_2 (with possible mechanical ventilation) and corticosteroids.
- **Pulmonary hypertension (PH)** is clinically defined as a mean PAP ≥ 25 mm Hg measured via right heart catheterization.
  - PH can be hereditary, idiopathic, or secondary to other conditions, including connective tissue disease, left heart disease, respiratory disease, and PE.
  - Compensated PH is characterized by normal cardiac output and RAP with right ventricular hypertrophy.

HELPFUL HINT:

In COPD, inflammation is mainly caused by neutrophils. In asthma, inflammation is caused by eosinophils and activated T cells. Corticosteroids are highly effective against eosinophilic inflammation but mostly ineffective against neutrophilic inflammation.

□ Decompensating PH is characterized by increased RAP and increased right ventricular hypertrophy.

□ Decompensated PH is characterized by decreased PAP and right-sided HF.

□ Treatment of PH focuses on treating the underlying etiology. Long-term management of PH includes selexipag, endothelin receptor antagonists, and calcium channel blockers.

QUICK REVIEW QUESTION

13. A 58-year-old patient is admitted to the critical care unit with a history of COPD. The patient is noncompliant with medical treatment (has continued smoking) and is being treated for bacterial pneumonia that has been worsening over the past 5 days despite antibiotic outpatient management. The patient presents with a diagnosis of acute exacerbation of COPD and is on BiPAP for hypercapnic failure after bronchodilators, IV methylprednisolone, and protocol-specific antibiotics. What signs and symptoms will indicate a worsening condition, and what therapies will the nurse anticipate next?

Pleural Space Abnormalities
Air-Leak Syndromes
Pathophysiology

Air-leak syndromes occur when air or gas enters the pleural space, resulting in extra-alveolar air accumulation and compression of the lung(s). There are two major categories of air-leak disorders: pneumothorax and pulmonary barotrauma. They have distinctly different pathophysiologies.

Pneumothorax occurs when air accumulates in the pleural space, collapsing the lung. Alveoli are underventilated, resulting in V/Q mismatch and intrapulmonary shunting. Hypoxia and respiratory failure may occur. The increased intrathoracic pressure may cause mediastinal shift, compressing the great vessels and decreasing cardiac output. Pneumothorax may be spontaneous or traumatic.

- **Primary spontaneous pneumothorax (PSP)** occurs spontaneously in the absence of lung disease and often presents with only minor symptoms.

- **Secondary spontaneous pneumothorax (SSP)** occurs in patients with an underlying lung disease and presents with more severe symptoms.

- **Traumatic pneumothorax** is caused by penetration of a blunt or sharp object. Common iatrogenic causes of pneumothorax include central line insertion, needle aspiration, or thoracentesis.

- **Tension pneumothorax**, a late progression of a pneumothorax, occurs when air enters the pleural space on inspiration and is unable to exit, causing increased pressure.

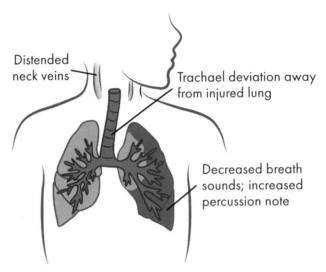

Distended neck veins

Trachael deviation away from injured lung

Decreased breath sounds; increased percussion note

Figure 2.8. Signs and Symptoms of Tension Pneumothorax

Pulmonary barotrauma occurs when the positive pressure from mechanical ventilation causes alveoli to rupture, leaking air into the interstitial space (pulmonary interstitial emphysema). Air may then travel into the mediastinum (pneumomediastinum), where it obstructs the airway and decreases venous return. Air may also travel to the pleural space (pneumothorax, as described above) or the pericardium (pneumopericardium), causing cardiac tamponade.

Signs and Symptoms

TABLE 2.6. Signs and Symptoms of Air-Leak Syndromes	
Disorder	**Signs and Symptoms**
Pneumothorax	dyspnea
	pleuritic chest pain
	tracheal deviation toward affected side
	hyper-resonance over affected area
	absent or diminished breath sounds over affected area
Tension pneumothorax	dyspnea
	agitation
	tracheal deviation away from unaffected side
	JVD
	hypotension
	tachycardia

Disorder	Signs and Symptoms
Pneumomediastinum	subcutaneous emphysema (palpable crepitus from face to upper chest)
	crunching/rasping sound over pericardium on auscultation (Hamman's sign)
	substernal stabbing pain with position changes
Pneumopericardium	friction rub
Tension pneumopericardium	signs and symptoms of cardiac tamponade

Diagnostic Findings

- CXR showing increased translucency on affected side

- in tension pneumothorax, CXR showing mediastinum and heart shift to unaffected side

Treatment and Management

- pneumothorax <15%: supplemental oxygen and monitoring

- pneumothorax >15%: percutaneous needle aspiration of air from pleural space and insertion of chest tube
  - □ small-bore chest tube (nonventilator patients); large-bore chest tube (ventilator patients)
  - □ insertion at fourth or fifth intercostal space mid-axillary line on affected side
  - □ water-seal drainage system or Heimlich valve
  - □ CXR to confirm lung re-expansion

- emergent treatment of tension pneumothorax: immediate percutaneous placement of large-bore needle (insertion at second intercostal space mid-axillary line on affected side) and chest-tube insertion

- tension pneumopericardium: immediate pericardiocentesis required

QUICK REVIEW QUESTION

14. A 68-year-old patient was intubated and placed on positive pressure mechanical ventilation. CXR post-intubation revealed a right main-stem placement of the ETT, which was pulled back appropriately. Later in the shift, the patient suddenly becomes highly agitated and hypotensive. The cardiac monitor shows tachycardia. The nurse observes JVD with tracheal and mediastinum deviation to the left. What interventions should the nurse anticipate?

PLEURAL EFFUSION

Pathophysiology

Pleural **effusion** is the buildup of fluid around the lungs in the pleural space. The fluid can displace lung tissue and inhibit adequate ventilation and lung expansion. There are two types of pleural effusions.

- **Transudative pleural effusions** are fluid leakages caused by increased systemic pressure in the vessels or low serum protein levels. The most common causes of transudative pleural effusions are heart failure (due to increased pulmonary capillary pressure) or cirrhosis (currently believed to be the result of fluid movement from the peritoneal cavity to the thorax).

- **Exudative pleural effusions** are the result of changes in capillary permeability resulting in exudate. They have widely varying etiologies, including malignancy (especially lung cancer), pulmonary embolism, and infections.

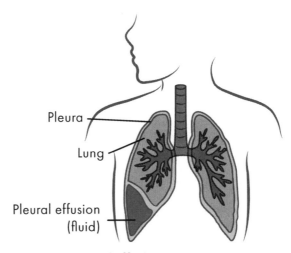

Figure 2.9. Pleural Effusion

Diagnosis

- dyspnea
- dullness upon percussion of the lung area
- asymmetrical chest expansion
- decreased breath sounds on affected side
- cough (dry or productive)
- pleuritic chest pain
- CXR showing white areas at the base of the lungs (unilaterally or bilaterally)

- CT scan to further diagnose the severity of the condition
- thoracentesis to determine the mechanism of effusion

Treatment and Management

- drainage of excess pleural fluid
- multiple thoracenteses necessary for reaccumulated fluid
- pleurodesis or indwelling pleural catheter for recurrent effusions
- medications based on underlying condition (e.g., diuretics, antibiotics)

QUICK REVIEW QUESTION

15. A nursing student requests assistance with understanding the difference between pulmonary effusion and ARDS. What is the response?

Status Asthmaticus

Pathophysiology

Asthma is a chronic obstructive pulmonary disease characterized by airway inflammation and bronchoconstriction. Asthma exacerbations may be triggered by allergens, infections, exercise, aspirin, and GERD. **Status asthmaticus** is a severe, progressively worsening asthma event that does not respond to bronchodilator therapy; the condition may develop into acute respiratory failure.

When the triggered response occurs, the airway becomes obstructed by a combination of bronchospasm, thick mucus, mucosal edema, and airway inflammation. The increased airway resistance increases the work of breathing. The lungs are hyperinflated, with the increased residual volume creating a V/Q mismatch and hypoxemia. Alveolar dead space increases, worsening hypoxia and leading to "air trapping" with hypercapnia and auto-PEEP (raised pressure in the distal airways).

Increased venous return causes blood to pool in the right ventricle. This distended right ventricle causes a shift of the intraventricular septum, compromising the left ventricle. Cardiac output and SBP drop.

Signs and Symptoms

- tachypnea and severe dyspnea
- bronchoconstriction
  - □ expiratory wheeze (early stage)

HELPFUL HINT:

Aspirin-exacerbated respiratory disease (aspirin-sensitive asthma) is asthma that develops after taking aspirin or other NSAIDs. It is a pseudoallergic reaction, meaning it is not antibody-mediated, seen in around 14% of people with severe asthma.

HELPFUL HINT:

During severe asthma exacerbations, lactate overproduction occurs in respiratory muscles, resulting in respiratory and metabolic acidosis.

- inspiratory and expiratory wheeze (late stage)
- wheezes may disappear with fatigue or if obstruction prevents wheezing
- increased use of accessory respiratory muscles
  - intercostal and subcostal retractions
  - use of abdominal muscles to overcome airway resistance
- decreased breath sounds in all lung fields (ominous sign, as patient is not moving enough air)
- hypoxia (early); hypercapnia (late)
- tachycardia and hypertension
- pulsus paradoxus >20 mm Hg
- with progression of disease
  - decreased cardiac output
  - hypotension and bradycardia
  - seizure
  - coma

Diagnostic Tests and Findings

- peak expiratory flow rate (PEFR) showing 20% drop from expected response to treatment or baseline best effort
- ABG
  - initial: respiratory alkalosis with hypoxemia
  - worsening: respiratory acidosis with hypercapnia
- ECG may show peaked P wave and right-axis deviation
- CXR to rule out other underlying diseases (e.g., pneumonia, pneumothorax)

Treatment and Management

- medications
  - inhaled bronchodilators (beta 2 agonists)
  - anticholinergics (synergistic effect with beta 2 agonists)
  - corticosteroids
- high-flow O_2 to keep SpO_2 >92%, or heliox to decrease airway resistance
- mechanical ventilation
  - larger ETT if possible (to decrease airway resistance and facilitate suctioning)
  - decrease ventilation rate to extend exhalation phase

- □ prolonged expiratory pause to reduce auto-PEEP from hyperinflated lungs
- □ lower V_T to reduce barotrauma
- □ sedation to reduce patient-ventilator dyssynchrony

QUICK REVIEW QUESTION

16. A critical care patient is admitted with a diagnosis of status asthmaticus. HR is 118 bpm, with diaphoresis, tachypnea, pulsus paradoxus >25 mm Hg, and an inspiratory and expiratory wheeze. Initial ABG shows hypoxia with respiratory alkalosis. One hour later, a repeat PEFR shows a 30% drop from the expected outcome of an initial albuterol treatment, and physical exam shows increased use of accessory muscles with abdominal and intercostal retractions. Although auscultation shows an absence of wheezes after nebulizer treatment, breath sounds are now diminished throughout all lung fields. How would the nurse interpret this change in breath sounds?

Thoracic Trauma

PATHOPHYSIOLOGY

Chest trauma, whether from blunt injury, sharp, invasive penetration, or thoracic surgical procedures, creates a wide range of respiratory complications. To prepare for the CCRN exam, focus on pulmonary contusion, rib fractures, and hemothorax. (Pneumothorax is reviewed above in "Air-Leak Syndromes.")

TABLE 2.7. Thoracic Injuries

Injury	Pathophysiology	Clinical Presentation
Pulmonary contusion	Bruising of the parenchyma of the lung. Capillary rupture causes blood and other fluid to leak into lung tissue, causes localized edema, and may result in hypoxia from diminished gas exchange. Fluid accumulation in alveoli and decreased pulmonary secretion clearance put patients at risk for ARDS and pneumonia.	• signs and symptoms may be delayed 24 – 72 hours until edema develops • hemoptysis (pink, frothy sputum) • crackles • tachypnea and tachycardia • hypoxia • chest wall bruising • pain • decreased $PaCO_2$ • decreased P/F ratio

continued on next page

TABLE 2.7. Thoracic Injuries (continued)

Injury	Pathophysiology	Clinical Presentation
Rib fractures	Commonly caused by traumatic crushing injury to chest or cancer; leads to altered ventilation and perfusion status. Most common fractures are ribs 4 – 8. Ribs 9 – 12 may cause splenic rupture and tears to the diaphragm and liver.	• pain with breathing • shallow breaths • splinting
Hemothorax	Blood in the pleural space, usually resulting from blunt or penetrating trauma to the chest wall. Damage to the lung parenchyma and great vessels causes alveoli collapse. May also present with pneumothorax (pneumohemothorax).	• symptomatic with blood volume >400 mL • absence of breath sounds on affected side • tracheal deviation toward unaffected side • dullness to percussion • tachypnea • hypovolemia • shock
Tracheal rupture (or perforation)	Occurs when there is injury to the structure of the trachea. The perforation can be caused by forceful or poor intubation efforts or by traumatic injury to the trachea such as in crush injuries or hanging injuries.	• hemoptysis • dyspnea • diffuse subcutaneous emphysema
Ruptured diaphragm	Injury to the diaphragm creates a negative pressure gradient, allowing abdominal viscera to enter the thoracic cavity. The shift compresses the lungs and mediastinum, causing decreased venous return and cardiac output.	• respiratory distress • bowel sounds in chest on auscultation • tracheal deviation
Flail chest	Multiple anterior and posterior fractures to 3 or more ribs.	• paradoxical movement of the chest wall (flail segment moves inward during inspiration and outward during exhalation)

Treatment and Management

- pain management as needed (intercostal nerve blocks, thoracic epidural analgesia, opioids, or NSAIDs)
- small contusions: heal in 3 – 5 days, often without treatment
- severe contusions
  - □ aggressive pulmonary care (e.g., ambulation, turning, incentive spirometry)
  - □ mechanical ventilation with PEEP
  - □ fluid management (to avoid overload)
  - □ infection prevention
- hemothorax: chest-tube insertion or thoracotomy (if bleeding cannot be managed)
- tracheal perforation: maintain airway and prepare for surgical repair
- ruptured diaphragm: prep patient for immediate surgical intervention
- flail chest: aggressive management with analgesics, pulmonary hygiene, and noninvasive positive pressure ventilation

HELPFUL HINT:

A sudden crush injury to the chest wall produces **traumatic asphyxia**. This specific crush injury results in an "ecchymotic mask" characterized by subconjunctival hemorrhage, facial edema, and petechiae and cyanosis of the head, neck, and upper extremities.

QUICK REVIEW QUESTION

17. A 46-year-old patient with A-fib who is on anticoagulant medication suffered a fall from a small step stool in the kitchen, with no head injury or loss of consciousness. Twenty-four hours later, the patient is admitted to the critical care unit with the following symptoms: pink frothy sputum, crackles in the lung fields, tachypnea, tachycardia, and pain. Ecchymosis is evident over ribs 4 – 8. ABG shows hypoxia. CXR has ruled out rib fractures but is not remarkable. The patient is sent for a chest CT scan. What diagnosis would the nurse expect, and why was a chest CT scan ordered?

ANSWER KEY

1. Bronchial breath sounds over the lung fields indicate consolidation and reflect pneumonia. The mixed venous blood gas analysis will show intrapulmonary shunting because of underventilated alveoli. The poor ventilation generates a V/Q mismatch. The results, which show how much venous blood participates in gas exchange, will help the nurse direct appropriate oxygen and possible mechanical therapy.

2. The patient has respiratory acidosis that is partially compensated, meaning the body is attempting unsuccessfully to restore acid-base balance.

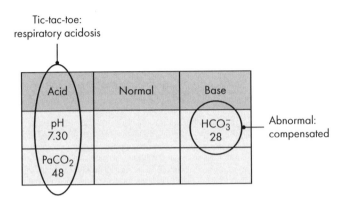

Tic-tac-toe: respiratory acidosis

Acid	Normal	Base
pH 7.30		HCO$_3^-$ 28
PaCO$_2$ 48		

Abnormal: compensated

3. Oxygen toxicity has been initiated, as evidenced by the patient's history of >24 hours on >60% FiO$_2$, clinical signs of substernal chest pain with deep breaths, dyspnea, cough, and bradycardia. Oxygen toxicity places the patient at high risk for ARDS.

4. The patient has developed pulmonary edema because >1000 mL fluid has been removed. This large amount of fluid removal has increased the negative intrapleural pressure, and the lung has not re-expanded to fill the space. The nurse should encourage immediate discontinuation of the procedure, administer oxygen, and evaluate for progression to mechanical ventilation. If the patient deteriorates because of an open pneumothorax, the nurse will prepare for chest tube insertion by the practitioner.

5. PEEP, or positive end-expiratory pressure, allows for more effective gas exchange by keeping the alveoli open especially at end expiration. Complications include barotrauma to the lungs, decreased blood pressure and cardiac output, and air-leak syndromes.

6. The nurse suspects post-extubation laryngeal edema.

7. (1) Elevate HOB 35 – 45 degrees; (2) oral care with chlorhexidine every 2 hours; (3) subglottic suctioning; and (4) low V$_T$ settings.

8. Definitive diagnosis of a PE is by pulmonary angiogram. Because the patient is stable, a faster but less definitive test is unlikely to be ordered.

9. LPV includes low tidal volumes (V$_T$), higher RR settings, permissive hypercapnia, and PEEP settings at the lowest possible amount to decrease intrapulmonary shunting while improving P/F ratio. Research has shown that a reasonable goal for reversing hypoxemia and preventing oxygen toxicity is a PaO$_2$ of 55 – 65 mm Hg.

10. The patient will likely receive noninvasive mechanical ventilation via BiPAP. NIV is the standard of care for acute hypercapnia due to COPD because it effectively manages hypercapnia while preventing risks associated with invasive ventilation.

11. The nurse should administer oxygen to the patient, establish IV access, and anticipate drawing blood cultures, collecting a sputum culture from the patient, and administering antibiotics after collection of blood cultures, per facility protocols.

12. Pulmonary aspiration (or aspiration pneumonitis) is the likely diagnosis, and sepsis protocol should be immediately instituted. Priorities should be obtaining blood cultures before the initiation of antibiotic therapy, and anticipating possible mechanical intubation to prevent respiratory collapse.

13. The nurse will monitor for increasing respiratory distress, signs of hemodynamic compromise, worsening acidosis on ABGs, and mental status changes and will plan for emergent intubation.

14. The patient has a tension pneumothorax with evidence of decreased cardiac output. Cardiac deterioration requires immediate percutaneous placement of a large-bore needle at the second intercostal space mid-axillary line on the affected side to relieve pressure from air trapped within the chest. The nurse knows the needle will need stabilization in place until a large-bore chest tube is inserted at the fourth or fifth intercostal space mid-axillary line and connected to either a water-seal drainage system or a Heimlich valve.

15. Pulmonary effusion and ARDS differ in which lung structures are affected. In pulmonary effusion, fluid collects in the pleural space that surrounds the lung and limits the ability of the lungs to expand. In ARDS, pulmonary capillary permeability is compromised, and fluid fills the alveolar sacs within the lungs. The fluid limits the ability of the lungs to exchange oxygen and carbon dioxide.

16. The decrease in breath sounds in all lung fields is an ominous sign, as the increased work of breathing requires more physical effort (recruitment of accessory muscles and abdominal and intercostal retractions) to overcome increasing airway obstruction. The patient is too obstructed or fatigued to overcome the narrowed airways, and wheezing disappears, while diminished breath sounds may indicate impending respiratory failure or arrest.

17. The more sensitive chest CT scan will confirm a diagnosis of pulmonary contusion.

3 ENDOCRINE REVIEW

Adrenal Insufficiency

Pathophysiology

Adrenal insufficiency is an endocrine disorder characterized by a decrease in circulating corticosteroids (both glucocorticoids and mineralocorticoids). **Primary adrenal insufficiency** (Addison's disease) is caused by the inability of the adrenal glands to produce corticosteroids. **Secondary adrenal insufficiency** is caused by low production of **adrenocorticotropic hormone (ACTH)** in the pituitary gland. (ACTH stimulates corticosteroid production.)

The condition can be chronic or acute. The most common cause of **chronic adrenal insufficiency** is autoimmune conditions that damage the adrenal cortex.

Acute adrenal insufficiency (**adrenal crisis**) causes distributive shock and is a medical emergency that requires immediate care. It usually occurs when infection or trauma exacerbate chronic adrenal insufficiency, but may occur following damage to the adrenal or pituitary glands. Rarely, it may be caused by withdrawal from long-term glucocorticoid use.

During an adrenal crisis, low levels of aldosterone cause vasodilation, increased excretion of sodium, and retention of potassium, resulting in volume depletion and hypotension. Low levels of glucocorticoids lead to hypoglycemia and further depress blood pressure.

The information below describes the diagnosis and management of adrenal crisis.

Signs and Symptoms

HELPFUL HINT:

Fever caused by infection may precipitate an adrenal crisis, or the fever itself may be caused by low corticosteroid levels.

- shock (e.g., hypotension, tachycardia, oliguria)
- abdominal pain/tenderness
- nausea, vomiting, or diarrhea
- fever
- hyperpigmentation (from chronic adrenal insufficiency)

Diagnostic Findings

- low cortisol or aldosterone levels
- ACTH stimulation test shows low cortisol level
- elevated renin
- low serum Na^+
- high serum K^+
- low blood glucose

Treatment and Management

- IV fluid resuscitation
- empiric administration of IV glucocorticoids (usually hydrocortisone or dexamethasone)
- replacement of mineralocorticoids may be required (e.g., fludrocortisone)
- management of hypoglycemia and electrolyte imbalances as needed

QUICK REVIEW QUESTION

1. A patient with refractory hypotension and a fever of unknown origin has the following laboratory results:

   sodium 130 mmol/L

potassium 4.2 mmol/L

plasma cortisol 25 mmol/L

What diagnostic test should the nurse anticipate will be ordered for this patient?

Antidiuretic Hormone Imbalances

Diabetes Insipidus

Pathophysiology

Antidiuretic hormone (**ADH**, also called **vasopressin**) is produced by the hypothalamus and stored in the posterior pituitary gland. When released, ADH constricts blood vessels and signals the kidneys to hold on to water. **Diabetes insipidus (DI)** occurs when an imbalance of ADH prevents the body from regulating blood volume and maintaining a normal serum osmolality. **Central diabetes insipidus** occurs when the body is unable to secrete an adequate amount of ADH; **nephrogenic diabetes insipidus** occurs when the kidneys cannot respond appropriately to ADH.

Excessive excreted free water causes a decrease in urine osmolality and specific gravity, while serum osmolality and serum sodium rise. Because the kidney tubules cannot concentrate urine or hold on to water, extracellular dehydration occurs, leading to hypotension and hypovolemic shock. Continued severe polyuria may lead to decreased cerebral perfusion, seizures, coma, and death.

Etiology

- central DI
  - TBI
  - infection (e.g., meningitis, encephalitis)
  - pituitary or hypothalamic dysfunction
  - increased ICP (can be life-threatening)
- nephrogenic DI
  - medications (e.g., lithium, phenytoin, demeclocycline)
  - hypercalcemia
  - hereditary

Signs and Symptoms

- marked polydipsia
- marked polyuria
- highly dilute urine

Diagnostic Findings

- high urine output (6 – 24 L/day)
- low urine osmolality (<300 mOsm/kg)
- low urine specific gravity (1.001 – 1.005)
- high serum Na^+ (>145 mEq/L)
- high serum osmolality (>295 mOsm/kg)
- low ADH (generally not measured in ICU settings)

Treatment and Management

- primary goals: rapid fluid resuscitation, ADH replacement, and identification and treatment of the underlying condition
- IV or subcutaneous ADH
- IV fluids to increase intravascular volume
  - Initiate with hypotonic IV fluids.
  - Correct fluid volume status slowly over 2 – 3 days.

HELPFUL HINT:

Patients with high calcium levels are unresponsive to ADH administration.

- monitoring
  - ADH administration increases risk of vasospasm of cardiac, cerebral, and mesenteric arteries
  - cardiac monitoring for ischemia and hypertension
  - overhydration possible after administration of ADH or analogue
  - daily weights and strict I&O
  - urine specific gravity and electrolytes balance (especially Na^+ and K^+).

QUICK REVIEW QUESTION

2. A 72-year-old patient is post-op neurosurgery for head trauma from an MVC. The patient's LOC has been variable. Urine output has been 6 L/24 hr, with specific gravity of 1.005. Serum Na+ is 145 mEq/L, with serum osmolality 295 mOsm/kg. The patient is given a diagnosis of CDI. Why should the nurse plan to monitor for angina?

SYNDROME OF INAPPROPRIATE SECRETION OF ANTIDIURETIC HORMONE (SIADH)

Pathophysiology

In **syndrome of inappropriate secretion of antidiuretic hormone (SIADH)**, excess secretion of ADH causes water retention and dilutional hyponatremia (low serum sodium is the result of excess water, not a sodium deficiency). The hallmark signs of SIADH are hyponatremia with decreased serum osmolality (dilute blood) and increased urine osmolality (concentrated urine). Neurological symptoms may occur as a result of cerebral edema caused by hyponatremia.

Etiology

- trauma to head (hypothalamus or posterior pituitary gland)
- oat cell carcinoma (lung cancer)
- infection (pneumonia, meningitis, Guillain-Barré syndrome)
- medications (e.g., chlorpropamide)
- surgery (particularly to pituitary gland)

Signs and Symptoms

- patients may be euvolemic or have signs and symptoms of fluid overload
- signs and symptoms of hyponatremia (see chapter 6, Renal and Genitourinary Review)

Diagnostic Findings

- low serum Na^+ (<120 mEq/L)
- low urine output
- decreased serum osmolality (<275 mOsm/kg)
- high urine osmolality (>100 mOsm/kg)
- high urine specific gravity (>1.030)

Treatment and Management

- primary goals: restore fluid/sodium balance and treat the underlying cause
- manage fluid overload
  - fluid restriction
  - loop diuretics (watch for hypokalemia)
  - daily weights and strict I&O

HELPFUL HINT:

DI is the result of **too little ADH**, causing polyuria. It results in dilute urine, concentrated serum, and high serum Na^+.

SIADH is the result of **too much ADH**, causing water retention. It results in concentrated urine, dilute serum, and low serum Na^+.

- slow correction of Na^+
  - Rapid correction can cause permanent neurological damage.
  - Limit Na^+ replacement to 8 – 12 mEq/L in 24 hours.
  - Stop Na^+ replacement when serum sodium is 130 mEq/L.
- hypertonic IV solutions (3% normal saline) for severe or refractory hyponatremia
  - reduces cerebral edema
  - monitor respiratory status for crackles, increased effort of breathing, and decreases in O_2 saturation
- declomycin inhibits ADH and promotes diuresis (off-label use)

> **QUICK REVIEW QUESTION**
>
> **3.** An authorized prescriber has ordered a vasopressin continuous IV infusion per ICU protocol for a neurological ICU patient with a secondary diagnosis of SIADH. Why should the nurse question this order?

Diabetes Mellitus

- **Diabetes mellitus (DM)** is a metabolic disorder affecting insulin production and insulin resistance. It is classified as type 1 or type 2.
  - **type 1:** an acute-onset autoimmune disease most prominent in children, teens, and adults <30. Beta cells in the pancreas are destroyed and are unable to produce sufficient amounts of insulin, causing blood sugar to rise.
  - **type 2:** a gradual-onset disease most prominent in adults 30. Individuals develop insulin resistance, which prevents the cellular uptake of glucose and causes blood sugar to rise.
- Diagnosis includes polyuria, polyphagia, and polydipsia; fasting blood glucose ≥126 mg/dL; 2-hour plasma glucose ≥200 mg/dL (75 g OGTT); and A1C ≥6.5%.
- DM is correlated to poor outcomes in critical care settings, particularly for patients with comorbid cardiovascular conditions. Patients with diabetes are more likely to develop complications (e.g., sepsis) while in the ICU, and are also more likely to be hyper- or hypoglycemic.
- Regular blood glucose monitoring is required for critical care patients, with closer monitoring for patients with DM.
  - Protocols will vary, but current guidelines suggest moderate glycemic controls (140 – 180 mg/dL) that may be tightened for individual patients (e.g., acute MI, neurosurgery post-op).

- Tight glycemic controls (e.g., 80 – 110 mg/dL) place patients at higher risk of hypoglycemia and sequelae such as seizure and dysrhythmias.

- Patients with type 2 diabetes require insulin management in critical care settings, even if their blood glucose is well managed at home. Insulin type and dosage depend on individual patient characteristics.

  - Patients may receive a combination of long-acting (basal) insulin, short-acting insulin following meals, and rapid-acting insulin to manage acute hyperglycemia.

  - Insulin may be given subcutaneously or via IV infusion.

  - Patients with DM who are being fed via TPN or enteral feedings require insulin. It may be delivered IV, subcutaneously, or as part of the nutritional solution (depending on the needs of the patient).

- Patients with type 1 diabetes require regular insulin administration, even if feedings are discontinued. These patients usually receive continuous IV insulin and IV dextrose (to prevent hypoglycemia).

- Oral anti-diabetic agents are usually discontinued in critical care settings because they are contraindicated or only indicated for postprandial use.

HELPFUL HINT:

Use of metformin is contraindicated in patients with renal or hemodynamic dysfunction; sulfonylureas may cause severe hypoglycemia.

QUICK REVIEW QUESTION

4. A patient with a history of type 2 diabetes is being fed via TPN during treatment for necrotizing pancreatitis and is on a continuous IV insulin infusion. The nurse is currently preparing the patient for surgery. Why is it important for the TPN to be discontinued gradually?

Hyperglycemia

Pathophysiology

HELPFUL HINT:

Stress-induced hyperglycemia is often seen in critical care settings, even in patients with no previous DM diagnosis. It should be managed with insulin to maintain normoglycemic levels.

Diabetic ketoacidosis (DKA) occurs when the body does not produce insulin. The elevated glucose levels increase the serum osmolality, resulting in osmotic diuresis that causes polyuria, with significant water loss. Simultaneously, the body also begins to break down fat cells for fuel, producing a buildup of serum ketones, resulting in acidosis. As acidosis worsens, potassium is shifted out of cells, resulting in an initial presentation with hyperkalemia. However, continued osmotic diuresis eventually leads to hypokalemia in most patients.

Hyperosmolar hyperglycemic state (HHS), also called **hyperglycemic hyperosmolar nonketotic syndrome (HHNK)**, is a slow-onset, high-mortality complication of type 2 DM. It occurs when the pancreas produces insufficient insulin. As with DKA, blood glucose levels become high, resulting in osmotic diuresis and hypovolemia. With decreased kidney perfusion and oliguria from dehydration, less glucose is removed and serum hyperosmolality increases. Serum potassium may be elevated, but total body potassium will be depleted due to osmotic diuresis. In HHS, insulin production is sufficient to prevent ketoacidosis, differentiating it from DKA.

HHS is often mistaken for a neurological event as intracerebral dehydration may cause profound CNS symptoms, including coma. Hemoconcentration also increases the risk of thromboemboli and possible cardiac, cerebral, and pleural infarctions.

HELPFUL HINT:

Look out for questions about HHS that involve an uncharacteristic patient (e.g., a teenager with Crohn's disease on home TPN infusion).

TABLE 3.1. DKA and HHS

DKA	HHS
Etiology	
• undiagnosed/ineffectively managed type 1 DM • destabilized type 2 DM (less common) • acute illness (e.g., MI, pancreatitis) • medications (e.g., steroids, epinephrine, thiazide diuretics, atypical antipsychotics) • stress of critical illness • endocrine disorders (e.g., hyperthyroidism, Cushing's syndrome)	• most common in older adult patients with obesity, type 2 DM, and underlying cardiovascular disease • patients who control diabetes through diet only • TPN • use of steroids or thiazides • pancreatitis • serious illness or infection (e.g., MI, pneumonia)
Signs and Symptoms	
• rapid onset • polyuria (early); oliguria (late) • signs and symptoms of hypovolemia • Kussmaul respirations and fruity breath odor • polyphagia and polydipsia • nausea, vomiting • abdominal pain • malaise and weakness • decreased LOC	• slow onset • polyuria • signs and symptoms of hypovolemia • rapid, extremely shallow breaths • polydipsia • mild nausea or vomiting • weight loss • diplopia • malaise and weakness • stupor or coma

DKA	HHS
Diagnostic Findings	
• elevated blood glucose (250 mg/dL)	
• metabolic acidosis	• elevated blood glucose (>600 mg/dL)
• pH <7.3	• high serum osmolality (>350 mOsm/kg)
• HCO_3^- <18 mEq/L	• no diagnostic findings of acidosis (i.e., normal pH and serum HCO_3)
• anion gap 10	
• increased serum ketones	• serum K^+ normal or high
• low serum Na^+ and Ca^{++}	• elevated BUN and creatinine
• increased serum K^+	• fluid deficit may be as high as 150 mL/kg total body weight
• elevated BUN and creatinine	
• fluid deficit (negative 50 – 100 mL/ kg common)	

Treatment and Management

- IV fluid protocols
  - first hour: 1 – 3 L of isotonic fluids (lactated Ringer's or 0.9% normal saline)
  - second hour: 1 L of hypotonic fluids (0.45% normal saline)
  - when blood glucose reaches 250 mg/dL: 1 L of hypertonic fluids with dextrose (D5 in half-normal saline).
- IV K^+ replacement if K^+ <5.3 mEq/L
- continuous IV insulin (0.1 units/kg/hr)
  - initiate only when K^+ 3.3 mEq/L
  - slow blood glucose reduction (decrease by 50 – 75 mg/dL/hr)
- monitoring
  - risk of ventricular dysrhythmias due to hypo- or hyperkalemia (especially in patients with renal insufficiency)
  - blood glucose every hour
- HHS may require management of type 2 DM insulin resistance (due to high levels of stress hormones)
  - High-dose insulin may be used.
  - After IV insulin is discontinued, administer oral agents specific to reducing insulin resistance.

HELPFUL HINT:

For fluid resuscitation in DKA, think "Oh, oh, ease off": isOtonic, hypOtonic, hypErtonic.

Hypoglycemia

Pathophysiology

Hypoglycemia is the sudden fall of blood glucose below normal levels. The decreased glucose levels result in neurological dysfunction. In addition, the adrenal medulla is triggered to release adrenaline (also called epinephrine) to restore normal glucose levels, leading to increased sympathetic nervous system activity.

Etiology

- use of insulin (IV or subcutaneous)
- interruption of oral, enteral, or parenteral feedings
- adrenal insufficiency
- infection
- pancreatitis
- vomiting
- drinking excess alcohol, or liver disease

Signs and Symptoms

- cardiovascular
  - tachycardia
  - diaphoresis
  - irritability, restlessness
  - cool skin
- neurological
  - lethargy
  - weakness
  - slurred speech or blurred vision
  - anxiety or confusion
  - seizure (at blood glucose 20 – 40 mg/dL)
  - coma (at blood glucose <20 mg/dL)

HELPFUL HINT:

Beta blockers may hide cardiovascular symptoms in patients with hypoglycemia.

Diagnostic Findings

- serum glucose <70 mg/dL

Treatment and Management

- overall treatment goal: maintain blood glucose level 70 mg/dL
  - □ blood glucose 60 – 70 mg/dL: 4 oz of juice if oral intake is not contraindicated
  - □ blood glucose 40 – 60 mg/dL: D50 via IV push (12.5 g = 0.5 ampule)
  - □ blood glucose <40 mg/dL: D50 via IV push (25 g = 1.0 ampule)
- refractory hypoglycemia
  - □ continuous infusion of D10 (dextrose 10% solution) via peripheral IV
  - □ continuous infusion of D20 (dextrose 20% solution) via central line
- longer-acting carbohydrates (oral intake, tube feeding, or TPN) after patient is stabilized
- seizure prophylaxis
- identify and treat underlying cause

QUICK REVIEW QUESTION

6. What hormone is released from the adrenal gland to restore glucose levels in hypoglycemia?

Thyroid Disorders
HYPERTHYROIDISM
Pathophysiology

Hyperthyroidism (thyrotoxicosis) occurs when the thyroid produces an excess of the thyroid hormones triiodothyronine (T3) and/or thyroxine (T4). Chronic hyperthyroidism presents with a characteristic set of symptoms, including anxiety, weakness, palpitations, tremor, and weight loss.

Thyroid storm is a severe form of thyrotoxicosis usually seen in patients with hyperthyroidism after a precipitating event (e.g., trauma, infection). Thyroid storm has a high mortality rate and requires immediate treatment.

The information below describes the diagnosis and management of thyroid storm.

Signs and Symptoms

- tachycardia (140 bmp)
- hypotension
- hyperpyrexia
- altered mental status (agitation, confusion)
- decreased LOC (progressing to coma)

Diagnostic Findings

- elevated T4 and/or T3
- low TSH

Treatment and Management

- pharmacological suppression of thyroid hormones (e.g., thionamides, iodine, and glucocorticoids)
- beta blockers (for cardiac symptoms)
- respiratory support as needed
- aggressive cooling measures (e.g., ice packs)

QUICK REVIEW QUESTION

7. A patient is admitted to the ICU with new onset of thyroid storm. Which physiological system should be a main focus of symptom management?

HYPOTHYROIDISM
Pathophysiology

HELPFUL HINT:

Myxedema coma caused by hypotha- lamic-pituitary disease may present with secondary adrenal insufficiency (caused by reduced secretion of ACTH).

Hypothyroidism is characterized by low levels of the hormones T3 and T4. **Primary hypothyroid** disease results from damage to the thyroid. **Secondary hypothyroidism** is the result of a hypothalamic-pituitary disease. Symptoms of chronic hypothyroidism are related to slowing of metabolic process and include fatigue, bradycardia, cold intolerance, weight gain, and localized non-pitting edema (myxedema).

Myxedema coma is severe hypothyroidism usually seen in patients with chronic hypothyroidism after a precipitating event (e.g., MI, infection). It is a medical emergency that requires immediate treatment.

The information below describes the diagnosis and management of myxedema coma.

Signs and Symptoms

- decreased LOC (confusion and lethargy progressing to coma)
- hypothermia
- bradycardia
- hypotension

Diagnostic Findings

- low serum T4
- low serum Na^+
- ABGs show respiratory acidosis

Treatment and Management

- empiric administration of IV levothyroxine (T4) and liothyronine (T3)
- glucocorticoids (usually hydrocortisone)
- fluids and vasopressors
- passive rewarming

QUICK REVIEW QUESTION

8. Why would a patient with suspected myxedema coma be administered glucocorticoids?

ANSWER KEY

1. The patient has symptoms of adrenal insufficiency. The provider will likely order an ACTH stimulation test to diagnose primary or secondary adrenal insufficiency.

2. DI is treated with vasopressin, which can cause vasospasm of cardiac, cerebral, and mesenteric arteries. Coronary artery spasm may precipitate an angina episode, resulting in a myocardial ischemic event.

3. SIADH is a condition of too much ADH in the patient's system. Vasopressin is an ADH. The nurse would know that giving additional ADH would exacerbate this condition.

4. Abruptly discontinuing TPN may lead to hypoglycemia, particularly in patients with DM. The TPN should be tapered and the patient's insulin dose recalculated to match the patient's changing carbohydrate intake.

5. The preferred diagnostic indicator is serum osmolality: patients with HHS will have a higher serum osmolality (350 mOsm/kg) than with DKA. HHS also presents with higher blood glucose (600 mg/dL) than DKA, and patients may have a higher fluid deficit (as high as 150 mL/kg of body weight). Because no ketoacidosis is present with HHS, there will be no significant serum ketones or findings associated with acidosis.

6. Adrenaline (epinephrine) increases blood glucose levels and increases cardiac output.

7. Patients with thyroid storm typically have severe cardiac disturbances and need supportive care to maintain hemodynamic stability. The patient should be placed on cardiac telemetry and the nurse should be prepared for emergent cardioversion and treatment with beta blockers.

8. Myxedema coma is often concomitant with secondary adrenal insufficiency. Because adrenal crisis requires immediate treatment with glucocorticoids, they are often administered to patients with myxedema coma until adrenal insufficiency has been ruled out.

4 HEMATOLOGY AND IMMUNOLOGY REVIEW

Overview of the Hematologic System

- **Plasma**, the liquid part of blood, includes albumin (which maintains osmotic pressure), serum globulins, and clotting factors.

- **Red blood cells (RBCs or erythrocytes)** transport oxygen (and, to a lesser extent, CO_2).
  - High RBC counts may indicate chronic hypoxia, dehydration, bone marrow overproduction, or kidney disease.
  - Low RBC counts indicate anemia caused by disease processes that result in underproduction or destruction of RBCs.
  - **Erythropoiesis**—the production of RBCs—is triggered by the release of erythropoietin from the kidneys. RBCs grow to maturity within the bone marrow.

- RBCs are broken down in the liver and spleen through **phagocytosis**; waste products are excreted as bilirubin and biliverdin in bile.
- **White blood cells (WBCs** or **leukocytes)** fight infection.
  - High WBC counts occur during infections, physiological distress, and steroid use.
  - Low WBC counts occur during bone marrow suppression and chemotherapy.
- A **WBC differential** includes the percentage or absolute number of different types of WBCs.
  - **Left shift** refers to an increased presence of band neutrophils in the peripheral blood. This shift may be due to inflammation, infection, steroids, or stress.
  - Viral infections show a decreased overall WBC count and high lymphocytes.
  - Malignancies show a high count of one type of WBC or high counts of numerous immature WBCs.

TABLE 4.1. CBC With Differential

Test	Description	Normal Range
Complete Blood Count (CBC)		
White blood cells (WBCs)	cells that fight infection; a high WBC count can indicate inflammation or infection	4,500 – 10,000 cells/µL
Red blood cells (RBCs)	cells that carry oxygen throughout the body and filter carbon dioxide	men: 5 – 6 million cells/µL women: 4 – 5 million cells/µL
Hemoglobin (HgB)	protein that binds oxygen in the blood	men: 13.8 – 17.2 g/dL women: 12.1 – 15.1 g/dL
Hematocrit (Hct)	percentage of the blood composed of red blood cells	men: 41% – 50% women: 36% – 44%
Mean corpuscular volume (MCV)	average size of RBCs	80 – 95 fL
Mean corpuscular hemoglobin (MCH)	average amount of HgB in RBCs	27.5 – 33.2 pg

Test	Description	Normal Range
Complete Blood Count (CBC)		
Mean corpuscular hemoglobin concentration (MCHC)	average concentration of HgB in RBCs	334 – 355 g/L
Platelets	blood components that play a role in clotting	150,000 – 450,000 platelets/µL
WBC Differential		
Neutrophils	first responders that quickly migrate to the site of infection to destroy bacterial invaders	2,000 – 7,000/µL (40% – 60%)
Band neutrophils	immature neutrophils (also called bands)	<700/µL (<5%)
Lymphocytes	B cells, T cells, and natural killer cells; all 3 types develop from common lymphoid progenitors	1,000 – 3,000/µL (20% – 40%)
Monocytes	cells that engulf and destroy microbes and cancer cells	200 – 1,000/µL (2% – 8%)
Eosinophils	cells that attack parasites and regulate inflammation	20 – 500/µL (1% – 4%)
Basophils	cells responsible for inflammatory reactions, including allergies	20 – 100/µL (0% – 2%)

- **Hemostasis**, the process that stops bleeding, occurs through vasoconstriction and coagulation.
  - During **coagulation**, a semisolid **clot** forms from platelets and red blood cells held together by the protein **fibrin**.
  - **Fibrinolysis** is the disintegration of blood clots.
- Coagulation is a cascade of reactions involving proteins called **clotting factors.**
  - Platelet aggregation is initiated by exposure to **von Willebrand factor (vW)** and **tissue factor (TF).**
  - During coagulation, the protein **fibrinogen** (clotting factor I) is converted to fibrin by the enzyme **thrombin** (clotting factor IIa).

HELPFUL HINT:

The liver is highly involved in the synthesis and removal of clotting components. Chronic liver disease often leads to coagulation disorders caused by decreased synthesis of clotting factors and poor clearance of activated factors.

□ **Prothrombin** (clotting factor II) is a precursor to thrombin.

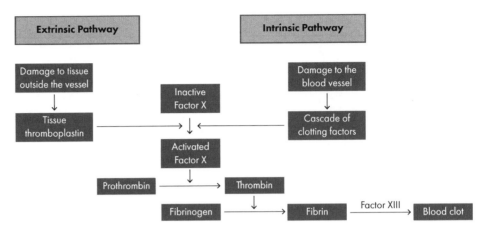

Figure 4.1. The Coagulation Cascade

■ Coagulation can follow two possible pathways:
  □ The intrinsic pathway is activated via damage within a blood vessel.
    ❑ This pathway is monitored by measuring the aPTT.
    ❑ Heparin disrupts the intrinsic pathway.
  □ The extrinsic pathway is activated by damage outside the vasculature.
    ❑ This pathway is monitored by measuring the PT.
    ❑ Warfarin disrupts the extrinsic pathway.
  □ Both pathways activate clotting factor X and produce a fibrin clot.

TABLE 4.2. Coagulation Studies and Clotting Factors

Test	Description	Normal Range
Prothrombin time (PT)	how long it takes blood to clot	10 – 13 seconds
International normalized ratio (INR)	ratio of a patient's PT and a standardized PT for patients taking anticoagulants	healthy adults: <1.1 patients taking anticoagulants: 2.0 – 3.0
Partial thromboplastin time (PTT)	the body's ability to form blood clots	60 – 70 seconds
Activated partial thromboplastin time (aPTT)	the body's ability to form blood clots using an activator to speed up the clotting process	20 – 35 seconds
D-dimer	protein fragment produced during fibrinolysis	negative

Test	Description	Normal Range
Fibrin split products (FSP) or fibrin degradation products (FDP)	components produced during fibrinolysis	<10 mg/L
Fibrinogen	amount of fibrinogen (clotting factor I)	200 – 400 mg/dL
Plasminogen	substrate involved in fibrinolysis	10 – 16 mg/dL

QUICK REVIEW QUESTION

1. Congenital hypofibrinogenemia is an inherited condition characterized by low circulating levels of fibrinogen (<150 mg/dL). What signs and symptoms should a nurse expect to see in a patient with severe hypofibrinogenemia?

Anemia

Pathophysiology

Anemia is a reduction in RBCs, usually diagnosed via low levels of HgB and Hct. Anemia can result from destruction or underproduction of RBCs.

- **Hemolytic anemia** is caused by premature destruction of RBCs. Underlying causes of hemolytic anemia may include autoimmune conditions, trauma, infection, and drugs or toxins.

- **Decreased erythropoiesis** can result from dietary deficiencies (e.g., iron deficiency, vitamin deficiency secondary to alcohol abuse) and bone marrow disorders.

Signs and Symptoms

- tachycardia and tachypnea
- weak pulse
- lethargy
- pallor

Diagnostic Tests and Findings

- decreased RBC, HgB, and Hct
- men
  □ HgB <13.5 g/dL
  □ Hct <41.0%

- women
  - □ HgB <12.0 g/
  - □ Hct <36.0%

Treatment and Management

- treat underlying cause
- blood products (PRBCs)
- erythropoiesis-stimulating agents

QUICK REVIEW QUESTION

2. An ICU patient recently diagnosed with chronic lymphocytic leukemia has lab values flagged with a critical HgB of 6.5. What intervention will the physician most likely order?

Coagulopathies
DISSEMINATED INTRAVASCULAR COAGULOPATHY
Pathophysiology

Disseminated intravascular coagulopathy (DIC) is a coagulation disorder with simultaneous intervals of clotting and bleeding. DIC occurs when injury exposes blood to TF, causing a rapid increase in circulating thrombin and fibrin. Microclots cascade throughout the vascular system, causing hypoxia and ischemia in multiple organs. The use of platelets in clot formation results in thrombocytopenia, decreased fibrinogen, and overall increased clotting time. Subsequent fibrinolysis of the clots leads to elevated D-dimer and FSP.

Acute (or decompensated) DIC occurs when the presence of large amounts of TF cause rapid depletion of platelets and clotting factors, resulting in severe bleeding. **Chronic (or compensated)** DIC is the result of long-term exposure to TF. The body is able to compensate for lost platelets and clotting factors, but the risk of thromboembolic complications is high.

Etiology

- sepsis
- trauma
- cancers (especially leukemia and brain tumors)
- blood transfusion reaction
- recent procedure or surgery with anesthesia

- obstetrical complications (e.g., preeclampsia)
- cardiac arrest

Signs and Symptoms

- bleeding (e.g., spontaneous hemorrhage, petechiae)
- thromboembolic event (e.g., PE, DVT)

Diagnostic Tests and Findings

- acute DIC
  - decreased platelets (moderate to severe)
  - prolonged PT and PTT
  - decreased fibrinogen
  - severely elevated D-dimer and FSP
- chronic DIC
  - decreased platelets (mild)
  - normal or slightly prolonged PT and PTT
  - normal or slightly decreased fibrinogen
  - elevated D-dimer and FSP

Treatment and Management

- identify and treat underlying cause
- IV fluid resuscitation
- vasopressors
- transfusion of blood products (FFP, PRBCs, platelets, or cryoprecipitate)
- heparin for chronic DIC

QUICK REVIEW QUESTION

3. What findings would confirm a diagnosis of acute DIC in a patient recovering from postpartum hemorrhage?

THROMBOCYTOPENIA

- **Thrombocytopenia** is an abnormally low platelet level that can lead to severe bleeding or thrombosis. It can generally be classified by the number of platelets:
  - mild: 100,000 – 150,000/μL
  - moderate: 50,000 – 100,000/μL
  - severe: <50,000/μL

- Thrombocytopenia has a diverse etiology. In the ICU, it is commonly seen in patients with cancer, bone marrow disorders, sepsis, chronic liver disease, and autoimmune diseases.

- **Heparin-induced thrombocytopenia (HIT)** is acute-onset thrombocytopenia in patients receiving heparin therapy.
  - causes platelet activation, significantly increasing risk of thrombosis
  - thrombocytopenia and thrombosis occur 5 – 10 days after exposure to heparin
  - more common after exposure to unfractionated heparin
  - if HIT is suspected, immediately discontinue heparin and administer anticoagulants

- **Idiopathic thrombocytopenic purpura (ITP**, also called **immune thrombocytopenia)** is an autoimmune disorder that causes the destruction of platelets.
  - Signs and symptoms include mild bleeding (e.g., petechiae, purpura); severe GI bleeding and hematuria are rarer.
  - Treatment includes corticosteroids and IV immunoglobulin.
  - Because platelet destruction occurs in the spleen, refractory ITP is treated with splenectomy.

HELPFUL HINT:

Heparin is neutralized with protamine sulfate. Warfarin is neutralized with vitamin K.

QUICK REVIEW QUESTION

4. A patient with sepsis after a complicated PE has been in the ICU for 2 weeks. The nurse calls the physician because the patient has frank blood in the stool and is oozing from around the PICC lines. Why should the nurse consider thrombocytopenia as the cause?

Immune Deficiencies and Leukopenia

Pathophysiology

Immune deficiencies can be primary disorders (i.e., inherited) or secondary to disease, medications, or malnutrition. Immune deficiencies commonly seen in critical care are discussed below.

- **Leukopenia** is the general term for a WBC <4000/μL. It can occur as the result of impaired production or rapid use of WBCs.

- **Acquired immunodeficiency syndrome (AIDS)** is the end-stage progression of HIV. Patients with AIDS have a depletion of

T lymphocytes and are susceptible to opportunistic and sometimes emergent infections.

- **Leukemia**, cancer of the WBCs, occurs in the bone marrow and disrupts the production and function of WBCs. In the absence of functioning WBCs, the patient becomes immunocompromised. The types of leukemia are differentiated by which WBCs are affected (lymphocytes or myeloid cells).

- Patient who have received **organ transplants** are started on a high-intensity regimen of immunosuppressants perioperatively and are at high risk of infection during recovery.

- **Chemotherapy** is conducted with a class of cytotoxic medications that destroy cancer cells by disrupting cell mitosis and DNA replication. A side effect of chemotherapy is severe **neutropenia** (a decrease in circulating neutrophils).

- Poorly managed **diabetes mellitus** and associated hyperglycemia increases the risk of infection. In the critical care setting, patients with diabetes are more prone to postoperative infections and skin infections.

Treatment and Management

- Patients with immune deficiencies require specialized care to prevent opportunistic infections.

- Maintain skin integrity.

- Ensure adequate nutrition and hydration.

- Ensure that patient, providers, and visitors use adequate hand hygiene.

- Place patients in isolation rooms, per hospital policy.

- High-risk patients may receive prophylactic antibiotics.

QUICK REVIEW QUESTION

5. A patient receiving chemotherapy presents with onset of cough and fever. A CBC reveals a WBC count of 20,000/μL and a left shift. Blood cultures are drawn, with results pending, and the patient's lactic acid level is 2.9 mmol/L. CXR shows bilateral pulmonary infiltrates. What diagnosis does the nurse anticipate?

Oncologic Complications

- Patients with cancer may be admitted to the ICU for conditions directly related to the malignancy or for complications of treatment.

- Common oncologic complications include pericardial effusion/cardiac tamponade (see chapter 1, Cardiovascular Review), PE or respiratory failure (see chapter 2, Respiratory Review), hypercalcemia (see chapter 6, Renal and Genitourinary Review), and sepsis (see chapter 11, Multisystem Review).

- **Tumor lysis syndrome** occurs when tumor lysis releases large amounts of potassium, phosphate, and nucleic acids into circulation. The resulting hyperuricemia and hyperphosphatemia lead to acute kidney injury and high risk for dysrhythmias.
  - □ The condition is most common in patients with hematological cancers, particularly non-Hodgkin lymphoma and acute lymphoblastic leukemia.
  - □ Patients present with signs and symptoms of hyperkalemia, hyper-phosphatemia, and hypocalcemia.
  - □ Management calls for allopurinol, febuxostat, or rasburicase (to reduce uric acid levels), pharmacological management of electrolyte imbalances (see chapter 6, Renal and Genitourinary Review), and 108cardiac monitoring.

- **Superior vena cava syndrome** occurs when a malignancy obstructs the superior vena cava either by invading or compressing the vein.
  - □ The condition is most common in patients with lung cancer and non-Hodgkin lymphoma.
  - □ Patients present with facial edema, dyspnea, and chest pain. Severe symptoms may include cerebral edema, hemodynamic instability, and airway obstruction.
  - □ Management involves stabilization (ABCs) and stent placement.

QUICK REVIEW QUESTION

6. Why would a patient with tumor lysis syndrome be administered allopurinol?

Transfusion Reactions

- Whole blood and blood products are **transfused** to replace lost volume or to replace specific components such as RBCs, platelets, or clotting factors.

TABLE 4.3. Uses of Blood Products

Blood Product	Uses	Notes
Packed red blood cells (PRBCs)	to treat hypovolemia due to hemorrhage to treat anemia for low HgB (<7 – 8 g/dL)	One unit of PRBCs raises hematocrit by 3% and HgB by 1 g/dL.
Platelets	to stop or prevent bleeding in patients with thrombocytopenia	Blood type match is not required but is preferred. One unit increases platelet count by 5,000 – 10,000 platelets/μL.
Fresh frozen plasma (FFP)	to replace clotting factors to reduce bleeding to prevent bleeding in patients with abnormal coagulation tests (e.g., low INR) for massive transfusion of PRBCs	Crossmatching is not required.
Cryoprecipitate	to replace fibrinogen and clotting factors VIII and XIII	Cryoprecipitate has a higher concentration of clotting factors than does FFP.
Whole blood	for massive hemorrhage	Whole blood is used rarely and only as an emergent treatment.
Albumin	for hypovolemic shock to treat hypotension during hemodialysis	Diuretics are often given with albumin.

- In an **exchange transfusion**, the patient's blood is slowly removed in cycles and simultaneously replaced with donor whole blood or plasma. Exchange transfusion is used to treat sickle cell disease, polycythemia vera, and malaria.

- **Plasmapheresis** is similar to dialysis and filters antibodies from blood. It is used for autoimmune disorders such as lupus, myasthenia gravis, and thrombotic thrombocytopenic purpura.

- A blood **type and screen (T&S)** or **type and crossmatch (T&C)** is necessary for the transfusion of some blood products to avoid immunological reactions.

- For suspected transfusion reactions, the nurse should:
  - □ Immediately stop transfusion.

HELPFUL HINT:

Leukocyte-reduced RBCs should be used for patients at high risk for transfusion reactions, including patients with a history of transfusion complications.

- ☐ Infuse with normal saline.
- ☐ Notify physician and blood bank.
- ☐ Continue to monitor vital signs.
- ☐ Return blood products to blood bank for investigation.

HELPFUL HINT:

Febrile reactions are the most common complication of blood transfusions. They occur more often in children and in patients receiving RBCs or platelets. Transfusion-associated circulatory overload is the most common cause of transfusion-related death in the United States.

TABLE 4.4. Complications of Blood Transfusions

Complication	Signs and Symptoms	Intervention
Immunological Reactions		
Acute hemolytic reaction (onset <15 minutes)	fever, chills, back pain, hypotension, tachycardia, elevated JVP, pink or dark-brown urine, DIC	normal saline and diuretic to maintain urine output at 100 mL/hr for 24 hours
Delayed hemolytic reaction (onset >24 hours)	dark urine, jaundice, decreased HgB	usually mild symptoms that do not require intervention monitor renal function
Febrile nonhemolytic reaction (onset 1 – 6 hours)	slight fever, chills, rigor, dyspnea	rule out hemolytic reaction and sepsis antipyretics
Allergic reaction	mild: urticaria, itching severe: anaphylaxis	mild: antihistamines severe: ACLS protocols
Other Complications		
Transfusion-associated circulatory overload (TACO)	signs and symptoms of CHF or pulmonary edema	diuretics slow the transfusion rate
Transfusion-related acute lung injury (TRALI)	signs and symptoms of ARDS or acute lung injury	discontinue transfusion O$_2$ and hemodynamic support per ARDS protocols

QUICK REVIEW QUESTION

7. The nurse began an infusion of PRBCs 30 minutes ago and reassesses the patient. The patient is experiencing lower back pain, diaphoresis, and tachycardia. What is the first thing the nurse should do?

ANSWER KEY

1. Fibrinogen (clotting factor I) is a substrate necessary for coagulation. Patients with very low fibrinogen levels are at risk for severe bleeding and will have prolonged PTs, INRs, PTTs, and aPTTs.

2. The nurse should expect the physician to order an immediate infusion of PRBCs.

3. Obstetrical complications are a common cause of DIC. Diagnostic findings that would confirm this diagnosis include thrombocytopenia, prolonged clotting times (PT and PTT), decreased fibrinogen, and increased levels of fibrinolysis products (D-dimer and FSP).

4. The patient would have been administered heparin to treat the PE, so heparin-induced thrombocytopenia should be considered as a cause of the bleeding.

5. The nurse should suspect septic pneumonia. Chemotherapy immunocompromises patients, making them more susceptible to infection.

6. Tumor lysis syndrome is characterized by the release of large amounts of nucleic acids, which metabolize to form uric acid, leading to hyperuricemia. Allopurinol is a hypouricemic agent that prevents the formation of uric acid.

7. The nurse should immediately stop the blood transfusion, run normal saline wide open through the line, and then notify the physician.

5 GASTROINTESTINAL REVIEW

CCRN TEST PLAN: GASTROINTESTINAL

- Abdominal compartment syndrome
- Acute abdominal trauma
- Acute GI hemorrhage
- Bowel infarction, obstruction, perforation (e.g., mesenteric ischemia, adhesions)
- GI surgeries (e.g., Whipple, esophagectomy, resections)
- Hepatic failure/coma (e.g., portal hypertension, cirrhosis, esophageal varices, fulminant hepatitis, biliary atresia, drug-induced)
- Malnutrition and malabsorption
- Pancreatitis

Gastrointestinal Assessment

1. Inspection: Look for distention, bulges, color, hernias, ascites, and/or pulsations.

2. Auscultation: High-pitched gurgling sounds are normal. Normal bowel sounds can be documented as normal, hypoactive, or hyperactive. Other types of bowel sounds include:

   □ **Borborygmi** are loud, rumbling sounds caused by the shifting of fluids or gas within the intestines; these sounds are a normal finding.

   □ **High-pitched bowel sounds** are often described as tinkling or rushing sounds and may indicate an early bowel obstruction.

☐ **Absent bowel sounds** are an indication of an **ileus**, where no peristalsis is occurring. Bowel sounds may be temporarily absent in certain cases (e.g., after surgery), but their absence, combined with abdominal pain, indicates a serious condition.

3. Percussion: **Tympany** (air) sounds are normal, and **dull sounds** are heard over solid organs (liver and spleen).

4. Palpation: Check for guarding, rigidity, masses, and/or hernias.

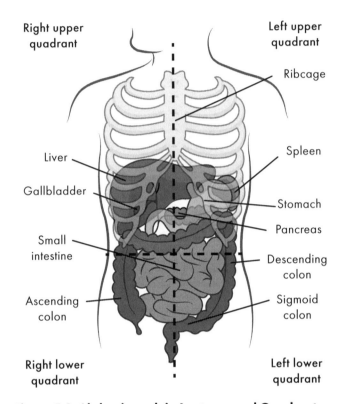

Figure 5.1. Abdominopelvic Anatomy and Quadrants

TABLE 5.1. GI Signs

Name	Description	Indication
Kehr sign	referred left shoulder pain caused when the diaphragm irritates the phrenic nerve	splenic rupture diaphragm irritation
Rovsing sign	pain in the RLQ with palpation of LLQ (indicates peritoneal irritation)	appendicitis
Cullen sign	a bluish discoloration to the umbilical area	retroperitoneal hemorrhage

Name	Description	Indication
Grey Turner sign	ecchymosis in the flank area	retroperitoneal hemorrhage
Psoas sign	abdominal pain when right hip is hyperextended	appendicitis, Crohn's disease
McBurney's point	RLQ pain at point halfway between umbilicus and iliac spine	appendicitis
Murphy sign	pain and cessation of inspiration when RUQ is palpated	acute cholecystitis
Markle test (heel drop)	pain caused when patient stands on tiptoes and drops heels down quickly or when patient hops on one leg	appendicitis, peritonitis

- Diagnostic studies for GI assessment
  - A **focused assessment sonography for trauma (FAST)** exam is a quick bedside exam that uses ultrasound to assess for bleeding after trauma.
  - **Esophagogastroduodenoscopy (EGD or upper endoscopy)** is an endoscopic procedure that uses a scope to visualize the linings of the upper GI tract.
  - **Colonoscopy** is an endoscopic procedure that uses a scope to visualize the linings of the lower GI tract.
  - **Flexible sigmoidoscopy** is endoscopy of the rectum and sigmoid colon.
  - **Balloon-assisted enteroscopy** is used to assess areas of the GI tract that are hard to access, particularly the small intestine.
  - **Ultrasound** is frequently used to visualize the gallbladder, liver, pancreas, spleen, and abdominal aorta.
  - A **CT scan** is frequently used to diagnose or rule out a cause of abdominal pain.
  - **X-rays** are taken to visualize free air, gas, obstructions, foreign bodies, and dilatation.
- Common laboratory tests for GI conditions
  - liver function panels
  - tests for pancreatic enzymes

→
CONTINUE

TABLE 5.2. GI Laboratory Tests

Test	Description	Normal Range
Liver Function Tests		
Albumin	protein made in the liver; low levels may indicate liver damage	3.5 – 5.0 g/dL
Alkaline phosphatase (ALP)	enzyme found in the liver and bones; increased levels indicate liver damage	45 – 147 U/L
Alanine transaminase (ALT)	enzyme in the liver; helps metabolize protein; increased levels indicate liver damage	7 – 55 U/L
Aspartate transami-nase (AST)	enzyme in the liver; helps metabolize alanine; increased levels indicate liver or muscle damage	8 – 48 U/L
Total protein	low levels may indicate liver damage	6.3 – 7.9 g/dL
Total bilirubin	produced during the breakdown of heme; increased levels indicate liver damage or anemia	0.1 – 1.2 mg/dL
Gamma-glutamyl-transferase (GGT)	enzyme that plays a role in antioxidant metabolism; increased levels indicate liver damage	9 – 48 U/L
L-lactate dehydroge-nase (LD or LDH)	enzyme found in most cells in the body; increased levels may indicate liver damage, cancer, or tissue breakdown	adults: 122 – 222 U/L
Pancreatic Enzymes		
Amylase	enzyme that breaks down carbohy-drates	23 – 140 U/L
Lipase	enzyme that breaks down fats	<160 U/L

QUICK REVIEW QUESTION

1. A patient presents with severe upper GI bleeding. What diagnostic study will likely be ordered to locate the source of the bleeding?

Nutrition

■ **Enteral nutrition (EN)** delivers formula through a tube and is indicated for patients with a functioning GI tract but who cannot maintain oral intake.

- Total enteral nutrition (TEN) delivers all required components of nutrition.
- Feedings should start within 48 hours of admission for hemodynamically stable patients who require EN.
- Prepyloric tubes (tip ending in stomach) can be nasogastric (NG tube), orogastric (OG tube), or gastrostomy (G-tube).
- Postpyloric tubes feed into the duodenum or jejunum.
- Gastric residuals should be monitored per protocols.
- Keep HOB raised at least 30° during administration and for 30 minutes afterward to prevent aspiration.
- Administer metoclopramide to improve motility, as ordered.

- **Parenteral feedings** deliver nutrition via IV catheter and are indicated for patients with GI disorders that prevent the absorption of nutrients (e.g., malabsorption, bowel obstruction, ileus).
  - Total parenteral nutrition (TPN) delivers all the required components of nutrition via a central venous catheter. TPN must be delivered via central line to prevent phlebitis or thrombosis.
  - Peripheral parenteral nutrition (PPN) delivers more-dilute nutrition through peripheral veins.
  - Monitor strict input/output when starting, with assessment of cardiac and respiratory to assess for fluid overload.
  - Monitor the patient for signs of hypoglycemia or hyperglycemia.
  - Feedings must not be stopped abruptly; give dextrose 5% if TPN is interrupted.

HELPFUL HINT:

Gastric residual volume (GRV or **gastric residuals)** is the amount of fluid aspirated from the stomach after enteral feedings. High GRV (250 mL) may put the patient at risk for aspiration.

QUICK REVIEW QUESTION

2. A patient receiving TPN has become diaphoretic and shaky and complains of blurred vision. What should the nurse consider?

Abdominal Compartment Syndrome

Pathophysiology

Abdominal compartment syndrome is organ dysfunction caused by increased **intra-abdominal pressure (IAP)**. For most patients, normal IAP will be 5 to 7 mm Hg. Intravesical (bladder) pressure is most commonly used to monitor IAP. Saline is inserted into the bladder via a Foley catheter, and expiration pressure is measured.

HELPFUL HINT:

Chronic obesity increases IAP, and bariatric patients may have elevated IAP with no symptoms.

Intra-abdominal hypertension is IAP >12 mm Hg (although this will vary by patient). Compartment syndrome is usually monitored using **abdominal perfusion pressure (APP)** where APP = MAP – IAP. The goal for adequate abdominal perfusion is APP 60 mm Hg.

Sequalae to intra-abdominal hypertension and abdominal compartment syndrome can be seen in most organ systems.

- Increased IAP displaces the diaphragm, reducing ventricular compliance, venous return, and cardiac output.
- Diaphragm displacement also compresses the lungs.
- Hypoperfusion of the intestines may lead to infarction or infection.
- Increased IAP may lead to increased ICP.

Etiology

- intraperitoneal or retroperitoneal bleeding
- extensive fluid resuscitation
- abdominal packing
- ascites
- burns

Signs and Symptoms

- distended abdomen
- increased peak inspiratory pressure
- oliguria
- JVD
- peripheral edema
- signs and symptoms of hemodynamic instability

Diagnostic Tests and Findings

- IAP >20 mm Hg
- APP <60 mm Hg

Treatment and Management

- definitive treatment: surgical decompression of abdomen (laparotomy) or percutaneous catheter decompression
- noninvasive management
  - fluid restriction
  - supine position (raising head of bed increases IAP)

HELPFUL HINT:

Applying excess PEEP will further reduce cardiac output in patients with IAP.

- ☐ nasogastric or rectal decompression
- ☐ analgesics, sedation, and/or pharmacological paralysis to improve abdominal wall compliance
- ■ mechanical ventilation: reduced tidal volume, permissive hypercapnia to lower airway pressures

QUICK REVIEW QUESTION

3. A patient is sedated and on mechanical ventilation after surgical repair of a pelvic fracture that required aggressive resuscitation with fluids and blood products. Monitoring shows increasing IAP, with IAP of 15 mm Hg and APP of 60 mm Hg. If the patient is currently hemodynamically stable, what interventions should the nurse anticipate?

Acute Abdominal Trauma

Pathophysiology

Acute abdominal trauma can be caused by a penetrating injury such as a gunshot or knife wound or by blunt force trauma from a motor vehicle injury or a fall. Abdominal trauma usually involves injury to multiple organs.

- ■ Trauma to the liver and spleen can cause massive hemorrhage because of the high volume of blood that circulates through them.

- ■ Blunt or penetrating trauma can cause rupture of the diaphragm, leading to dyspnea and possible herniation of abdominal organs into the thoracic cavity.

- ■ Hollow viscus perforation may cause leakage of gastric acids or biliary secretions, leading to peritonitis, SIRS, infection, or sepsis.

Signs and Symptoms

- ■ The following physical assessments indicate visceral injuries.
    - ☐ Grey Turner sign (ecchymosis in the flank area): retroperitoneal bleeding or pancreatic injury
    - ☐ Cullen sign (purple discoloration at umbilicus or flank): blood in the abdominal wall
    - ☐ Kehr sign (referred pain to left shoulder): ruptured spleen or irritated diaphragm from bile in peritoneum
    - ☐ hematoma in the flank: kidney trauma
    - ☐ abdominal distension: accumulated fluid, gas, or blood from ruptured blood vessels or perforated organs

HELPFUL HINT:

All undifferentiated trauma patients should be treated as having hemorrhagic shock until proven otherwise. Fluid resuscitation is the recommended initial treatment following rapid primary and (when possible) secondary survey.

- □ auscultation of friction rub over spleen or liver: may indicate rupture
- □ rebound tenderness and rigidity during abdominal palpation: peritoneal inflammation
- □ subcutaneous emphysema: free air from ruptured bowel
- Signs and symptoms of retroperitoneal bleeding (or hematoma) include hypotension; bradycardia; Grey Turner sign; and abdominal, back, or flank pain.

Diagnostic Findings

- FAST: assess for abdominal fluid, blood, and hemoperitoneum
- abdominal CT: gold standard specific for retroperitoneal hemorrhage
- Foley catheter: assess for frank blood
- NG tube: assess for frank or occult blood (also used for effective gastric decompression)
- diagnostic peritoneal lavage (DPL): invasive insertion of catheter through abdominal wall after bladder emptied
  - □ frank blood: immediate surgery
  - □ no blood: if lab analysis positive for occult blood, immediate surgery is necessary; 1L 0.9% NaCl or LR infused through abdominal catheter and fluid drained back into dependent-position IV bag
- hemoconcentration distorts HgB/Hct results (use serial labs to monitor status)

Treatment and Management

- Common conditions requiring management following abdominal trauma include:
  - □ pre- and post-op hemorrhage (especially with liver injury) and hypovolemic shock
  - □ coagulopathy (deterioration in serial values may warrant rapid surgical exploration)
  - □ hypothermia (caused by large cavity wounds, DPL, fluid resuscitation with non-warmed fluids, or massive transfusion protocol)
  - □ infection and sepsis
- Multiple visceral organ injury generally requires a 3-phase "damage control" surgical plan.

HELPFUL HINT:

A hemodynamically unstable trauma patient with a positive FAST will likely require emergency surgery.

HELPFUL HINT:

Removal of the spleen compromises the immune system and places patients at high risk of infection and **postsplenectomy sepsis**. Patients who have undergone full or partial splenectomy should receive vaccinations per hospital policies (usually pneumococcal, meningococcal, and influenza).

QUICK REVIEW QUESTION

4. A patient is admitted to the ICU after a motor vehicle accident that included blunt force trauma to the abdomen. What signs and symptoms would the nurse look for to assess for retroperitoneal hemorrhage?

Acute GI Hemorrhage

UPPER GI BLEEDING

Pathophysiology

An **upper GI bleed** is bleeding that occurs between the esophagus and duodenum. Bleeding may be severe and require immediate hemodynamic management.

Etiology

- **Peptic ulcers** and **esophagitis** (secondary to GERD) are the most common causes of upper GI bleeding.

- **Esophageal varices** occur when veins in the esophagus rupture because of portal hypertension (usually caused by hepatic cirrhosis). Bleeding may be severe and is likely to recur.

- **Esophageal perforation** or **rupture** may be iatrogenic, secondary to trauma, or caused by the severe effort of vomiting (**Boerhaave syndrome**).

- **Mallory-Weiss tears** occur at the gastroesophageal junction and result from forceful vomiting.

- NSAIDs and chronic gastritis can cause or worsen upper GI bleeding.

Signs and Symptoms

- upper abdominal pain

- hematemesis (may be in nasogastric aspirate)

- melena

- coffee-ground emesis

- hematochezia (if hemorrhaging)

- signs and symptoms of hypovolemia (after significant blood loss)

Diagnostic Tests and Findings

- decreased HgB, Hct, and platelets

> **HELPFUL HINT:**
>
> **Acid suppressive therapy** in the critical care setting is aimed at reducing stress-related peptic ulcer formation and subsequent bleeding. Acid suppression includes a PPI or an H_2 receptor blocker.

HELPFUL HINT:

Elevated BUN-creatinine ratio is associated with decreased kidney function and increased breakdown of protein. It is often seen with upper GI bleeds (due to digestion of blood) but not with lower GI bleeds.

- longer PT and aPTT
- electrolyte imbalances (due to hypovolemia)
- elevated BUN and BUN-creatinine ratio
- positive hemoccult
- diagnosed via appropriate endoscopy or angiogram (EGD to locate source of bleeding)

Treatment and Management

- O_2 therapy
- manage hemodynamic status: IV fluids, blood products, and management of coagulopathies
- medications to constrict vasculature: vasopressin, octreotides, and beta blockers
- endoscopic or surgical repair if bleeding persists
  - esophageal varices: endoscopic variceal band ligation (EVL) or esophageal balloon tamponade (e.g., Sengstaken-Blakemore tube)
  - PPI to prevent post-procedure ulcers

QUICK REVIEW QUESTION

5. The physician has ordered an octreotide drip for a patient diagnosed with esophageal varices. The critical care nurse knows that this medication is appropriate for this diagnosis because it has what type of action?

LOWER GI BLEEDING

Pathophysiology

A **lower GI bleed** is any bleeding that occurs below the duodenum. Lower GI bleeds occur less frequently than do upper GI bleeds, are typically less emergent, and may stop on their own.

Etiology

- disease of the colon (e.g., diverticulitis, IBD, colitis)
- colon polyps, cancer, or tumors
- abscess or inflammation of rectum
- hemorrhoids
- anal fissures

Signs and Symptoms

- abdominal or chest pain
- hematochezia
- melena
- bleeding from rectum
- signs and symptoms of hypovolemia (after significant blood loss)

Diagnostic Tests and Findings

- positive hemoccult
- decreased HgB and Hct
- PT and aPTT may be longer
- diagnosed via appropriate endoscopy, CT scan, or angiogram

Treatment and Management

- manage hemodynamic status: IV fluids, blood products, and management of coagulopathies
- endoscopic or surgical repair if bleeding persists

QUICK REVIEW QUESTION

6. What signs and symptoms would the nurse expect to see in a patient with a lower GI bleed?

Bowel Infarction

Pathophysiology

Bowel infarction, necrosis of part of the intestinal wall, occurs when decreased blood flow causes ischemia in the small bowel (**mesenteric ischemia**) or large bowel (**colonic ischemia**). The most common cause of mesenteric ischemia is embolus or thrombus in the mesenteric artery. Colonic ischemia is usually nonocclusive and is associated with low flow states (e.g., MI, CHF).

Signs and Symptoms

- abdominal pain, cramping, and distension
- nausea and vomiting

- diarrhea
- hematochezia
- altered mental status (in patients 65 years old)

Diagnostic Tests and Findings

- elevated WBC count
- ABG may show metabolic acidosis
- elevated L-lactate or serum amylase
- diagnosed via CT scan of abdomen

Treatment and Management

- fluid resuscitation
- gastric decompression
- anticoagulant therapy and possible angioplasty for arterial occlusion
- broad-spectrum antibiotics
- surgery required to resect necrotic bowel

HELPFUL HINT:

Vasopressors and digitalis should be used cautiously in patients with bowel infarction, as these medications may worsen the ischemia.

> **QUICK REVIEW QUESTION**
>
> 7. A patient with infective endocarditis complains of severe abdominal pain, diarrhea, and vomiting. Why should the nurse suspect a bowel infarction?

Bowel Obstruction and Perforation

Pathophysiology

A **bowel obstruction** occurs when normal flow through the bowel is disrupted. **Mechanical obstructions** are physical barriers in the bowel. The most common mechanical obstructions in the small bowel are **adhesions, hernias,** and **volvuli** (twisting of the bowels). The most common obstruction in the large bowel are tumors.

Paralytic ileus is the impairment of peristalsis in the absence of mechanical obstruction. It is most common in postoperative patients and can also be caused by endocrine disorders or medications (e.g., opioids).

Increased pressure proximal to the obstruction can lead to **perforation** of the bowel wall. Other common causes of bowel perforation include surgery, abdominal trauma, and neoplasm (in large bowel).

Signs and Symptoms

- nausea and vomiting
- diarrhea
- distended and firm abdomen
- abdominal pain (cramping and colicky)
- unable to pass flatus
- high-pitched bowel sounds (early); absent bowel sounds (late)
- tympanic percussion
- pain, often sudden onset (perforation)

Diagnostic Tests and Findings

- increased WBCs
- elevated BUN and decreased electrolytes from dehydration/vomiting
- abdominal X-ray may show dilated bowel loops
- CT scan to diagnose

Treatment and Management

- bowel rest (NPO) or nutritional support distal to obstruction
- fluid resuscitation
- bowel decompression via tube (NG or Miller-Abbott) with low, intermittent suction
- antibiotics as needed
- medications for GI signs and symptoms: antiemetics, simethicone, and/ or magnesium hydroxide
- surgical intervention for obstructions that do not resolve within 48 hours
- surgical closure of perforation

QUICK REVIEW QUESTION

8. A patient presents with abdominal pain, nausea, and vomiting. A bowel obstruction is suspected and then confirmed by CT scan. What priority interventions should the nurse anticipate for this patient?

Gastric Surgeries

- Resection of portions of the GI tract may be required in patients with Crohn's disease, ulcers, tumors, polyps, or cancers affecting the bowels.

  - **Colectomy** is the surgical partial or full resection or removal of a portion of the large intestine.

  - **Ileal pouch anal anastomosis** occurs after a total colectomy and creates a pocket from the distal end of the ileus by surgically attaching it to the anus to preserve bowel function.

  - **Abdominoperineal** (or rectal) **resection** is the removal of the sigmoid colon, rectum, and anus.

  - **Small bowel resection** is the removal of a diseased portion of the small intestine and reattachment of healthy tissue.

  - **Gastrectomy** is the resection of part or all of the stomach, usually because of cancer.

- **Ostomies** divert fecal matter from its normal path through the GI tract by connecting the intestines to an opening in the anterior abdominal wall.

  - Ostomies are commonly performed with resections.

  - An **ileostomy** bypasses the large intestine.

  - A **colostomy** bypasses the distal colon, anus, and rectum.

  - Waste is collected in an **ostomy pouch**.

- **Bariatric surgeries** are performed to resect, bypass, or band the stomach to promote weight loss. Common complications of bariatric bypass surgery include malabsorption, bowel obstruction, anastomotic leaks, and GI bleeding. (See Ch. 11 Multisystem Review for more detailed information on management of bariatric surgery patients.)

- An **abdominal wall hernia** is an area of weakness within the abdominal cavity; organs or tissue can protrude through this weak area.

  - Large hernias can become incarcerated or trapped, which will lead to **strangulation** and ischemia.

  - Hernias with a large diameter or strangulation need surgical repair.

HELPFUL HINT:

Anastomotic leaks should be considered when patients recovering from GI surgery develop s/s of infection.

QUICK REVIEW QUESTION

9. A patient recovering from a partial colectomy is having loose stools several times a day. What intervention should the nurse expect to provide?

_____

Hepatic Failure

Hepatic (liver) failure can be acute (onset <26 weeks) or chronic. Common causes of acute liver failure (also called **fulminate hepatitis**) include acetaminophen overdose and viral hepatitis; the most common cause of chronic liver failure is alcohol abuse.

Liver failure leads to dysfunction in multiple organ systems.

- **Hepatic encephalopathy** is impaired cognitive function caused by increased serum ammonia (NH_3) levels. NH_3 is produced by bacteria in the bowels and is normally broken down by healthy liver tissue before it enters circulation. Increased NH_3 levels may also cause neuromuscular symptoms, including asterixis and bradykinesia.

- Coagulopathies are caused by impaired synthesis of clotting factors in liver tissue.

- **Jaundice** is caused by hyperbilirubinemia.

- Acute kidney injury occurs in approximately 50% of patients with liver failure. (The mechanism is unknown.)

- Infections and sepsis develop secondary to decreased and defective WBCs.

- Metabolic imbalances may include hypokalemia, hyponatremia, and hypoglycemia.

- Lowered peripheral vascular resistance decreases BP and increases HR.

Chronic liver failure leads to **cirrhosis**—the development of fibrotic tissue in the liver. Cirrhosis in the liver increases resistance in the portal vein, causing **portal hypertension**. Common conditions that occur secondary to portal hypertension include esophageal varices, **ascites**, and **splenomegaly**.

Biliary atresia, a rare condition that affects the hepatic and biliary ducts, presents between 2 and 8 weeks of age. Most individuals require a liver transplant in early childhood. However, approximately 35% of people affected reach adulthood before needing liver transplants.

Signs and Symptoms

- cognitive changes or motor dysfunction
- jaundice
- petechiae or purpura
- spider angiomas
- ascites
- RUQ pain

- palmar erythema
- nausea and vomiting

Diagnostic Tests and Findings

- elevated AST, ALT, and/or bilirubin
- elevated NH_3 levels
- decreased protein, albumin, and fibrinogen
- decreased WBCs, HgB, Hct, and platelets
- longer PT and PTT, and increased INR
- CT scan or MRI may show fibrosis of liver

Treatment and Management

- IV fluid resuscitation
- lactulose and neomycin to reduce ammonia levels
- diuretics for ascites
- prophylactic treatment for stress ulcers
- monitor ICP
- tight glucose control for nonalcoholic fatty liver disease
- shunt to reduce portal hypertension
  - ☐ transjugular intrahepatic portosystemic shunt (TIPS): portal vein to a hepatic vein
  - ☐ distal splenorenal shunt (DSRS): splenic vein to the left kidney vein

QUICK REVIEW QUESTION

10. A nurse is providing care to a patient with acute liver failure. What should the nurse expect to see in the patient's CBC and coagulation tests?

Malabsorption

Pathophysiology

Malabsorption is a dysfunction of the small intestine resulting in the inability to effectively absorb the micro- and/or macronutrients that are needed for health. Malabsorption may be global (inability to absorb any nutrients) or specific to certain nutrients.

Etiology

- impairment of digestive enzyme production (e.g., cirrhosis, resection of pancreas)
- bacterial overgrowth
- small intestine dysmotility
- chronic bowel disease (e.g., Crohn's disease)
- bowel resection
- rapid gastric emptying
- medications that affect the lining of the small intestine
- fluid overload

Signs and Symptoms

- steatorrhea
- diarrhea
- abdominal distention
- signs and symptoms related to malabsorption of specific nutrients (e.g., anemia, edema, peripheral neuropathy)

Diagnostic Tests and Findings

- blood tests for low levels of micro- and macronutrients (e.g., iron, calcium)
- CT scan to look for changes in the wall of small intestine

Treatment and Management

- treat primary illness
- antimotility medications
- investigate possible causes of diarrhea
    - enteral feeding (e.g., osmolality, fiber content, contamination)
    - *Clostridium difficile* (C. diff)
    - medications (e.g., PPIs, NSAIDs, diabetes medications, antibiotics)

QUICK REVIEW QUESTION

11. A patient has been treated for severe sepsis with antibiotics and fluid resuscitation. The patient remains on mechanical ventilation, and enteral feeding has been started. The nurse notes that the patient has increased diarrhea. What should the nurse consider to prevent malabsorption?

Pancreatitis

Pathophysiology

Pancreatitis is caused by the release of digestive enzymes into the tissues of the pancreas. The condition causes autodigestion, inflammation, tissue destruction, and injury to adjacent structures and organs. Pancreatitis can be acute or chronic, but its onset is usually sudden. The most common causes of pancreatitis are gallstones and alcohol abuse.

The tissue damage caused by pancreatitis increases capillary permeability, resulting in fluid shifts into interstitial spaces that cause edema and systemic inflammatory responses (e.g., ARDS). Inflammation may also limit diaphragm movement and cause atelectasis. Severe damage to the pancreas may cause retroperitoneal bleeding.

Signs and Symptoms

- steady, severe pain abdominal pain; usually in the LUQ and may radiate to the back or shoulder
- guarding
- nausea and vomiting
- decreased bowel sounds
- steatorrhea
- fever
- tachycardia and hypotension
- dyspnea
- Cullen sign
- Grey Turner sign

Diagnostic Tests and Findings

- elevated amylase and lipase
- hypocalcemia
- decreased total protein
- hypoglycemia
- elevated Hct, BUN, and CRP
- increased WBCs
- imaging (MRI or CT scan with contrast) to diagnose

Treatment and Management

- fluid resuscitation, including electrolyte replacement

- pain management (usually opioids)

- enteral nutritional support (postpyloric)

- endoscopic retrograde cholangiopancreatography (ERCP) for gallstones and bile duct inflammation

- monitor for respiratory complications, including ARDS and atelectasis

---

QUICK REVIEW QUESTION

12. The nurse is caring for a patient who is complaining of sudden, severe abdominal pain in the mid-epigastric area that spreads to the left shoulder. What complications should the nurse assess for?

ANSWER KEY

1. EGD is the diagnostic study most commonly used to visualize sources of upper GI bleeding.

2. The patient may be hyperglycemic or hypoglycemic. The nurse should perform a capillary or serum blood glucose check immediately. If the blood glucose is outside the normal range, protocol to treat for hyperglycemia or hypoglycemia should be followed, and the physician and pharmacy should be notified to adjust the composition of additives.

3. The patient has intra-abdominal hypertension but does not currently have symptoms of abdominal compartment syndrome. The nurse should expect to implement noninvasive interventions to manage IAP, including fluid restriction and supine positioning, and to continue monitoring IAP.

4. Retroperitoneal hemorrhage can lead to ecchymosis (Grey Turner sign, Cullen sign); abdominal, back, or flank pain; and signs or symptoms of hypovolemia (e.g., hypotension).

5. Because octreotide is a vasoconstrictor, it constricts the dilated vessels present in esophageal varices and reduces bleeding.

6. Early signs of a lower GI bleed include hematochezia, abdominal pain, and fatigue. Decreased HgB, decreased Hct, tachycardia, and hypotension may occur after a significant amount of blood loss and would be seen as late signs of a lower GI bleed.

7. Arterial embolus is a common complication of infective endocarditis. When the embolus occludes the mesenteric artery, the resulting hypoperfusion in the bowels may cause ischemia and infarction.

8. Patients with bowel obstructions need IV fluids. During a bowel obstruction, severe vomiting and fluid sequestration in the bowel lumen lead to hypovolemia and electrolyte imbalances.

9. Diarrhea is a common complication of a partial colectomy and is usually temporary. The large intestine is the organ primarily responsible for water absorption, so resection of the colon often results in loose stools. The patient's diet should be adjusted, and the patient may be given an antimotility agent.

10. Patients with liver failure will be pancytopenic with low levels of RBCs, platelets, and WBCs. They will also have prolonged PT and aPTT/PTT, an increased INR, and low fibrinogen.

11. The nurse should collaborate with dietary staff to determine if the correct formula is being used for the patient's needs. Loperamide may help slow the diarrhea. The nurse should also keep in mind that fluid overload may be affecting absorption rates. Finally, because the patient received high-dose antibiotics for sepsis, a diagnosis of *C. diff* should be ruled out with a stool sample.

12. The patient has symptoms of acute pancreatitis. Atelectasis and other respiratory problems are common in patients with acute pancreatitis. The nurse should thoroughly assess lung sounds and note any adventitious or diminished breath sounds, look for signs of orthopnea or other dyspnea, and monitor oxygen saturation levels.

6 RENAL AND GENITOURINARY REVIEW

CCRN TEST PLAN: RENAL AND GENITOURINARY

- Acute genitourinary trauma
- Acute kidney injury (AKI)
- Chronic kidney disease (CKD)
- Infections (e.g., kidney, urosepsis)
- Life-threatening electrolyte imbalances

Renal Physiology and Assessment

- The renal system consists of the kidneys, ureters, bladder (KUB), and urethra. Functions include:
  - □ fluid balance
  - □ blood pressure monitoring and homeostasis
  - □ electrolyte regulation
  - □ metabolic waste excretion
  - □ acid-base balance
  - □ secretion of erythropoietin

- **Nephrons** are the functioning portion of the kidney within the renal cortex. The **glomerulus**, the network of small capillaries within the nephron, is where filtration occurs. This filtration is a result of hydrostatic and oncotic pressure differences across the capillary bed.

HELPFUL HINT:

ACE inhibitors have a greater vasodilatory effect on efferent arterioles than on afferent arterioles in the glomerulus. This imbalance reduces the intraglomerular pressure that drives filtration and reduces the GFR.

HELPFUL HINT:

Acidosis increases bicarbonate reabsorption from the tubular fluid and increases hydrogen ion secretion from the collecting ducts.

Alkalosis increases bicarbonate excretion and decreases hydrogen ion secretion.

- □ The **basement membrane** prevents large particles (e.g., proteins) from entering the filtrate.
- □ Filtrate from the glomerulus travels through the **proximal tubule, loop of Henle**, and **distal convoluted tubule**, where water, electrolytes, and bicarbonate are reabsorbed to maintain fluid, electrolyte, and acid-base balance.

- Kidney function is assessed by measuring the rate of filtration and buildup of metabolic waste in the blood.
  - □ The **glomerular filtration rate (GFR)** is the approximate volume of fluid filtered from the glomeruli per minute.
  - □ **Creatinine clearance (CrCl)** is the volume of plasma cleared of creatinine per minute. (Normal rate is 90 – 140 mL/min for men and 80 – 125 mL/min for women.)
  - □ **Blood urea nitrogen (BUN)** and **serum creatinine** tests assess the levels of metabolic waste products that are normally cleared by the kidneys.
  - □ During renal hypoperfusion, urea may be reabsorbed in the proximal tubules because of compensating increases in the reabsorption of sodium and water. Creatinine is not reabsorbed, so an increased **BUN-to-creatinine ratio** indicates hypoperfusion.

TABLE 6.1. Kidney Function Tests

Test	Description	Normal Range
Serum Tests		
BUN	byproduct of ammonia metabolism; filtered by the kidneys; high levels can indicate insufficient kidney function	7 – 20 mg/dL
Creatinine	product of muscle metabolism; filtered by the kidneys; high levels can indicate insufficient kidney function	0.6 – 1.2 mg/dL
BUN-to-creatinine ratio	increased ratio indicates dehydration, AKI, or GI bleeding; decreased ratio indicates renal damage	10:1 – 20:1
GFR	volume of fluid filtered by the renal glomerular capillaries per unit of time; decreased GFR indicates decreased renal function	men: 100 – 130 mL/min/1.73 m^2 women: 90 – 120 mL/min/1.73 m^2 GFR <60 mL/min/1.73 m^2 is common in adults 70 years

Test	Description	Normal Range
Serum Tests		
Potassium (K$^+$)	helps with muscle contraction and regulates water and acid-base balance	3.5 – 5.2 mEq/L
Sodium (Na$^+$)	maintains fluid balance and plays a major role in muscle and nerve function	135 – 145 mEq/L
Calcium (Ca^{2+})	plays an important role in skeletal function and structure, nerve function, muscle contraction, and cell communication	8.5 – 10.3 mg/dL
Chloride (Cl$^-$)	plays a major role in muscle and nerve function	98 – 107 mEq/L
Magnesium (Mg^{2+})	regulates muscle, nerve, and cardiac function	1.8 – 2.5 mg/dL
Urinalysis		
Leukocytes	presence of WBCs in urine indicates infection	negative
Nitrate	presence in urine indicates infection by gram-negative bacteria	negative
Protein	presence in urine may indicate diabetic neuropathy, nephritis, or eclampsia	negative
pH	decreased (acidic) pH may indicate systemic acidosis or diabetes mellitus; increased (alkali) pH may indicate systemic alkalosis or UTI	4.5 – 8
Blood	presence in urine may indicate infection, renal calculi, a neoplasm, or coagulation disorders	negative
Specific gravity	concentration of urine; decreased concentration may indicate diabetes insipidus or pyelonephritis; increased concentration may indicate dehydration or syndrome of inappropriate antidiuretic hormone secretion (SIADH)	1.010 – 1.025
Urine osmolality	concentration of urine; more accurate than specific gravity	300 – 900 mOsm/kg
Ketones	produced during fat metabolism; presence in urine may indicate diabetes, hyperglycemia, starvation, alcoholism, or eclampsia	negative

QUICK REVIEW QUESTION

1.   Why do patients with upper GI bleeding often have a high BUN-to-creatinine ratio?

Renal Therapeutic Interventions

- **Renal replacement therapies** are considered when the GFR is <30 mL/min; options include dialysis and kidney transplantation.

- Filtration may occur via diffusion or convection.
  - Diffusion occurs when blood is exposed to a **dialysate fluid** with water, electrolytes, and osmotic agents. The composition of the dialysate fluid creates an osmotic gradient that moves water and metabolic waste out of the blood.
  - During convection, hydrostatic pressure forces water and permeable molecules out of the blood.

- During **intermittent hemodialysis**, blood is pumped through an external dialyzer.
  - standard method of dialysis for hemodynamically stable patients
  - access through a temporary or permanent dialysis catheter or a surgically created fistula
  - treatments take 3 –5 hours
  - heparin administered to prevent microemboli formation
  - complications usually related to shifts in fluid volume; include hypotension, angina, dyspnea, and dysrhythmias

- **Continuous renal replacement therapy (CRRT)** uses an extracorporeal blood pump to continuously move blood through a hemofilter.
  - used in patients who cannot tolerate changes in water and electrolyte levels during intermittent hemodialysis
  - can be used to remove larger particles than those removed by intermittent hemodialysis
  - requires large-bore double-lumen central catheter

- During **peritoneal dialysis**, the dialysate fluid is infused into the peritoneal cavity and allowed to remain there for several hours.
  - preferred method for hemodynamically unstable patients who cannot tolerate hemodialysis
  - requires percutaneous or laparoscopic insertion of catheter into abdominal cavity

HELPFUL HINT:

Continuous venovenous hemofiltration (CVVH) is a type of CRRT that uses convection to remove excess water from the blood.

- □ patients with diabetes require careful monitoring to ensure stability of blood-glucose level
- □ most common complication: peritonitis
- □ signs and symptoms: abdominal pain, cloudy peritoneal effluent, and fever
- **Dialysis disequilibrium syndrome (DDS)** is a set of neurological symptoms that occur during dialysis, due to cerebral edema. Signs and symptoms include headache, blurred vision, and altered LOC or mental status.

QUICK REVIEW QUESTION

2. Why is intermittent hemodialysis contraindicated for patients with TBI or increased ICP?

Acute Genitourinary Trauma

Pathophysiology

Genitourinary (GU) trauma can cause injury to the kidneys, bladder, urethra, or external genitalia. GU trauma symptoms can be nonspecific and can be masked by or related to other injuries. Trauma may occur from blunt or penetrating injury.

- Renal: The majority of renal trauma occurs from blunt trauma such as direct impact into the seatbelt or steering wheel in frontal MVCs or from body panel intrusion in side-impact crashes. Renal injuries are ranked graded from 1 to 5 based on severity. Grade 5 renal injuries are referred to as **shattered kidney** and include severe renal vascular laceration.

- Bladder: The majority of bladder trauma occurs from blunt trauma, usually occurring with a pelvic fracture. Bladder rupture can also result from lap belt restraint. Leakage from ruptures may lead to peritonitis or sepsis.

- Urethral: Urethral injuries are more common in males and may result from trauma and pelvic fracture or from iatrogenic injuries resulting from catheterization.

Signs and Symptoms

- pain (suprapubic, abdominal, groin/genital, or flank)
- urinary symptoms (e.g., hematuria, dysuria)
- bleeding at meatus

- ecchymosis
- distended bladder
- abdominal distention
- foul-smelling vaginal discharge

Diagnostic Tests and Findings

- urinalysis (for hematuria)
- decreased hemoglobin and hematocrit
- monitor for
  - elevated BUN and creatinine
  - fluid and electrolyte status
- diagnostic imaging (CT scan, KUB X-ray)

Treatment and Management

- low-grade renal trauma may be admitted for monitoring (Hct, hemodynamic)
- use angioembolization for persistent bleeding
- keep bladder decompressed via Foley catheter (if no urethral injury present)
- manage sequalae (e.g., acute kidney injury, hemorrhage)

QUICK REVIEW QUESTION

3. A patient with grade 4 blunt renal injury is admitted to the ICU for monitoring. What symptoms and diagnostic findings should the nurse expect to monitor?

★ Acute Kidney Injury

Acute kidney injury (AKI), previously called acute renal failure, is an acute decrease in kidney function characterized by increased serum creatinine (**azotemia**) with or without decreased urine output. Changes in kidney function may result in multiple systemic conditions that require intervention. These conditions include:

- fluid imbalance (hypo- or hypervolemia)
- electrolyte imbalance
- acid-base imbalance
- hematological abnormalities (e.g., anemia, low platelet count)

AKI has a diverse etiology and is characterized as prerenal, intrarenal, or postrenal, based on the cause of injury. Questions on the CCRN will focus on intrarenal disease.

PRERENAL DISEASE

Pathophysiology

Prerenal disease is renal hypoperfusion caused by hemodynamic compromise (e.g., hypovolemia, systemic vasodilation) or renal ischemia. Prerenal disease presents with no damage to renal tubules and can usually be reversed by treating the underlying condition.

Diagnostic Findings

- increased creatinine and BUN
- elevated BUN-to-creatinine ratio (20:1)
- low urine Na^+ (<20 mEq/L)
- increased urine osmolality and specific gravity
- normal finding on urine microscopy (no casts)
- serum creatinine returns to normal value after fluid repletion

Treatment and Management

- treat underlying cause to maintain MAP 65 mm Hg
  □ fluids to rehydrate
  □ vasopressors as needed to manage vasodilation

QUICK REVIEW QUESTION

4. A patient with sepsis has received 3 L of normal saline over the past 24 hours and currently has maintenance fluids at 125 mL/hr. The nurse notes that urine output is at 250 mL for the past 4 hours. The last serum creatinine is 1.8 mg/dL, and BUN is 38 mg/dL. What interventions should the nurse anticipate?

INTRARENAL DISEASE

Pathophysiology

Intrarenal (or intrinsic) disease is caused by damage to the kidneys. The most common intrarenal condition in critical care settings is **acute tubular necrosis (ATN)**, the destruction of the renal tubular epithelium. ATN may be ischemic (usually caused by severe prerenal disease) or nephrotoxic. Common nephrotoxic substances include contrast dyes, NSAIDs, ARBs, ACE inhibitors,

HELPFUL HINT:

NSAIDs, ARBs, and ACE inhibitors can cause or worsen prerenal disease and ATN.

and aminoglycosides. ATN may also occur secondary to rhabdomyolysis or after cardiovascular surgery.

Intrarenal disease and recovery occurs in 4 phases.

1. The **onset phase** occurs immediately after the triggering event but before cell injury. Patients may have reduced urine output but few other symptoms.

2. During the **oliguric phase** (1 – 2 weeks), urine output is reduced to <400 mL/day, and creatinine and BUN serum levels will increase. In rare cases, patients may become **anuric** (urine output <100 mL/day). The inability of the kidneys to excrete urine may cause fluid overload, electrolyte imbalances (particularly hyperkalemia), and metabolic acidosis.

3. The **diuretic phase** (1 – 2 weeks) begins when the underlying cause of AKI has been corrected and GFR begins to increase. This phase is characterized by increased urine output (3 L/day). Patients should be monitored for hypovolemia and electrolyte depletion.

4. The **recovery phase** may last up to a year as kidney function slowly returns.

HELPFUL HINT:

Infection is the most common cause of death for patients with AKI.

Diagnostic Findings

- increased creatinine and BUN
- BUN-to-creatinine ratio <20:1
- oliguric phase
  - increased urine osmolality and specific gravity
  - urine Na^+ <10 mEq/L
- diuretic phase
  - decreased urine osmolality and specific gravity
  - urine Na^+ <40 mEq/L
- casts seen through urine microscopy
- serum creatinine does not respond to fluid repletion

Treatment and Management

- treat underlying cause
- discontinue or minimize use of nephrotoxic medications
- fluid volume management
  - IV fluids for hypovolemia
  - loop diuretics for hypervolemia (if not anuric)
  - daily weights and strict monitoring of fluid I/O

- correct electrolyte imbalances and monitor for related complications (including cardiac monitoring)
- sodium bicarbonate for metabolic acidosis
- indications for urgent dialysis in patients with AKI
  - severe or symptomatic hyperkalemia
  - severe metabolic acidosis
  - volume overload
  - pulmonary edema
  - uremia

QUICK REVIEW QUESTION

5. Several days after a cardiac catheterization, a patient is suspected of having intrarenal disease related to the imaging contrast dye used. The patient's I/O are being monitored closely, with outputs of approximately 500 mL per shift charted. The patient's assessment is as follows: BP 165/92, HR 85 bpm, 3+ pitting edema, auscultation of crackles in the bases of lungs, and SpO_2 92%. What condition should the nurse suspect, and what intervention will be required?

POSTRENAL DISEASE

Pathophysiology

Postrenal conditions are characterized by the blocked drainage of urine, usually because of prostatic hypertrophy or renal calculi. Treatment addresses the underlying cause of obstruction.

Diagnostic Findings

- oliguria
- increased serum creatinine and BUN
- normal BUN-to-creatinine ratio
- possible pain or hematuria

QUICK REVIEW QUESTION

6. What lab values can be used to differentiate between pre- and postrenal failure?

Chronic Kidney Disease

Pathophysiology

Chronic kidney disease (CKD) is long-term (3 months) kidney damage or dysfunction caused by destruction of nephrons. Like AKI, the etiology of CKD can be categorized as pre-, intra-, or postrenal. Common causes of CKD include:

- decreased perfusion due to heart failure or cirrhosis
- hypertensive nephrosclerosis
- diabetic nephropathy
- renal artery stenosis (usually due to atherosclerosis)
- glomular or tubulointerstitial disease
- chronic urinary obstruction

The kidneys initially compensate by hyperfiltration in individual nephrons, so patients are initially asymptomatic and present only with abnormal creatinine or BUN values. As the kidneys' ability to remove excess fluid and metabolic waste is further impaired, patients show signs and symptoms related to hypervolemia and decreased GFR. Related conditions that may require acute care include pulmonary edema and electrolyte imbalances. Other sequalae include anemia, hypertension, nausea/vomiting, pericarditis, peripheral neuropathy, weakness/lethargy, and altered mental status.

HELPFUL HINT:

Patients with CKD have an elevated risk of CAD and worse outcomes after MI, CABG, and PCI.

Diagnostic Findings

- decreased GFR
  - Stage 1: 90 mL/min
  - Stage 2: 60 – 89 mL/min
  - Stage 3: 30 – 59 mL/min
  - Stage 4: 15 – 29 mL/min
  - Stage 5: <15 mL/min (**end-stage renal disease [ESRD]**)
- increased serum creatinine and BUN
- increased K^+ and decreased Ca^{2+}
- decreased HgB
- increased serum bicarbonate

Treatment and Management

- reverse initial cause of kidney injury
- sodium restriction and diuretics for hypervolemia

- sodium bicarbonate for acidosis
- ACE inhibitors or ARBs for hypertension
- erythropoietin for anemia
- renal replacement therapy (hemodialysis, peritoneal dialysis, or transplant)

QUICK REVIEW QUESTION

7. Why would diuretics be prescribed for a patient with CKD?

Electrolyte Imbalances

TABLE 6.2. Electrolyte Imbalances

Imbalance	Clinical Manifestation	Treatment and Management	Etiology
Sodium (normal: 135 – 145 mEq/L)			
Hyponatremia	tachycardia hypotension weakness dizziness headache abdominal cramping cerebral edema increased ICP	sodium replacement, ≤12 mEq/L/24 hr in a 24-hour period PO sodium replacement as tolerated isotonic IV solutions (lactated Ringers or 0.9% normal saline) restrict fluid intake and monitor fluid I/O	dilutional depletion of Na⁺ CHF diarrhea diaphoresis use of thiazides
Hypernatremia	hypotension tachycardia polydipsia lethargy or irritability edema warm, flushed skin hyperreflexia seizures	restrict dietary sodium increase PO fluid or free-water intake diuretics D5W or other hypotonic IV solutions	sodium overload volume depletion impaired thirst renal or GI loss inability to replace fluid losses

continued on next page

TABLE 6.2. Electrolyte Imbalances (continued)

Imbalance	Clinical Manifestation	Treatment and Management	Etiology
Potassium (normal: 3.5 – 5 mEq/L)			
Hypokalemia	dysrhythmias • flat or inverted T waves • prominent U waves • ST depression • prolonged PR interval hypotension altered mental status leg cramps or muscle cramps hypoactive reflexes flaccid muscles	potassium replace-ment PO or IV • IV administration ≤20 mEq/hr • not to exceed 40 – 80 mEq/24 hr in a 24-hour period • stop infusion if urine output <30 mL/hr cardiac monitoring necessary presents with hyper-calcemia	acid-base shifts alkalosis true depletion or deficits IV dextrose use diarrhea alcoholism Cushing's syndrome medications • steroids • diuretics • amphotericin • insulin
Hyperkalemia	dysrhythmias or cardiac arrest • tall, peaked T waves • prolonged PR interval • wide QRS complex • absent P waves • ST depression abdominal cramping and diarrhea anxiety	medication or IV solution, depending on severity of symptoms • calcium gluconate • IV insulin and D50 • loop diuretics • sodium polystyrene sulfonate • sodium bicarbonate • beta 2 agonists • hypertonic IV solution (3% normal saline) ECG and continued cardiac monitoring restrict PO intake of potassium-containing foods may require dialysis	increased intake of salt substitutes or potassium-sparing medications hemolysis, burns, crushing injury, or rhabdomyolysis decreased urine output

Imbalance	Clinical Manifestation	Treatment and Management	Etiology
Magnesium (normal: 1.3 – 2.1 mEq/L)			
Hypomagnesemia	dysrhythmias • torsades de pointes • flat or inverted T waves • ST depression • prolonged PR interval • widened QRS complex hypertension Chvostek sign Trousseau sign seizures hyperreflexia	magnesium sulfate IV, 1 – 2 g over 60 minutes monitor for seizures, dysrhythmias, and magnesium toxicity	excessive excretion (from GI tract or kidneys) diuretic use alcoholism
Hypermagnesemia	dysrhythmias or cardiac arrest • prolonged PR interval • wide QRS complex • peaked T waves bradycardia (more common) or tachycardia bradypnea respiratory paralysis altered mental status, lethargy, or coma	calcium gluconate loop diuretics isotonic IV solutions (lactated Ringers or 0.9% normal saline) may require dialysis	increased magnesium intake renal dysfunction hepatitis Addison's disease

TABLE 6.2. Electrolyte Imbalances (continued)			
Imbalance	Clinical Manifestation	Treatment and Management	Etiology
Calcium (normal: 4.5 – 5.5 mEq/L)			
Hypocalcemia	dysrhythmias or cardiac arrest prolonged QT interval flattened ST segment hypotension third-space fluid shift decreased clotting time laryngeal spasm or broncho-spasm seizures Chvostek sign Trousseau sign hyperactive deep-tendon reflexes	PO or IV calcium replacement calcium gluconate, 10 – 20 mL, over 5 – 10 minutes dilute IV solution with D5W only, never with normal saline vitamin D supplements (to enhance absorption) seizure precautions	low serum proteins decreased calcium intake renal failure hypoparathyroid-ism vitamin D deficiency pancreatitis medications calcitonin steroids loop diuretics
Hypercalcemia	anxiety cognitive dys-function constipation nausea/vomiting shortened QT interval muscle weakness	loop diuretics isotonic IV solutions (0.9% normal saline) glucocorticoids and calcitonin	malignancies hyperthyroidism and hyperparathy-roidism Paget's disease medications lithium androgens tamoxifen excessive vitamin D excessive thyroid replacement therapy

Imbalance	Clinical Manifestation	Treatment and Management	Etiology
Phosphate (normal: 1.8 – 2.3 mEq/L)			
Hypophosphatemia	respiratory distress or failure tissue hypoxia chest pain seizures decreased LOC increased susceptibility to infection nystagmus	PO or IV phosphate replacement replace slowly if on TPN seizure precautions	increased renal excretion
Hyperphosphatemia	tachycardia Chvostek sign Trousseau sign hyperreflexia soft-tissue calcifications	saline and loop diuretics phosphate binders (e.g., aluminum hydroxide) limit dietary intake of phosphates dialysis may be appropriate	decreased renal excretion

QUICK REVIEW QUESTION

8.   A patient receiving enteral feedings has had severe diarrhea. The patient becomes irritable and is twitching. The nurse's assessment reveals the following vital signs: BP 92/53 mm Hg, HR 108 bpm, RR 20 breaths/min, and oral temperature 38.3°C (100.9°F). What condition should the nurse suspect?

Infections

- Urinary tract infections (UTIs) include **pyelonephritis** (infection of the kidney or upper urinary tract) and **cystitis** (infection of the bladder or lower urinary tract).

- Most UTIs in critical care settings are associated with urinary catheters (**catheter-associated urinary tract infection [CAUTI]**).

- Signs and symptoms of UTI include costovertebral pain, fever, and dysuria. Patients 65 years old may present with delirium.

- Signs and symptoms are often absent or nonspecific in ICU patients. Patients with catheters or an altered LOC may not be able to communicate signs or symptoms.

- UTIs are diagnosed via urinalysis and culture.

- Symptomatic UTIs (with fever or obstruction) should be treated with antibiotics.

QUICK REVIEW QUESTION

9. A patient in the ICU for a subdural hematoma has ICP monitoring in progress and is receiving mannitol. I/O of fluid is being strictly monitored with an indwelling Foley catheter for output collection. The patient's urine is cloudy and has a foul odor. What is the best action for the nurse to take?

ANSWER KEY

1. The BUN-to-creatinine ratio increases because of hypovolemia. Urea is reabsorbed in the proximal tubules when reabsorption rates of water and sodium (to which urea is passively linked) are increased. Creatinine is not reabsorbed at the same rate. BUN levels are also increased by the breakdown of blood proteins in the GI tract.

2. The rapid removal of urea from the blood can lower plasma osmolality, which results in fluid shift to the intracellular space. For patients at risk for ICP, the resulting cerebral edema can cause neurological deterioration. While cerebral edema may occur with any type of dialysis, it is more common with intermittent dialysis.

3. Patients with kidney injury are at high risk for hemorrhage. The nurse should monitor for signs of bleeding (e.g., serial hematocrit) and shock (e.g., hypotension).

4. The patient is likely experiencing sepsis-induced prerenal disease. The nurse should ensure optimal perfusion through continued fluid replacement and titrating vasopressors to keep MAP 65 mm Hg. The physician should be notified if the patient does not respond with improving urine output.

5. These symptoms may indicate pulmonary edema. The nurse should immediately inform the physician and prepare the patient for hemodialysis.

6. In prerenal disease, the BUN-to-creatinine ratio will be 20:1. In postrenal disease, the ratio will be normal (10:1 – 20:1).

7. Diuretics are prescribed to manage conditions related to hypervolemia in patients with CKD; these conditions include PE and hypertension. Diuretics may also be used to lower K^+ levels (loop diuretics).

8. The patient's history and symptoms suggest hypernatremia, likely due to the dehydration associated with diarrhea and possibly insufficient free water administered with the enteral feedings.

9. The nurse should remove the Foley catheter, obtain a clean-catch urine sample, and monitor for fever and elevated WBCs. The physician should be notified for alternative output monitoring, such as weighing linens or an external female catheter.

7 INTEGUMENTARY REVIEW

Integumentary Interventions

- **Negative-pressure wound therapy (NPWT)** devices, also known as **vacuum-assisted wound closure (VACs)**, apply a controlled suction to the wound bed to promote healing.
  - □ Wound VACs promote healing by improving circulation to the wound bed, decreasing fluid in the wound bed, and promoting formation of granulation tissue.
  - □ Wound VACs are commonly used for wounds with high-volume drainage or that are high risk for infection, surgical wounds, burns, and chronic wounds (e.g., pressure ulcers).
  - □ Wound VACs should not be used on wounds with necrotic or cancerous tissue, exposed nerves or organs, or underlying coagulopathies.

- A **fecal management device** is a closed system that collects and contains liquid or semiliquid stools.
  - □ The goals of using a fecal management device are to prevent cross-contamination by virulent stool pathogens and to reduce the threat to skin integrity posed by diarrhea.

HELPFUL HINT:

Suction pressure that is too strong (less than −175 mm Hg) may reduce perfusion in the tissue under the wound and slow healing.

- Contraindications to use of fecal management devices include rectal/anal injury, bleeding, tumor, or stenosis; fecal impaction; recent large bowel surgery; and antithrombic therapy (requires caution).
- Potential adverse outcomes of fecal management include pressure necrosis, leakage of fecal material, and abdominal distension.

QUICK REVIEW QUESTION

1. A patient is 2 days post-op. The patient's left trochanter surgical site has high-volume drainage requiring application of NPWT to promote wound healing. While changing the dressing, the nurse notes purulent discharge and erythema at the wound site. What should the nurse do next?

Cellulitis

Pathophysiology

Cellulitis is a bacterial infection that has compromised the skin through to the hypodermis. The infection is caused by bacterial entry wounds in the skin. While it can develop anywhere on the body, the lower extremities are most commonly affected in adults.

The infection is usually localized at first but may quickly progress to sepsis if not treated promptly. Patient populations with chronic comorbidities such as diabetes, heart failure, and autoimmune diseases are more susceptible to serious complications.

Signs and Symptoms

- erythema, warmth, and tenderness at site
- lymphadenopathy of affected side
- fever

Diagnostic Findings

- elevated WBCs
- culture and sensitivity (most commonly group A *Streptococcus*)

Treatment and Management

- antibiotics
- debridement and drainage
- pain management

QUICK REVIEW QUESTION

2.   The nurse is conducting a skin assessment on a patient admitted with DKA. She notes a localized area of erythema on the left lower extremity that is warm and tender. The patient states that it started as a bug bite. How should the nurse manage this patient's risk for cellulitis?

IV Infiltration/Extravasation

Pathophysiology

IV infiltration is the infusion of fluids into the tissue around a venipuncture site. **Extravasation** is infiltration of a chemotherapeutic drug or vesicant fluid into the tissue around the venipuncture site. **Vesicants** can cause pain, tissue sloughing, loss of mobility in the surrounding areas, blisters, erythema, and infection. Mild symptoms of extravasation may appear immediately, but more serious symptoms may take days or weeks to develop.

Drugs classified as vesicants include:

- electrolyte solutions
- vasopressors
- antineoplastics
- most antibiotics (e.g., doxycycline, nafcillin, and vancomycin)
- radiocontrast infusions
- D10
- phenytoin

Signs and Symptoms

- immediate (at insertion site)
  - tingling, burning, or pruritus
  - swelling
- later (at insertion site)
  - erythema
  - pain
  - discoloration
  - blistering, ulceration, or necrosis

Treatment and Management

- Immediately stop infusion.
- Assess patency of IV ports to determine need for alternative IV access sites.
- Aspirate the infusing medication from the catheter until blood return and waste amount is achieved (hospital-specific policy).
- Flush catheter (hospital-specific protocol).

HELPFUL HINT:

Use of hyaluronidase for extravasations of parenteral nutrition and calcium chloride can be beneficial. Hyaluronidase should not be used for extravasation of vasoconstrictive agents.

> **QUICK REVIEW QUESTION**
>
> 3.   An intubated patient is hemodynamically stabilizing on a titrated infusion of norepinephrine, with propofol and fentanyl, via a triple-lumen internal jugular venous catheter. The nurse assesses an area of erythema and slight puffiness around the catheter insertion site and sees a scant amount of clear liquid pooling under the transparent dressing during palpation. What should the nurse do first?

Necrotizing Fasciitis

Pathophysiology

Necrotizing soft-tissue infections (NSTIs) are fast-spreading infections that cause soft tissue death. **Necrotizing fasciitis** is an NSTI that affects the muscle fascia and hypodermis. It may spread quickly without noticeable skin symptoms, making it difficult to diagnose. Patients with diabetes or compromised immune systems are at higher risk of NSTIs. Prompt treatment of necrotizing fasciitis is necessary to prevent tissue necrosis, amputation, or death.

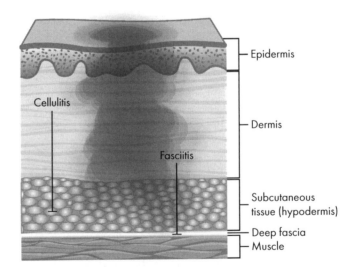

Figure 7.1. Cellulitis and Fasciitis

Signs and Symptoms

- erythema, warmth, and tenderness at site
- progression of necrosis on skin (red to blue to black)
- tingling or lack of sensation in affected area
- significant pain
- crepitus
- hematic or gas bullae
- fever
- sepsis

Diagnostic Findings

- elevated WBCs

Treatment and Management

- prompt surgical exploration and debridement (should not be delayed for diagnostic labs)
- empiric administration of broad spectrum antibiotics
- IV fluids and vasopressors as needed to maintain hemodynamic stability
- pain management
- hyperbaric oxygen therapy

> **QUICK REVIEW QUESTION**
>
> 4. An immunocompromised patient is recovering from a hemicolectomy in the ICU. Three days post-op, the nurse notes new areas of erythema and edema on both flanks. The patient is started on IV antibiotics, but the erythema continued to spread and the patient reports significant pain. Four days post-op, the patient presents with fever and decreased LOC, and wound crepitus is observed. What intervention should the nurse anticipate for this patient?

HELPFUL HINT:

Fournier gangrene is a necrotizing infection of the perineum. It is most common in patients with DM, and is a rare side effect of SGLT2 inhibitors.

HELPFUL HINT:

During hyperbaric O_2 treatment, patients with history or increased risk of seizures are at a higher risk for repeat seizure.

Pressure Injury

Pressure injuries (also known as pressure ulcers, decubitus ulcers, or bedsores) are wounds occurring secondary to tissue ischemia. Unrelieved pressure is the most common cause, with most wounds occurring over a bony prominence. Unrelieved pressure compromises the blood flow to the skin and underlying tissue, which deprives the tissue of oxygen and nutrients and limits waste removal. Pressure ulcers are described as stage 1 through stage 4. They can also be labeled as a deep-tissue injury or unstageable. (Staging of pressure ulcers is not tested on the CCRN.)

Treatment and Management

- Measures to prevent pressure ulcers include systematic position changes and use of positioning devices.

- Stage 1: Begin preventive measures, including repositioning and transparent film.

- Stage 2: Dress wound to maintain moist environment.

- Stages 3 and 4: Debride necrotic tissues (surgical or hydrogel dressing).

- Other interventions include NPWT and topical antibiotics.

QUICK REVIEW QUESTION

5.   An ICU patient is intubated 24 hours post-insertion of an IABP. During a skin assessment, the nurse notices a non-blanchable area of redness on the left heel of the patient. What should the nurse do next?

_____

ANSWER KEY

1.   The wound shows signs of infection, so the nurse should discontinue use of NPWT. The wound will need to be cleaned and a wound culture taken so that the patient can receive the appropriate antibiotics.

2.   The nurse should note the patient's risk for cellulitis and document the wound size, shape, and location. The circumference of the area should be marked with a skin-safe pen to assess for progression. The physician should be notified, and the nurse should expect a culture and sensitivity and empiric antibiotics to be ordered while awaiting results.

3.   The nurse should stop the IV infusions through the central IJ line and begin a quick assessment of each individual port for patency. A quick evaluation, per hospital policy, will indicate whether it is safe to restart vesicant infusions or whether the nurse needs to obtain other IV access. The results of these assessments and interventions can then be communicated to the physician.

4.   The patient has symptoms of necrotizing fasciitis. The nurse should anticipate that the patient will undergo immediate surgical exploration and debridement.

5.   A non-blanchable red area on the heel is likely a stage 1 pressure ulcer. Because the patient has an IABP and is intubated, they cannot be repositioned laterally. The nurse should use a positioning device, such as a pillow or heel lift device, to reduce pressure on the heel.

8 MUSCULOSKELETAL REVIEW

CCRN TEST PLAN: MUSCULOSKELETAL

- Compartment syndrome
- Fractures (e.g., femur, pelvic)
- Functional issues (e.g., immobility, falls, gait disorders)
- Osteomyelitis
- Rhabdomyolysis

Compartment Syndrome

Pathophysiology

Compartment syndrome is the result of increased intracompartmental pressure, usually due to a fracture or crush injury. When the increased pressure in the closed compartment exceeds the pressure of perfusion, blood circulation is impaired, resulting in ischemia of the nerves and muscle tissue. Oxygen deficiency and the buildup of waste irritate the nerves, resulting in pain and a decrease in sensation. As ischemia progresses, muscles become necrotic, which can lead to rhabdomyolysis, hyperkalemia, and infection if left untreated.

HELPFUL HINT:

The most common cause of compartment syndrome is extremity fractures.

Signs and Symptoms

- the 6 Ps
  - pain (not proportional to injury and does not respond to opioid medications)
  - paresthesia
  - pallor

     ☐ paralysis

     ☐ pulselessness

     ☐ poikilothermia

- decreased urine output

- hypotension

- tissue tight on palpation

- edema with tight, shiny skin

- intracompartmental pressure 30 mm Hg or within 20 to 30 mm Hg of MAP

Treatment and Management

- Remove casts or dressings to relieve pressure.

- Push IV fluids to maintain urine output >30 cc/hr.

- If intracompartmental pressure >30 mm Hg, prepare patient for fasciotomy.

- If intracompartmental pressure is 10 – 30 mm Hg, monitor pressure and hemodynamic status.

> **QUICK REVIEW QUESTION**
>
> 1. A patient admitted to the ICU following an MVC has a cast on their right wrist for a Salter-Harris fracture. The patient reports acute onset of paresthesia and pain in the distal fingers. The nurse observes pallor in the extremities and is unable to obtain a radial pulse. What should the nurse do first?

FRACTURES

- While most fractures are uncomplicated and may be treated in an acute care setting, traumatic fractures of the pelvis or femur are often managed in the ICU. These fractures require complex stabilization and place patients at high risk of complications, including internal hemorrhage, organ perforation, hematoma formation, and lipid embolisms.

- Acute care for both pelvic and femur fractures focuses on hemodynamic stabilization and surgical stabilization of the fracture.

- **Pelvic fractures** are caused by high-energy trauma (e.g., MVC) and usually occur alongside injuries to the chest, abdomen, or vertebral column.

     ☐ Pelvic fractures are classified by the location of the fracture. Patients with unstable pelvic ring fractures (fractures that disrupt the integrity of the pelvic ring) are at the highest risk for complications.

□ Patients with pelvic fractures (particularly open fractures) are at high risk of hemorrhage from venous or arterial bleeding, which is the most common cause of mortality related to pelvic fractures.

HELPFUL HINT:

Patients with pelvic fractures should be closely monitored for signs and symptoms of retroperitoneal bleeding.

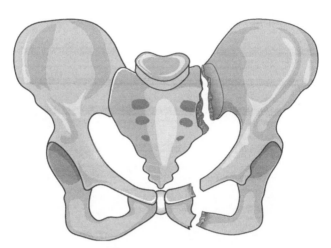

Figure 8.1. Example of an Unstable Pelvic Ring Fracture (Vertical Shear Injury)

□ Soft tissue injuries that may accompany pelvic fractures include ruptured bladder, perforation of abdominal organs, and lacerations of the reproductive organs.

□ Diagnostic imaging may include pelvic X-rays, pelvic CT scan, pelvic angiogram (when patient has an unstable pelvic ring with ongoing hemorrhage), cystogram (for suspected urinary bladder injury), or retrograde urethrogram (for suspected urethral tears).

□ Perforation of the GI tract places the patient at high risk for infection and sepsis, the second most common cause of mortality related to pelvic fractures. Patients may require a temporary colostomy or ileostomy to prevent wound contamination.

□ Immobility and hemodynamic disruption in the lower extremities create a high risk of DVT.

□ Postoperative care includes hemodynamic monitoring, aggressive DVT prophylaxis, pain management, and care for related injuries.

■ **Femur fractures** may be caused by high-energy trauma (e.g., MVC) in young patients, or by low-energy trauma (e.g., falls) in patients 65 years old. Life-threatening complications of femur fractures include hemorrhage, compartment syndrome, fat embolism syndrome, and respiratory distress (ARDS caused by fat embolism or PE).

■ **Fat embolism syndrome (FES)** is caused by fat in the pulmonary circulatory system.

□ A cardinal cutaneous sign of fat emboli is reddish-brown non-palpable petechiae that appear over the upper body (particularly in the axilla region) 24 – 36 hours after the trauma event.

□ Other symptoms include hypoxemia, dyspnea, altered mental status/decreased LOC, and fever.

□ The development of progressive altered mental status, restlessness, confusion, seizures, and coma indicate cerebral fat emboli.

□ Care is supportive and includes respiratory support and IV fluids.

QUICK REVIEW QUESTION

2. A 28-year-old patient has been receiving supportive care for a closed femur fracture caused by an MVC. After being hemodynamically stable with a GCS of 15 for two days post-injury, the patient is now unable to follow commands. His vital signs are: HR 122 bpm, RR 30, temperature 101°F (38.5°C). What condition should the nurse suspect, and how will it be diagnosed?

 # Functional Issues

Falls and Gait Disorders

Falls are less common in critical care environments than in acute care settings, but the critical care nurse should be active in fall prevention. Patients should be assessed for fall risk and appropriate precautions put in place. Common risk factors in critical care settings include:

- altered LOC

- agitation or delirium

- medications (particularly analgesics, sedatives, and antipsychotics)

    Gait disorders affect patients' ability to walk; they may be neurological or non-neurological. Common causes of gait disorders in critical care settings include stroke, dementia, encephalopathy, injury or infection in limbs, and chronic neurological disorders (e.g., Parkinson's disease).

Treatment and Management

- Assess patients' fall risk each shift with a screening tool (e.g., Morse Fall Scale, Johns Hopkins Fall Risk Assessment Tool).

- Universal fall precautions are designed to provide a safe environment for all patients.

- Always place nonslip footwear or socks on patients before ambulating or transferring.
- Keep environment free from fall hazards (e.g., cords or other items that could trip the patient).
- Ensure patient's call light and personal possessions are within reach.
- Lower bed to lowest setting and leave bed rails up.

- Moderate and high fall risk precautions should be tailored to individual patients.
  - Consult physical therapy to collaborate on early mobilization plans.
  - Encourage use of mobility aids like gait belts, walkers, etc.
  - Use chair and bed alarms.
  - Consider using a patient safety companion for confused patients.
  - Consider restraints only as the last option.

QUICK REVIEW QUESTION

3. A patient who is normally independent at home has gait issues and is deemed a moderate fall risk. What fall precautions should the nurse put in place?

IMMOBILITY

Immobility is common in critical care settings and can have negative short- and long-term effects on patient health. Possible side effects of prolonged immobilization include pressure ulcers, muscle atrophy, bone demineralization, and reduced respiratory and cardiac function. Mitigating these side effects during critical care can prevent future complications and shorten recovery time.

Nursing Interventions

- Regularly assess ROM and strength.
- Assess nutritional needs.
- Implement DVT prevention measures.
- Maintain skin integrity.
- Mobilize patient as early as possible.
  - Use the minimum sedation necessary.
  - Limit use of neuromuscular blockers.
  - Collaborate with PT for passive and active ROM exercises.
  - Encourage patient to participate in their own care as much as they can.

HELPFUL HINT:

Neuromuscular weakness in ICU patients is sometimes referred to as **ICU-acquired weakness**, particularly when there is no obvious underlying cause for the weakness.

QUICK REVIEW QUESTION

4. How can a nurse alleviate the effects of immobility on a patient who is vented and sedated?

OSTEOMYELITIS

Pathophysiology

Osteomyelitis is an infection in bone, most commonly caused by *Staphylococcus aureus*. Non-hematogenous osteomyelitis is the result of infection from adjacent tissues or penetrating injuries; hematogenous osteomyelitis is a result of bacteremia. In adults it is most common in the spine, but may affect other areas such as the clavicle, pelvis, or long bones.

Signs and Symptoms

- signs and symptoms of local infection
- musculoskeletal pain
- fever

Diagnostic Findings

- MRI or CT scan
- positive blood culture or culture of bone biopsy

Treatment and Management

- surgical debridement
- IV antibiotics

QUICK REVIEW QUESTION

5. A patient is admitted to the ICU with bacteremia and sepsis with an unknown cause of infection. The health history reveals that the patient suffers from chronic back pain and has recently received an epidural steroid injection. What diagnostic tests should the nurse anticipate?

Rhabdomyolysis

Pathophysiology

Rhabdomyolysis is muscle necrosis that leads to the release of intracellular components into circulation, including CK, electrolytes, and myoglobin. The resulting serum abnormalities result in organ dysfunction, particularly AKI.

Etiology

- trauma (crush or compartment syndrome)
- sepsis
- cardiac or vascular surgery
- alcohol or drug use

Signs and Symptoms

- myoglobinuria (red-brown urine)
- myalgia
- muscle weakness

Diagnostic Findings

- elevated CK (>5x normal levels)
- urinary myoglobin >250 mcg/mL
- hyperuricemia
- electrolyte abnormalities (hyperkalemia, hypo- or hypercalcemia, hyperphosphatemia)

Treatment and Management

- IV fluids
- correct electrolyte imbalances
- treat underlying condition

QUICK REVIEW QUESTION

6. The nurse is reviewing labs from a patient who is 2 days post-op of mitral valve repair. The chemistry panel returns with CK 1200 IU/L, myoglobulin 390 mcg/mL, and K+ 6.8. What treatment would be expected for this patient?

ANSWER KEY

1. Remove the cast as soon as possible and reassess circulation, sensation, movement, and neurovascular status. If compartment syndrome is suspected, prepare for emergent fasciotomy or surgery.

2. The patient has signs and symptoms of FES. FES is a clinical diagnosis, so the nurse should assess for other symptoms (e.g., petechial rash) and anticipate a CXR to rule out a PE.

3. The nurse should assess the patient to determine if a mobility device should be used, provide the patient with nonslip footwear and encourage their use whenever the patient is out of bed, ensure the environment is free from fall hazards, and provide stand-by assistance as needed. The nurse should ensure the call light is within reach and encourage the patient to use it rather than getting out of bed.

4. The nurse should determine the patient's prior status and assess their current strength and flexibility. A care plan should incorporate measures to maintain skin integrity and maintain or improve flexibility through passive and active ROM exercises. It should also include collaboration with nutritional services to ensure an optimal diet. The nurse should discuss DVT risk with the interdisciplinary team and use anticoagulation devices and administer medications as ordered.

5. The nurse should suspect osteomyelitis caused by introduction of bacteria to the spine via epidural spinal injections. An MRI or CT scan will be ordered. If imaging shows osteomyelitis, a bone biopsy may be performed to identify the pathogen.

6. The patient is experiencing rhabdomyolysis, which is affecting the efficacy of the kidneys. The nurse can expect to provide supportive care through IV fluid administration and hemodialysis to correct the critical value of potassium.

9 NEUROLOGY REVIEW

HELPFUL HINT:

"Time is brain" is a guiding principle in critical care neurology. The sooner care is initiated, the more brain function can be preserved.

Neurological Anatomy, Physiology, and Assessment

BRAIN ANATOMY AND PHYSIOLOGY

- Blood supply to the brain comes by two arterial sources: the internal carotid artery and the vertebral arteries.

- The **internal carotid artery** branches off from the subclavian artery and divides into the middle cerebral artery (MCA), the anterior cerebral artery (ACA), and the posterior cerebral artery (PCA). Together, these arteries provide 80% of blood to the brain.
- The **vertebral arteries** come up through the brainstem area and fuse together to form the basilar artery just below the pons. In the midbrain area, the basilar artery merges into the posterior cerebral arteries. The vertebral arteries supply blood to the spinal cord, cerebellum, and brainstem.

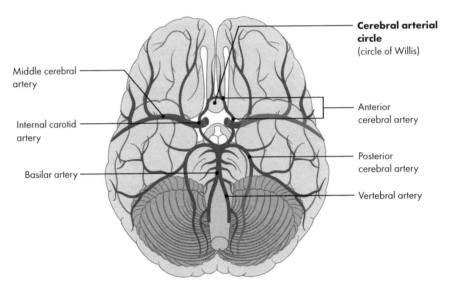

Figure 9.1. Vasculature in the Brain

- Blockage in any of these arteries causes intense temporary or permanent damage to each area of the brain they supply.
- Each area of the brain has specific functions that are affected by localized tissue damage.
    - frontal lobe: thinking, speaking, movement, memory
    - parietal lobe: touch, language
    - temporal lobe: emotions, hearing, learning
    - occipital lobe: vision, color perception
    - cerebellum: balance, coordination
    - brainstem: breathing, heart rate, temperature regulation
    - thalamus: sleep, alertness, sensory processing
- The cerebrum and thalamus have 2 hemispheres, the right and left. Each hemisphere controls movement and sensory processing on the contralateral side of the body.
- **Cerebral spinal fluid (CSF)** is a clear, colorless fluid that circulates around the brain and spinal cord.

- CSF cushions the brain and transports nutrients and waste.
- The normal volume of CSF is 125 – 150 mL.
- CSF is produced and circulated by 4 **ventricles** in the brain. The 2 lateral ventricles are found in the 2 cerebral hemispheres; the third ventricle is located midline between the thalami; and the fourth ventricle is surrounded by the pons and medulla oblongata.
- Fluid drains from the fourth ventricle into the subarachnoid space and the spinal cord.

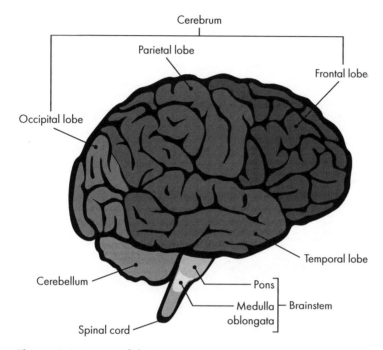

Figure 9.2. Areas of the Brain

QUICK REVIEW QUESTION

1. What type of focal neurological deficits would indicate likely damage to the occipital lobe?

NURSING NEUROLOGICAL ASSESSMENT

- Neurological assessment should be done continuously to obtain baseline data and to assess for neurological deterioration or improvements related to treatment.
    - level of consciousness (LOC): earliest indication of neurological deterioration
    - pupillary response: late indication of neurological deterioration
    - mental status

- ☐ motor function
- ☐ sensation/touch perception
- ☐ vision changes
- ☐ speech changes
- ☐ Glasgow Coma Scale (GCS) (Table 9.1)

TABLE 9.1. Scoring on the Glasgow Coma Scale

Eye Opening (E)	Verbal Response (V)	Motor Response (M)
4 = spontaneous 3 = to sound 2 = to pressure 1 = none	5 = oriented 4 = confused 3 = inappropriate words 2 = incomprehensible sounds 1 = no response	6 = obeys command 5 = localizes 4 = normal flexion 3 = abnormal flexion 2 = extension 1 = none
15: fully awake <8: severe brain injury 3: coma or death		

- ☐ cranial nerve assessment (Table 9.2)

TABLE 9.2. Cranial Nerve Function and Assessment

Cranial Nerve	Function
I. Olfactory	sense of smell
II. Optic	central and peripheral vision
III. Oculomotor	constriction of pupils
IV. Trochlear	downward eye movement
V. Trigeminal	facial sensation and motor control of mouth
VI. Abducens	sideways eye movement
VII. Facial	movement and expression
VIII. Vestibulocochlear	hearing and balance
IX. Glossopharyngeal	tongue and throat
X. Vagus	sensory and motor
XI. Accessory	head and shoulder movement
XII. Hypoglossal	tongue position

Other Cranial Nerve Assessments	
Doll's eyes reflex	assessment of oculocephalic function (cranial nerves III, IV, VI) in an unconscious patient: **normal** (both eyes roll/move to opposite side of head position) **abnormal** (eyes roll/move in opposite directions of each other): indicates a brainstem injury **absent** (eyes remain midline/move with head position): indicates significant brainstem injury
Consensual response	assessment of CN II and III: constriction of pupil when light shined into opposite eye

- postural indicators of brain damage
    - □ **decorticate** (patient brings arms to the CORE of the body): damage to cerebral hemispheres (<u>COR</u>tex)
    - □ **decerebrate** (extended position): ominous sign of brainstem damage and possible brain herniation

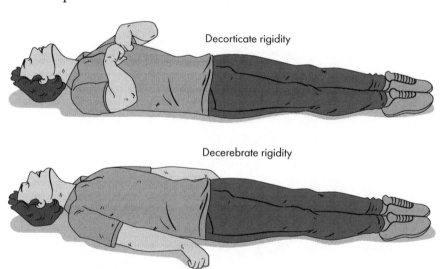

Figure 9.3. Decorticate and Decerebrate Postures

- medical signs of possible brain damage
    - □ **Kernig's sign** (indicator of meningitis): patient in supine position with the hips and knees flexed, unable to straighten leg due to hamstring pain
    - □ **Brudzinski's sign** (indicator of meningitis): passive flexion of the neck elicits automatic flexion at the hips and knees
    - □ **nuchal rigidity** (indicator of meningitis): inability to place the chin on the chest (neck flexion) due to muscle stiffness

- **Babinski sign** (indicator of damage to corticospinal tract): a single, firm stroking of the sole of the foot from the heel to toes causes big toe to point up and toes to fan out

- **Cushing's triad** is a late, ominous sign of increased ICP and possible brain herniation.
    - widening pulse pressure (elevated SBP and decreased DBP)
    - bradycardia
    - decreased/abnormal RR (Cheyne-Stokes respiration)

QUICK REVIEW QUESTION

2. A patient is being assessed with the GCS. There is a slight reaction to pressure, incoherent verbal responses, and decorticate positioning. What would the GCS result be, and what does it indicate?

Acute Spinal Cord Injuries

- **Spinal cord injuries (SCIs)** are injuries to the vertebral column.
    - The **primary injury** is caused by trauma, including compression, hyperextension, contusion, or shearing.
    - **Secondary injuries** are caused by resulting physiological processes such as hypoxia and ischemia; they may lead to neurological dysfunction that presents hours or days after the initial trauma.

- SCIs may be **complete** (meaning all sensory and motor function is lost below the level of injury) or **incomplete** (meaning some sensory and motor function is retained).

- The location and severity of sensory/motor loss depends on the type of injury.
    - **Anterior spinal cord syndrome** occurs when the blood flow to the anterior spinal artery is disrupted, resulting in ischemia in the spinal cord and complete loss of motor and sensory function below the lesion.
    - **Brown-Séquard syndrome** is an SCI caused by complete cord hemitransection, typically at the cervical level. Symptoms include ipsilateral motor loss below the lesion and contralateral loss of sensation of pain and temperature.
    - **Cauda equina syndrome** is an SCI typically caused by compression of, or damage to, the cauda equina, the nerve bundle that innervates the lower limbs and pelvic organs, most notably the bladder. Symptoms include sensory loss in the lower extremities, bowel and

bladder dysfunction, numbness in saddle area, and loss of reflexes in upper extremities.

- □ **Central cord syndrome** is caused by spinal cord compression and edema, both of which cause the lateral corticospinal tract white matter to deteriorate. Symptoms include greater motor function loss in the upper extremities than in the lower extremities and paresthesia in the upper extremities.

- ■ Assessment of SCIs: anteroposterior and lateral spinal cord X-rays (to assess lesions), CT of cervical spine and top of T1 (to rule out cervicothoracic junction injury), initial/ongoing spinal cord assessment (American Spinal Injury Association [ASIA] exam)

- ■ Respiratory compromise due to SCI is determined by lesion level.

TABLE 9.3. Respiratory Compromise in SCIs	
Level of Lesion	**Description**
C1 or C2 (high cervical lesions)	vital capacity 5% – 10% of normal cough absent ventilator dependent
C3 – C6	vital capacity 20% of normal ineffective cough variable ventilator support/weaning ability
T2 – T4 (high thoracic lesions)	vital capacity 30% – 50% of normal cough weak compromised respiratory function
Below T4 – T10	vital capacity 50% of normal respiratory function improved
T11	vital capacity normal cough strong minimal respiratory dysfunction

- ■ Management of SCIs
  - □ goals of management: prevent life-threatening complications, maximize organ system functions, prevent secondary spinal cord damage, and address neurological deficits
  - □ immediate spinal cord stabilization (tongs, halo traction braces, kinetic therapy beds, body casts)
  - □ methylprednisolone IV (bolus followed by 24 – 48 hour infusion)
  - □ monitor for, and treat, cardiac and respiratory complications (both common in SCIs)

HELPFUL HINT:

The use of methylpred-
nisolone following SCI
remains controversial
because of the high
risk of infection in
already compromised,
sepsis-prone trauma
patients.

HELPFUL HINT:

Spinal shock refers to
depressed or absent
reflexes that result from
SCIs. It is not related to
the circulatory system.

- □ temperature stabilization
- □ urinary catheterization (to avoid bladder distension)

- **Neurogenic shock** is a form of distributive shock caused by an injury or trauma to the spinal cord, typically above T6. The injury causes a decrease in sympathetic tone, leading to vasodilation and rapid onset of hypotension. The resulting decrease in SVR causes blood to pool in the lower extremities, and cardiac output is greatly reduced. Bradycardia occurs because of unopposed vagal tone exacerbated by hypoxia and suctioning (common in spinal injury patients). Unless rapidly recognized and treated, multisystem organ failure occurs with a very high mortality. This shock state may persist for more than a month from injury event.

  - □ Symptoms: rapid onset of hypotension, bradycardia, hypothermia; wide pulse pressure; skin warm, flushed, and dry; priapism
  - □ Management: IV fluids (first line); vasopressors/inotropes (second line); atropine or isoproterenol (for bradycardia)

- **Autonomic dysreflexia** is the overstimulation of the autonomic nervous system after SCIs above the T6 level. A sympathetic stimulation to the lower portion of the body leads to vasoconstriction below the area of injury and vasodilation above the injury, resulting in bradycardia and hypertension. If left untreated, cardiac status quickly deteriorates, and MI or stroke may occur.

  - □ Symptoms: flushing and sweating above the level of injury; cold, clammy skin below the level of injury; bradycardia; sudden, severe headache; hypertension
  - □ Management: anti-hypertensives; elevate HOB to 90°; have patient empty bladder and bowel; remove tight, restrictive clothing

QUICK REVIEW QUESTION

3. A 25-year-old patient was brought into the ED after a 20-foot fall at a construction site. Spinal immobilization was performed in the field. The patient was intubated in the ED, and a primary assessment showed HR 59 bpm, BP 84/50 mm Hg, SaO$_2$ 95%, GCS 6, and no other abnormalities. Secondary assessment showed diffuse abrasions over the back, torso, and extremities, but no abdominal ecchymosis or distension, pelvic instability, or extremity deformities. The patient arrives in the spinal cord ICU post-CT with a suspected partial lesion of the spinal cord at T2. What initial treatment plan would the CCRN expect to implement?

Brain Death

- **Brain death** is the irreversible cessation of all brain functions, including brainstem function. It is determined based on the American Academy of Neurology's clinical diagnosis guidelines, although US state and hospital policies vary.

- To declare brain death, the cause and irreversibility of the coma must be confirmed after all factors that might influence the results have been removed.

- Confirmation of management or absence of confounding conditions includes the following:
  - absence of hypotension: SBP >90 mm Hg; patient may be on vasopressors
  - absence of severe hypothermia (i.e., core temperature >32°C)
  - sedation, opioids, analgesics, intoxicants, and poisons cleared from system
  - absence of recent/current neuromuscular blockade (NMB): 4 twitches with maximal ulnar nerve stimulation by train-of-four peripheral nerve stimulator
  - absence of acid-base, endocrine, or electrolyte dysfunction

- The bedside exam includes the following components:
  - absence of cerebral motor reflexes (note that motor responses seen during apnea testing are considered spinal cord reflexes)
  - absence of brainstem reflexes (oculocephalic reflex, oculovestibular reflex, gag reflex, cough reflex, pupillary response, corneal reflex)
  - absence of respiratory drive (positive apnea test)

- Apnea test conducted to assess respiratory drive:
  - pulse oximeter on with 100% O_2 and 10-minute preoxygenation
  - reduce PEEP to 5 cm H_2O, and reduce vent rate to 10 breaths/minute
  - if O_2 saturation >90%, obtain ABG for baseline
  - disconnect ventilator, and insert insufflation catheter via ETT at level of carina
  - deliver 100% O_2 at 6 L/min flow
  - observe for spontaneous respiratory efforts over 8 – 10 minutes; monitor for abdominal or chest movements that produce adequate tidal volumes
  - abort test if SBP drops <90 mm Hg and if drop continues despite increasing vasopressor dose
  - abort test if O_2 saturation is <80% for >30 seconds

HELPFUL HINT:

Additional tests for confirming brain death include an EEG, somatosensory evoked potential (SSEP), and a cerebral perfusion evaluation (MRI, CT scan, or transcranial Doppler).

- □ if no respiratory drive seen, obtain ABG after 8 minutes
- □ if respiratory movements are absent and arterial pCO_2 is ≥ 60 mm Hg or if there is a 20 mm Hg increase in arterial pCO_2 over baseline, the apnea test result is positive (supports the clinical diagnosis of brain death)
- □ if patient breathes or gasps during test, return to pretest ventilator status and repeat apnea test in a few hours

QUICK REVIEW QUESTION

4. During an apnea test to determine brain death, the patient's BP decreases to 87/55 mm Hg. Norepinephrine is increased to maintain SBP >90. The BP continues to decrease, with the next reading at 78/52. What action should the nurse expect to take next?

Delirium

Delirium, an acute cognitive change from baseline, affects up to 80% of patients hospitalized in ICUs. The patient exhibits confusion and disorientation, with a decreased ability to focus and converse coherently. The delirium may be categorized as hypoactive, hyperactive, or mixed (with characteristics of both). Delirium is a common complication of underlying disease processes (e.g., pneumonia), particularly in the elderly. It may also be trigged by physiological conditions such as pain, fever, intoxication, sleep deprivation, severe burns or trauma, and idiosyncratic response to medications.

HELPFUL HINT:

Pain management is the first-line consideration in preventing delirium, especially in elderly at-risk patients.

Signs and Symptoms

- hypoactive
  - □ listless and lethargic
  - □ decreased response or nonresponsive
  - □ flat affect and slowed speech
- hyperactive
  - □ combative, agitated, or restless
  - □ unable to follow commands
  - □ repeatedly attempts to leave the bed, room, or hospital
  - □ labile moods

Treatment and Management

- assess for delirium every shift and whenever cognitive changes are observed, using cognitive assessment tools
  - Confusion Assessment Method for the ICU (CAM-ICU)
  - Intensive Care Delirium Screening Checklist (ICDSC)
  - Richmond Agitation-Sedation Scale (RASS)
- identify and treat underlying cause (THINK)
  - toxins
  - hypoxemia
  - infection
  - non-pharmacologic intervention (e.g., remove any unnecessary lines or tubes, reduce use or remove restraints)
  - K^+ (electrolyte imbalances)
- reduce number of medications
  - decrease sedative use and limit benzodiazepines
  - dexmedetomidine (Precedex) has a lower delirium risk than benzodiazepines
- nonpharmacological methods for preventing delirium
  - treating pain
  - maintaining routines and sleep schedule
  - introducing nutrition as soon as tolerated
  - refraining from use of restraints, if possible
  - discouraging the use of unnecessary equipment, tubing, and catheters
  - securing and concealing necessary lines
  - avoiding excessive environmental noise and clutter
  - providing cognitive stimulation (e.g., talking to patient during care)
  - increasing patient's mobility (passive range of motion progressing to baseline ability)

QUICK REVIEW QUESTION

5. An 88-year-old patient was admitted to the ICU with pneumonia and respiratory failure, requiring noninvasive positive-pressure ventilation. Over the past 2 days, the patient has become increasingly withdrawn and confused and is currently responding listlessly and incoherently to the nurse's questions. What interventions are appropriate to include in the care plan?

Dementia

Dementia is a broad term for progressive, cognitively debilitating symptoms that interfere with independent functioning. Patients may show decline in one or more cognitive domains, including language, memory, executive function, motor skills, and social cognition.

Etiology

- Alzheimer's disease (most common form of dementia in older adults)
- vascular dementia (from stroke)
- Lewy body dementia
- frontal temporal dementia
- other dementias (e.g., Huntington's disease, Parkinson's disease)
- mixed (multiple causes)

Treatment and Management

- Assess for dementia using the **mini-mental state exam (MMSE)**. A score less than 24 indicates dementia.
- Unless dementia is caused by a treatable disease process, its progression can be slowed but not cured.
  - antidementia medications: cholinesterase inhibitors (e.g., donepezil) and memantine
  - other medication, including antidepressants and analgesics, to help manage symptoms

---

QUICK REVIEW QUESTION

6. A patient in the ICU was recently diagnosed with Alzheimer's disease and began taking donepezil. The patient's spouse asks why the patient has not improved since starting the medication. How should the nurse respond?

Encephalopathy

Anoxic encephalopathy (hypoxic-ischemic brain injury) is a process that begins when **cerebral blood flow (CBF)** stops, resulting in global brain ischemia. In a hypoxic brain injury, restricted oxygen supply to the brain tissue causes the gradual death of brain cells; anoxic brain injuries lead to death of brain cells after 4 minutes without oxygen.

"Watershed" areas of injury (the destruction of cerebral white matter) affect significant parts of the brain and cause motor and sensory disturbances of varying severity. Major brain injury also occurs during reperfusion.

Etiology

- vascular injury
- poisoning (e.g., drug overdose, carbon monoxide)
- drowning
- cardiac or respiratory arrest
- shock
- severe asthma event
- suffocation/strangulation
- electric shock

Signs and Symptoms

- confusion or delirium
- altered LOC (diminished arousal/awareness, coma, or vegetative state)
- sensory impairment
    - eye movement deficit (CN III, IV, and VI)
    - changes in pupil size, shape, or reaction to light
    - impaired consensual response (CN II and III)
    - impaired equilibrium and hearing (CN VIII)
- motor impairment (muscle weakness, paraplegia, or quadriplegia)
- tremor, myoclonus, or asterixis
- recurrent partial or myoclonic seizures

Treatment and Management

- primary treatment goal: prevention of further neurological damage and management of symptoms
- monitor ICP and fluid balance
- manage risk for falls, aspiration, infection, and gastric ulcers
- provide nutritional support

HELPFUL HINT:

Targeted temperature management (therapeutic hypothermia) is used for post-cardiac-arrest patients to prevent neurological damage. Patients should have their core temperature kept at 32 – 36°C for at least 24 hours after resuscitation.

QUICK REVIEW QUESTION

7. A patient is brought into the ED unresponsive after a suicide attempt via hanging. The patient is intubated, vented, and stabilized. What nursing interventions are important for this patient when they are admitted to the ICU?

Increased Intracranial Pressure

Intracranial pressure (ICP) is the pressure within the intracranial compartment (the area enclosed by the cranium). A normal adult cranium encloses a fixed volume of around 1500 mL divided between brain tissue (80% of volume), CSF (10%), and blood (10%). Since the cranium does not expand or otherwise move, insults to brain tissue that increase intracranial volume will increase ICP. **Intracranial compliance** is the change in volume over the change in pressure. When the brain's compensation mechanisms fail, intracranial compliance is reduced, and even small changes in volume can produce large changes in ICP.

When ICP increases, immediate interventions must be implemented to maintain **cerebral perfusion pressure (CPP)**, the net pressure gradient that drives oxygen delivery to brain tissue. Increased ICP may also cause brain tissue to herniate downward through the tentorial notch and foramen magnum into the brainstem; herniation is rapidly fatal.

Normal ICP is 5 – 15 mm Hg. An ICP >20 mm Hg is a neurological emergency that requires immediate treatment. CPP is defined as the difference between MAP and ICP (i.e., MAP – ICP), and should be maintained at 50 – 70 mm Hg. ICP monitoring is always recommended for:

- large-territory acute ischemic stroke
- head injuries with a GCS score <8
- cerebral edema
- hydrocephalus
- when early recognition of ICP changes is needed

Several options are available for ICP monitoring:

- An **external ventricular drain (EVD)** or **intraventricular catheter** is the gold standard for continuous direct measurement of dynamic ICP.
  - the most invasive technique, with the catheter placed into ventricle of nondominant hemisphere
  - device both monitors ICP and drains CSF
  - transducer is placed at level of foramen of Monro
  - high risk for infection and CSF leakage at insertion site
- A subarachnoid "bolt" with intraparenchymal catheter provides subarachnoid access and fixation without penetration of brain tissue.
- Noninvasive monitoring may be done with a transcranial Doppler study (TCD), transcranial color-coded duplex sonography (TCCS), or a handheld infrared pupillometer, which provides a neurological pupil index (NPi).

HELPFUL HINT:

The **Monro-Kellie Doctrine**: The total volume of brain tissue, CSF, and blood in the cranium is constant. An increase in the volume of one of the three elements should cause a decrease in one or both of the others. If not, ICP will increase.

HELPFUL HINT:

An elevated tidal wave (P2) in an ICP waveform indicates reduced intracranial compliance.

- Under normal physiologic conditions, the ICP waveform has three peaks: P1 (percussion wave), P2 (tidal wave), and P3 (dicrotic wave or notch) with descending heights.
  - An elevated tidal wave (P2) indicates reduced intracranial compliance and increased ICP.
  - A single wave with a lack of distinct peaks indicates a critical increase in ICP that requires immediate intervention.

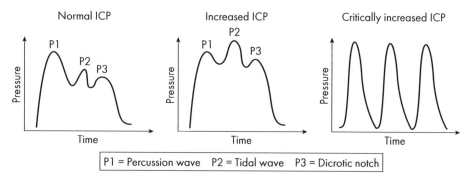

Figure 9.4. ICP Waveform

Etiology

- trauma (TBI, brain contusion)
- mass displacement of brain tissue by tumor, hematoma, or abscess
- hypoxic-ischemic brain injury
- intracranial hemorrhage
- increased CSF production (meningitis)
- blockages to CSF flow/reabsorption (hydrocephalus, meningeal disease)
- seizures
- hyperthermia (core temperature >37.5°C)

Signs and Symptoms

- change in LOC
- headache
- vomiting
- Cushing's triad
- irritability
- photophobia
- lethargy and impaired/slowed decision-making

HELPFUL HINT:

Hypoxia in brain tissue leads to edema and arterial vasodilation, both of which increase ICP. Hypercapnia may also increase ICP by increasing blood flow to the brain and reducing venous return.

Diagnostic Findings

ICP >20 mm Hg

Treatment and Management

- hyperosmolar/hypertonic fluid therapy
    - mannitol 20% (0.25 – 1 g/kg IV bolus)
    - loop diuretics (assess for hypokalemia)
    - hypertonic saline (2%, 3%, 5% NaCl)
- patient positioning: elevate HOB 30 – 35° with midline head alignment, and avoid hip flexion
- maintain normal body temperature
- limit activities that may raise ICP, including coughing, sneezing, vomiting, suctioning, PEEP, restraint use, and the Valsalva maneuver
- stabilize blood glucose: insulin therapy to maintain blood glucose ≤140 mg/dL
- decrease environmental stimuli, and minimize nursing care
- higher-level interventions for refractory ICP
    - mechanical ventilation with hyperventilation (keep PaO_2 at 35 – 40 mm Hg)
    - IV fentanyl (paradoxical ICP increase may occur) or IV morphine
    - sedation (avoid "sedation holidays"), possibly with neuromuscular blockade
    - barbiturate coma
    - decompressive craniotomy

QUICK REVIEW QUESTION

8. A patient is in the ICU after sustaining a head injury during a motorcycle accident. The patient's ICP has risen to 21 mm Hg, and the nurse alerts the physician. The following orders are received: mannitol 20% 0.5 g/kg IV bolus, furosemide 20 mg IV push, and 0.45% sodium chloride 125 mL/hr IV continuous infusion. Which order should the nurse question?

Stroke (Hemorrhagic)

A **hemorrhagic stroke**, the disruption of CBF, is caused by bleeding. The resulting hypoxia rapidly leads to brain cell death, and the excess blood in the cranium also increases ICP, increasing the risk of brain herniation. Bleeding

---

HELPFUL HINT:

Hypotonic solutions (D5W, 0.45% NaCl) should be avoided in patients with ICP. They decrease plasma osmolality and move water from extracellular to intracellular spaces in the brain, increasing ICP.

HELPFUL HINT:

Each 1°C increases cerebral O_2 demand by 7 – 10%, which in turn increases CBF and ICP.

may be caused by the spontaneous rupture of a blood vessel, head trauma, a brain mass, or uncontrolled anticoagulation conditions. The hemorrhage is classified by location as intracerebral or subarachnoid. **Intraventricular hemorrhage (IVH)** is bleeding in the ventricles; it rarely occurs alone and is usually seen with intracerebral and subarachnoid hemorrhages.

INTRACEREBRAL HEMORRHAGE

An **intracerebral hemorrhage (ICH)** is arterial bleeding directly into cerebral tissue. An ICH is most commonly caused by hypertensive rupture of a cerebral artery that has become damaged over time by atherosclerosis. The burst of blood from such a break in the artery causes a hematoma in the brain tissue around the rupture site. Patients with an ICH often present to EMS as unconscious and require immediate intubation for ventilatory support.

Signs and Symptoms

- acute onset of symptoms that gradually worsen over minutes or hours
- sudden loss of consciousness (hallmark differentiation from ischemic stroke)
- sudden focal deficit (determined by site of bleed)
- severe headache
- nausea and vomiting
- severe hypertension (200/100 – 250/150 mm Hg)
- seizures

Diagnostic Findings

- priority (interpreted in < 45 minutes): noncontrast CT scan of head to differentiate ischemic from hemorrhagic stroke

Treatment and Management

- priority goal: management of ABCs and reduction of BP
- intubation and mechanical ventilation usually necessary
- moderate BP reduction to reduce bleeding
  - □ MAP = 110 – 130 mm Hg
  - □ CPP >70 mm Hg
  - □ vasopressor therapy after fluid replacement if SBP <90 mm Hg
- treat increased ICP (per above)
- reverse or stabilize anticoagulation state
- management of seizures (prophylactic medication likely)

HELPFUL HINT:

Hypertension is the most important risk factor for all types of stroke. Other risk factors include hyperlipidemia, smoking, diabetes, and A-fib.

HELPFUL HINT:

Hematoma expansion is evident on repeat CT scans in nearly 40% of cases within the first 3 hours after onset of symptoms.

- DVT prophylaxis
- surgical removal of clot may be considered, depending on ICP and neurological condition

QUICK REVIEW QUESTION

9. A CT scan has determined a patient with stroke symptoms has had an intracerebral hemorrhage. The patient has a history of hypertension and A-fib and is currently taking hydrochlorothiazide, lisinopril, and warfarin. The patient's SBP was initially 200 mm Hg but has been stabilized to 170/86 mm Hg on a nicardipine IV infusion at 10 mg/hr. Results of coagulation labs find that the INR is 4.5. What medication should the nurse expect to administer?

SUBARACHNOID HEMORRHAGE

A **subarachnoid hemorrhage (SAH)** is bleeding into the subarachnoid space. About 85% of spontaneous SAHs are due to the rupture of a saccular **cerebral aneurysm**, most commonly located at the circle of Willis. When age-related or long-term hypertension places stress on the weakened arterial blood vessel, the dome of the outpouching aneurysm thins and ruptures. The mortality rate is 25 – 50% in the first 24 hours of the event.

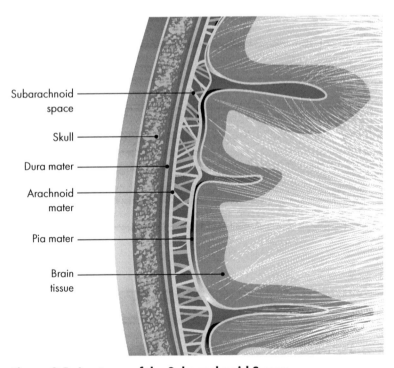

Subarachnoid space

Skull

Dura mater

Arachnoid mater

Pia mater

Brain tissue

Figure 9.5. Anatomy of the Subarachnoid Space

Around 6% of SAHs are caused by the rupture of an **arteriovenous malformation (AVM)**, a mass of arterial and venous blood vessels that shunt arterial blood directly into the venous system (bypassing the capillary system). Cerebral "feeder" arteries to the AVM become enlarged over time and increase the mass size of the AVM. The high pressure of arterial blood flow engorges the veins, which eventually rupture.

Signs and Symptoms

- abrupt onset of pain, often described as "the worst headache of my life"
- brief loss of consciousness that may progress to coma
- nausea and vomiting
- focal neurological deficits, especially CN III palsy
- nuchal rigidity
- meningeal irritation: positive Kernig's and Brudzinski's signs

Diagnostic Findings

- noncontrast CT scan: blood visualized in subarachnoid space if scan obtained within 48 hours of hemorrhage
- lumbar puncture (if initial CT scan is negative): CSF bloody with RBC >1000 cells/μL
- CT angiogram to locate cause of hemorrhage (for surgical intervention)
- Hunt and Hess Grading Scale

TABLE 9.4. Hunt and Hess Grading System for SAH

Asymptomatic, mild headache, slight nuchal rigidity	1
Moderate to severe headache, nuchal rigidity, no neurological deficit other than cranial nerve palsy	2
Drowsiness, confusion, mild focal neurological deficit	3
Stupor, moderate to severe hemiparesis	4
Coma, decerebrate posturing	5

Treatment and Management

- priority goal: management of ABCs and reduction of BP
- manage BP (SBP < 160 mm Hg)
- treat increased ICP (per above)
- reverse or stabilize anticoagulation state
- manage seizures (prophylactic medication likely)
- DVT prophylaxis

HELPFUL HINT:

Infectious vegetation from bacterial endocarditis can migrate to cerebral arteries, causing aneurysms that may rupture.

HELPFUL HINT:

Patients with SAH may describe sudden onset of headaches with vomiting in preceding weeks. These symptoms are the result of small amounts of blood leaking from aneurysms ("warning leaks" from preruptured aneurysms).

HELPFUL HINT:

Vasodilators (such as nitroprusside) should be avoided in patients with SAH because they raise ICP.

- surgical intervention (clipping, embolization, or endovascular coiling of aneurysm) within 48 hours
  - □ monitor post-op for reperfusion bleeding and embolic stroke
- prevention and treatment of secondary conditions
  - □ rebleeding: monitor for onset of neurological, respiratory, or hemodynamic changes
  - □ cerebral vasospasm: hypertensive, hypervolemic, hemodilution (HHH) therapy
  - □ hydrocephalus (due to slowed absorption of CSF) requires ventriculostomy; may require permanent ventriculoperitoneal shunt placement

HELPFUL HINT:

Cerebral vasospasm is a common cause of death after cerebral aneurysm rupture but is rare in SAH due to AVM rupture.

QUICK REVIEW QUESTION

10. A patient returns from CT guided intervention for SAH. What nursing interventions are required?

Stroke (Ischemic)

HELPFUL HINT:

Hemiplegic migraine headaches and severe hypoglycemia can mimic stroke.

During an **ischemic stroke**, blood flow to the brain is interrupted because of either a thrombotic or an embolic clot. Regardless of etiology, loss of CBF leads to hypoperfusion of brain cells, ischemic injury to a focal area, and brain death if anoxia is sustained.

Cerebral edema is expected with large-territory cerebral infarcts and is the leading cause of death in the week after an ischemic stroke. Around 10 – 20% of ischemic stroke patients develop cerebral edema sufficient to increase ICP, which reaches maximal levels at 4 days postevent. Other poststroke pathological sequelae include new-onset seizure disorder and hemorrhagic conversions at the stroke lesion site.

A **transient ischemic attack (TIA)**, a sudden, brief neurological deficit resulting from brain ischemia, does not cause permanent damage or infarction. Symptoms depend on the area of the brain affected. Most TIAs last less than 5 minutes and are resolved within 1 hour. A majority are caused by emboli in the carotid or vertebral arteries.

Signs and Symptoms

- focal neurological signs determined by location and size of the area of ischemia (lesion)

- dominant left hemisphere
  - aphasia or dysarthria
  - emotional lability and/or memory loss
  - vision changes (right hemianopia and conjugate gaze difficulties)
  - right hemiparesis
  - right-sided sensory loss
- nondominant right hemisphere
  - rambling speech or dysarthria
  - vision changes (left visual neglect or hemianopia)
  - left-sided sensory loss and stimuli extinction
  - spatial disorientation
  - difficulty in problem-solving
- posterior hemisphere, cerebellum, or brainstem
  - dysarthria
  - vision changes (nystagmus, disconjugate gaze, bilateral vision-field deficit)
  - sensory loss in all 4 limbs
  - ataxia or loss of fine motor movement control
- subcortical/brainstem (pure motor stroke): face/limb weakness on one side of body; no deficit in sensation, vision, or brain function
- subcortical/brainstem (pure sensory stroke): face/limb decreased sensation on one side of body; no deficit in motor function, vision, or brain function

Diagnostic Testing

- priority (interpreted in < 45 minutes): noncontrast CT scan of head to differentiate ischemic from hemorrhagic stroke
- National Institute of Health Stroke Scale (NIHSS)
  - LOC
  - eye deviation (CN III, IV, VI)
  - visual field loss (tests hemianopia and extinction)
  - facial palsy
  - motor arm (drift)
  - motor leg (drift)
  - limb ataxia (tests for unilateral cerebellar lesion)
  - sensory
  - best language (tests for comprehension/aphasia)

□ dysarthria (tests for speech ability)

□ extinction and inattention (tests for visual/spatial "neglect")

Treatment and Management

- IV or intra-arterial fibrinolytic therapy (alteplase)
  □ dosage: 0.9 mg/kg to a maximum of 90 mg; first 10% as IV bolus dose over 1 minute, with remaining 90% given as IV infusion over 1 hour
  □ must be initiated within 3 hours from "last seen normal"
  □ time window expanded to 4.5 hours for eligible patients (<80 years old, no history of diabetes/stroke, NIHSS score <25)
  □ hypertensive patients: BP should be lowered to <185/110 with anti-hypertensive medication before administration
  □ aspirin administered 24 hours after alteplase administration
  □ monitor for side effects, including bleeding, angioedema, ICH, pulmonary edema, DVT, seizure, and sepsis

- mechanical thrombectomy for fibrinolytic-ineligible patients or fibrinolytic-eligible patients with high likelihood of stroke due to LVO; may be done in conjunction with tenecteplase administration

- cardiac monitoring for post-reperfusion dysrhythmias

- regular neurological checks, and monitor ICP

- maintain normal body temperature

- maintain blood glucose of 140 – 180 mL/dL (do not administer D5W)

- supplemental O_2 for saturation below 94%

- DVT prophylaxis

QUICK REVIEW QUESTION

11. A patient recovering from TAVR presents with aphasia and right-sided hemiparesis. What is the priority diagnostic test for this patient?

Neurological Infectious Disease

- **Meningitis,** an acute inflammation of the meninges, is caused by bacterial, viral, or fungal pathogens that invade the subarachnoid space.

The infection triggers WBC accumulation and tissue damage, leading to swelling and purulent exudate within the cranium.

- □ Viral infection is the most common cause of meningitis; bacterial meningitis is a medical emergency because of the rapidity of deterioration and the high mortality rate.
- □ Diagnosis: headache, nuchal rigidity, fever, altered mental status, rash, positive Brudzinski's and Kernig's signs, photophobia, lumbar puncture to confirm
- □ CSF finding for viral meningitis: elevated protein and lymphocytes; clear fluid
- □ CSF finding for bacterial meningitis: very elevated protein, elevated WBCs and neutrophils, low glucose, cloudy fluid
- □ Management: empirical IV antibiotic therapy; corticosteroids; antivirals (as appropriate); monitor for sepsis, increased ICP, and SIADH/DI

- **Encephalitis**, an infection of the brain parenchyma, may be caused by bacteria, viruses, fungi, or parasites. It may present alone or alongside meningitis.
  - □ Diagnosis: altered mental status, seizures, focal neurological deficits; lumbar puncture shows elevated protein and WBC
  - □ Management: antibiotic, antiviral, or antifungal therapy (as indicated); manage seizures, including prophylaxis; monitor for increased ICP

- **Brain abscesses** are localized infections in the brain parenchyma. The infection can be caused by bacteremia or by direct spread from nearby tissues (e.g., otitis media, dental conditions).
  - □ Diagnosis: headache (on side of abscess), fever, focal neurological deficits, seizures; CT scan or MRI to confirm
  - □ Management: antibiotics, glucocorticoids; needle aspiration (via trephination) or surgical excision may be required

HELPFUL HINT:

Lumbar punctures are contraindicated for some patients with increased ICP because decompression of the CSF may lead to brain herniation.

QUICK REVIEW QUESTION

12. A 22-year-old college student arrives at the ED with complaints of headache, neck pain, fever, and sensitivity to light. On examination, the patient is positive for Brudzinski's and Kernig's signs. What test would be expected to help with diagnosis?

_____

CONTINUE →

Neuromuscular Disorders

- **Amyotrophic lateral sclerosis (ALS)** (Lou Gehrig's disease) is a neurodegenerative disorder that affects the neurons in the brainstem and spinal cord. Symptoms progressively worsen until respiratory failure occurs.
  - Symptoms: progressive asymmetrical weakness (can affect both upper and lower extremities); difficulty swallowing, walking, or speaking; muscle cramps
  - Management: supportive care for symptoms; respiratory support (high risk of aspiration)

- **Cerebral palsy (CP)** is a group of disorders characterized by permanent, nonprogressive muscle weakness. CP may present with a wide range of comorbidities, including intellectual disability, GI disorders, chronic lung disease, epilepsy, vision/hearing impairment, and chronic pain. Common reasons for ICU admission in patients with CP include infection, refractory seizures, and postoperative care.

- **Guillain-Barré syndrome** is an acquired demyelinating neuropathy believed to result from an immune reaction to recent infection. It is characterized by progressive symmetric muscle weakness, which may lead to respiratory dysfunction.
  - Symptoms: neuropathy and weakness ascending from lower extremities and advancing symmetrically upward; paresthesia in extremities; unsteady gait; absent or diminished deep tendon reflexes; autonomic dysfunction (hypertension, bradycardia, temperature instability)
  - Management: plasmapheresis, IV immunoglobulins; manage signs and symptoms of autonomic dysfunction

- **Multiple sclerosis (MS)** is a neurodegenerative disorder caused by patches of demyelination in the brain and the spinal cord. It has periods of both remission and exacerbation of symptoms, with gradually growing disability.
  - Symptoms: paresthesia; weakness of at least one extremity; visual, motor, or urinary disturbance; vertigo; fatigue; mild cognitive impairment; increased deep tendon reflexes; clonus
  - Management: corticosteroids for inflammation, baclofen or tizanidine for spasticity, gabapentin or tricyclic antidepressants for pain

- **Muscular dystrophy (MD)** is a genetic disorder in which a mutation in the recessive dystrophin gene on the X chromosome causes muscle fiber degeneration. It is usually first noted at 2 – 3 years of age and results in steady, progressive proximal-muscle weakness.

- Symptoms: steady progression of weakness; limb flexion and contraction; scoliosis; dilated cardiomyopathy, conduction abnormalities, or dysrhythmias; respiratory insufficiency
- Management: prednisone or deflazacort; monitor CO_2 levels; noninvasive ventilator support may be needed; supportive treatment of symptoms related to falls and cardiovascular disorders

- **Myasthenia gravis (MG)** is an autoimmune disorder that causes cell-mediated destruction of acetylcholine receptors, resulting in episodic muscle weakness and fatigue. **Myasthenic crisis** is an emergent condition in which MG symptoms rapidly worsen; weakening of the bulbar and respiratory muscles can cause respiratory dysfunction. (The information below is for myasthenic crisis.)
  - Symptoms: dyspnea, respiratory failure, tachycardia, hypertension, no cough or gag reflex, urinary and bowel incontinence
  - Management: IV fluids; IV immunoglobulin; anticholinesterase; respiratory support; long-term medications include pyridostigmine, steroids, muscle relaxants

QUICK REVIEW QUESTION

13. What type of weakness should a nurse expect to observe in a patient with ALS?

HELPFUL HINT:

Patients with myasthenia gravis are at risk for a cholinergic crisis if they are given high doses of anticholinesterase medications. Antidotes for anticholinesterase overdoes include atropine and pralidoxime.

Neurosurgery

- A **craniotomy** is the surgical opening of the skull to gain access to tissues inside the cranium.

- Common reasons for craniotomy include evacuation of hematoma or abscess, clipping or removal of an aneurysm or an AVM, brain tumor resection or removal, cerebral decompression, ICP monitoring, and placement of deep brain stimulators.

- Surgical access may be transcranial (through the skull) or transsphenoidal (through the nose).

- Patients should be closely monitored for the following post-op complications:
  - increased ICP
  - surgical hemorrhage: monitor for increased ICP (transcranial) or postnasal drip/external drainage (transsphenoidal)
  - CSF rhinorrhea: may require continuous lumbar drainage or surgical repair
  - SIADH or DI: monitor fluid balance

HELPFUL HINT:

A transsphenoidal craniotomy is used to remove a pituitary tumor. Patient teaching pre-op must include preparing the patient for nasal packing pressure; mouth breathing required; and the importance of avoiding sneezing, blowing nose, or coughing.

- infection: meningitis, surgical site infection, subdural empyema, or cerebral abscess
- injury to brain tissue: altered mental status, seizures

- **Burr hole trephination** is the drilling of small holes (trepanations) in the skull to drain fluid; the process usually includes the placement of a catheter in the hole.
  - Burr holes are used to drain hydrocephalus, hemorrhages, empyema/abscess, and subdural hematomas. They may also be used for some diagnostic procedures.
  - Postoperative complications of burr holes include infection, hemorrhage, embolism, and brain injury.

QUICK REVIEW QUESTION

14. After a transsphenoidal craniotomy to remove the pituitary gland, a patient experiences increased nasal discharge. What may this indicate, and what action should the nurse take?

Patients with a history of seizures are especially at high risk in the critical care setting because of a combination of sleep deprivation, poor nutrition, high levels of stimulation, medications that can lower seizure thresholds, and changes in the therapeutic level of antiepileptic drugs.

Seizure Disorders

Seizure disorders are caused by abnormal electrical discharges in the brain. During a seizure, brain neurons abnormally or excessively fire because the membrane potential is altered in a way that makes those neurons hypersensitive to stimuli. Seizures may be **focal** (limited to one part of the brain) or **generalized**.

Status epilepticus is a medical emergency in which seizure activity continues or recurs for more than 5 minutes. It has a high mortality rate (20 – 30%) and requires immediate intervention.

Etiology

- genetic/congenital
- trauma
- drug toxicity or withdrawal
- fluid or electrolyte imbalances
- hypoglycemia
- hypoxic-ischemic events
- cerebral edema
- sepsis
- tumors

Signs and Symptoms

- convulsive: tonic-clonic (grand mal) seizure pattern of extremities
  - tonic phase: loss of consciousness, rigidity of extremities, dilated pupils
  - clonic phase: rhythmic shaking, violent alternating contraction/relaxation, tachycardia, mouth frothing
  - postictal: impaired mental status and focal neurological deficits (Todd paralysis common)
  - nonconvulsive: EEG tracing of seizure activity with/without clinical signs

Treatment and Management

- manage ABCs
- finger-stick blood glucose: administer 50 mL D50W IV push if blood glucose <60 mg/dL
- prompt pharmacological treatment
  - first-line drugs: IV lorazepam, IV diazepam, or IM midazolam
  - second-line drugs (after 20 minutes of nonresponse to treatment): IV fosphenytoin, IV valproate, or IV levetiracetam
- After status epilepticus is aborted, determine etiology of seizure and begin antiepileptic drug therapy

QUICK REVIEW QUESTION

15. A patient with liver cirrhosis is being treated in the ICU for hepatic encephalopathy with refractory increased ICP. Lorazepam IV continuous infusion has been titrated up to 0.1 mg/kg/hr to manage agitation. The patient has a history of seizure, and current EEG monitoring shows a pattern consistent with status epilepticus. What medication should the nurse anticipate will be ordered for the patient?

Space-Occupying Lesions (Brain Tumors)

- **Brain tumors** are space-occupying lesions that, depending on their location, size, and rate of growth, create a range of symptoms.
- **Primary tumors** originate from brain tissue or immediately surrounding brain tissue; they are rare, and can be either benign or malignant.
  - The most common type of primary tumor is a **glioma**, which originates in the glia cells that surround the neurons in the brain.

- Common benign primary brain tumors include meningiomas, schwannomas, and pituitary adenomas.

- **Secondary**, or **metastatic**, **brain tumors** are malignant cancers that have originated elsewhere and migrated to the brain. Metastatic cancer may spread from the primary cancer in any part of the body, including the lungs, breasts, colon, skin, or kidneys.

- Symptoms of brain tumors will vary and may include headaches, seizures, unilateral weakness, and neurological deficits (related to tumor location).

- Disorders that occur secondary to brain tumors and that require critical care include encephalopathy, hemorrhage, and increased ICP (managed as discussed above).

- Patients with brain tumors may also be admitted to manage side effects of treatment, such as sepsis (due to chemotherapy's effects on the immune system) or cardiac disorders (a side effect of radiation therapy).

QUICK REVIEW QUESTION

16. A patient has metastatic pancreatic cancer and is admitted to the ICU because of a secondary brain tumor causing seizures. What lab value requires close monitoring for this patient?

★ Traumatic Brain Injury

PATHOPHYSIOLOGY AND GENERAL MANAGEMENT GUIDELINES

- **Traumatic brain injury (TBI)** results from a blunt or penetrating blow to the head or from a blast injury.
  - **Primary injuries** are caused by mechanical forces and can cause skull fractures, brain contusions and concussions, lacerations, hemorrhages, hematomas, or damage to white brain matter.
  - **Secondary injuries** occur days or weeks after the TBI event as a result of neurochemical cascades leading to chronic inflammation and vascular changes in the brain.

- In patients with TBI, decreased cerebral perfusion may lead to tissue ischemia and edema. Cerebral vasodilation occurs to compensate for decreased perfusion and to increase O_2 to cerebral tissue. This increased cerebral blood volume leads to increased intracranial volume and ICP.

- Severe cerebral edema causes loss of autoregulation, meaning CPP will vary with changes in MAP. Tight control of MAP is required to main adequate CPP.

- Hypotension is closely associated with poor outcomes in patients with TBI. Hypotension may be a direct result of brain tissue injury but often has other causes (e.g., hemorrhage). Hypotension requires immediate stabilization to maintain CPP.

- The goal of critical care management of TBI is to maintain CPP and decrease secondary injury to the brain.
  - ICP monitoring and management (discussed in detail above)
  - target CPP: minimum 60 mm Hg (70 mm Hg is optimal)
  - maintain MAP 60 mm Hg (fluid management)
  - fluids and vasopressors for hypotension
  - brain tissue oxygen monitoring may be implemented
  - capnography to identify hypo- or hypercapnia
  - serial ABGs to ensure adequate oxygenation
  - manage hyperthermia to reduce CV demand (target 36°C – 37°C)

HELPFUL HINT:

ETT Suctioning for TBI Patients

2 passes of suction catheter

each pass <10 seconds

hyperventilate patient before and after each pass

minimize stimulation of airway with suction

QUICK REVIEW QUESTION

17. A 36-year-old construction worker is admitted to ICU with TBI after falling from a ladder. The intubated, sedated patient has a subarachnoid screw for ICP and CPP monitoring. Arterial line shows MAP <60, ICP 30 mm Hg, and CPP 40 mm Hg. What interventions should the nurse anticipate?

_____

SPECIFIC TRAUMATIC BRAIN INJURIES

- The level of care for **skull fractures** depends on the type and severity of fracture.
  - Nondisplaced fractures generally do well with conservative treatment.
  - No treatment is usually required for a linear fracture, especially as the dura mater usually remains intact in adults.
  - Surgical decompression for a depressed fracture is necessary only when the depression is greater than the thickness of the skull (if the depression is ≥6 mm).
  - Basilar skull fractures require critical care monitoring and intervention.

- **Basilar skull fractures** affect the floor of the skull.
  - may cause rupture of meninges, resulting in pneumocephalus
  - likely injury to CN I, III, VII, and VIII

□ associated spinal cord injury common

□ signs and symptoms: Battle sign, raccoon eyes, otorrhea, and rhinorrhea

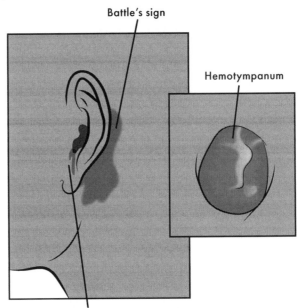

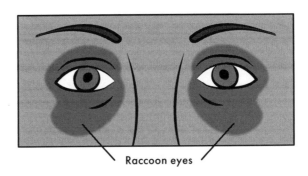

Figure 9.6. Signs and Symptoms of Basilar Skull Fracture

□ management: manage ABCs; manage ICP, hemorrhage, and meningeal injury (as described above); avoid NT and oral tube, oral suctioning, and positive-pressure support

■ **Diffuse axonal injury (DAI)** is a shearing injury that occurs during rapid acceleration–deceleration or rotational acceleration. These forces can shear axons in the brain and cause the death of the brain cells to which they were connected. Sufficient force will disconnect the cerebral hemisphere from the reticular activating system.

□ signs and symptoms: coma (GCS <8), decorticate or decerebrate posturing, cerebral edema, increased ICP, temperature elevation

□ management: manage ABCs; supportive treatment for symptoms; reduce secondary injury

- An **epidural hematoma (EDH)** is a traumatic collection of blood between the dura mater and the skull, usually because of a temporal- or parietal-region skull fracture that causes a laceration of the middle meningeal artery.

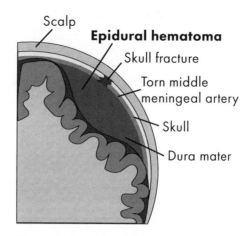

Figure 9.7. Epidural Hematoma

  - EDH is a neurosurgical emergency: a rapidly expanding hematoma will increase ICP and quickly progress to uncal herniation of brain tissue.
  - Diagnosis: CT scan or MRI; lucid interval followed by coma; agitation and confusion; nausea and vomiting; headache; ipsilateral pupil dilation; Cushing's triad
  - Management: manage ABCs; craniotomy or trephination for hematoma evacuation

- A **subdural hematoma (SDH)** is low-pressure venous bleeding between the dura mater and the arachnoid space. SDH is generally caused either by trauma or by anticoagulation therapy. SDH is categorized into 3 main types, based on the rate of bleed, symptom appearance, and rebleeding subsequent to the initial trauma/event.

  - Diagnosis: CT scan or MRI; decreasing LOC, headache, confusion, contralateral hemiparesis, increased ICP, ipsilateral pupil dilation
  - **Acute SDH:** symptoms appear immediately or <4 days from trauma/event
  - **Subacute SDH:** symptoms appear 4 – 21 days after trauma/event
  - **Chronic SDH:** symptoms appear 21 days after trauma/event
  - Management: manage ABCs; craniotomy or trephination for hematoma evacuation

HELPFUL HINT:

Older adults, individuals on antiplatelet therapy, and chronic dialysis patients are at greatest risk for both a spontaneous SDH and a fall-related bleed.

HELPFUL HINT:

Because symptoms of chronic SDH evolve slowly, the condition may be mistaken for dementia, strokes, or brain tumors.

QUICK REVIEW QUESTION

18. A 72-year-old patient is admitted to the ICU after emergent surgical repair of a hip fracture sustained during a fall. The patient remains sedated and vented post-surgery. Before the surgery, the neurology assessment noted that the patient was alert and oriented to person, place, and time (A&O×3) and within normal limits, except for a headache rated at 3/10. The postsurgical assessment shows that the patient is not responding to stimuli and exhibits ipsilateral pupil dilation. What would be appropriate action for this patient?

ANSWER KEY

1. Focal neurological deficits resulting from damage to the occipital lobe, which controls vision, include loss of vision, hallucinations, and cortical blindness.

2. The GCS score would be 7, indicating that the patient has severe brain injury (likely in the cerebral hemispheres, as suggested by decorticate positioning).

3. The immediate treatment for an undifferentiated trauma patient with spinal immobilization and a stabilized ventilatory status is fluid resuscitation. This unstable trauma patient should be considered to be in hypovolemic shock until proven otherwise. If the spinal cord injury is radiologically confirmed and neurogenic shock differentiated, the nurse should expect to administer vasopressors, atropine or isoproterenol, and methylprednisolone.

4. The patient is hypotensive and unresponsive to vasopressors. The apnea test should be aborted, and the ventilator delivery returned to pretest settings.

5. The nurse should review the patient's medications, especially any current or prior benzodiazepine use. The nurse should request an order for a chemistry panel to assess for electrolyte imbalances, replacing deficiencies per protocol. Because the patient has a known infection, a sepsis screen should be completed once per shift and when any changes are observed. A sleep protocol and grouping of care will prevent overstimulation and provide adequate rest. Family should be encouraged to visit and talk with the patient. Dietary staff must be consulted for appropriate nutritional intake.

6. The nurse should answer honestly and explain that the medication does not cure the disease and will not improve the patient's cognitive symptoms. However, the medication will slow the progression of the disease. The nurse should tell the spouse that the patient should continue the medication as directed by the physician, even if they see no obvious improvement.

7. The hanging action has caused a hypoxic-ischemic brain injury. The nurse should expect to obtain baseline readings (vital signs, GCS score, cranial nerves responses, and LOC) and to closely monitor the patient for changes in neurological status. The nurse will also need to closely monitor ICP and tightly manage the patient's fluid balance.

8. The nurse should question the hypotonic solution of 0.45% sodium chloride because it can further increase ICP. A hypertonic solution would be expected in a patient with increased ICP.

9. Phytonadione (vitamin K) 1 mg IV would be administered to reverse the anticoagulation effects of warfarin and prevent further bleeding in the brain. The provider may also order 4-factor PCC or FFP to encourage clotting.

10. Nursing interventions would include monitoring and treating hypertension and ICP per ordered parameters; completing neurological assessments, including NIHSS every 4 hours; and monitoring for signs and symptoms of rebleeding, including hemodynamic or respiratory changes.

11. The priority intervention for a patient with a suspected ischemic stroke is to immediately obtain a noncontrast CT scan of the head.

12. A lumbar puncture with fluid analysis would be completed to determine viral or bacterial meningitis.

13. A patient with ALS presents with a progressive, asymmetrical pattern of weakness that affects both upper and lower extremities.

14. The patient may have a CSF leak, which is a common complication of pituitary surgery done via transsphenoidal craniotomy. The nurse should confirm that the discharge is CSF and alert the physician.

15. The patient will be treated with a second-line antiepileptic medication, most likely IV fosphenytoin or phenytoin. (Note that valproate is hepatotoxic and would not be administered to a patient with liver cirrhosis.)

16. Because the primary cancer is pancreatic, this patient is at greater risk of hypoglycemia which may increase the likelihood of seizures. The patient should be monitored closely for signs and symptoms of hypoglycemia and treated according to facility policy.

17. Hypotension is not usual in TBI and needs to be corrected quickly. The nurse should notify the provider while rapidly assessing for additional trauma sources such as internal crush injuries or hemorrhage. The nurse should anticipate administration of fluids and vasopressors to increase MAP and CPP.

18. Given the history of the fall, the age of the patient, and the noted headache, this patient may be experiencing an SDH. A stat CT scan should be completed. The patient should be prepared for, and family notified of, possible surgery for hematoma evacuation.

10 BEHAVIORAL AND PSYCHOSOCIAL REVIEW

CCRN TEST PLAN: BEHAVIORAL AND PSYCHOSOCIAL

- Abuse/neglect
- Aggression
- Agitation
- Anxiety
- Depression
- Medical non-adherence
- PTSD
- Risk-taking behavior
- Suicidal ideation and/or behaviors
- Substance use disorders (e.g., withdrawal, chronic alcohol or drug dependence)

Abuse and Neglect

Characteristics

Patients presenting with concern for **abuse** and **neglect** generally fall into one of three categories: domestic abuse, child abuse/neglect, and geriatric abuse/neglect. Nursing assessment for each of these concerns begins at admittance, and patients should be screened for signs or indications of neglect. Abuse can include both physical and emotional abuse; neglect may be on the part of caregivers or self.

Diagnosis

- physical signs and symptoms: unexplained injuries, fractures, or bruising at different stages of healing, poor hygiene, weight loss or gain

- emotional signs and symptoms: severe mood swings or changes, agitation, depression, suicidal ideation

Treatment and Management

- Protected populations (including pediatric and geriatric patients) require obligatory reporting of suspected abuse and neglect.
- Priority treatment of the abused or neglected patient should focus on physical injuries.
- Consideration should be made for emotional needs that result from abuse and neglect.
  - Provide same-gender caregivers or a same-gender chaperone for exams.
  - Use organizational resources to provide support for the patient.
  - Ask permission to touch the patient or narrate the physical exam.
  - Warn the patient when and where they will be touched during the exam.

QUICK REVIEW QUESTION

1. A pediatric patient is admitted for acute asthma exacerbation. Upon assessment, the nurse discovers bruising to the abdomen, back, and arms that appears to be in different stages of healing. The patient's parent is at the bedside. What is the nurse's next action?

Agitation, Aggression, and Violent Behavior

Characteristics

HELPFUL HINT:

Urosepsis is a common cause of agitation and aggression in patients over 65 years old.

Agitation is a state of anxiety and restlessness. This is a common challenge in the ICU and must be monitored in patients who are mechanically ventilated, restrained, or otherwise impeded from normal freedom of movement or who are experiencing delirium or a crisis.

Aggression or **violent behavior** in patients may occur for many reasons. These include:

- crisis or psychosis
- influence of drugs or alcohol
- underlying organic processes (e.g., TBI)

Treatment and Management

- recognize early signs and attempt to control situation
- alert security and follow facility protocol
- de-escalation techniques
  - verbal redirection
  - allowing the patient to express needs
  - allowing the patient to exercise
  - decreased environmental stimulation (quiet room time)
  - PRN medication administration (as requested by patient)
- restraint protocols
  - should be used conservatively and only for patients whose behavior cannot be controlled through less restrictive measures
  - require a physician order and initial assessment
  - require frequent assessment
    - every 5 – 15 minutes, depending on organizational policy
    - check vitals; assess pain, circulation, and skin integrity of all restrained extremities; address restroom needs
  - should be removed as soon as they are deemed unnecessary for patient and staff safety
- opioids and benzodiazepines for sedation

The **Richmond Agitation-Sedation Scale (RASS)** is a widely accepted method to assess a patient's level of sedation within a critical care unit. The goal is to maintain an RASS score between −2 and 0.

TABLE 10.1. Richmond Agitation-Sedation Scale (RASS)	
Description	**Score**
Combative	+4
Very agitated	+3
Agitated	+2
Restless	+1
Alert and calm	0
Drowsy	−1
Light sedation	−2
Moderate sedation	−3
Deep sedation	−4
Unarousable sedation	−5

QUICK REVIEW QUESTION

2. A patient was placed in mechanical restraints after demonstrating violent and aggressive behavior toward nursing staff. It has been 15 minutes since the restraints were applied, and the nurse is preparing to assess the patient. What will the nurse include in the assessment?

Anxiety

Characteristics

Anxiety is feelings of fear, apprehension, and worry that can be characterized as mild, moderate, or severe (panic). Anxiety can affect the respiratory, cardiac, and gastrointestinal systems. A key nursing consideration is to assess for organic causes for reported symptoms, as other illnesses, some life-threatening, may present with similar symptoms (e.g., palpitations, dizziness, dyspnea).

Treatment and Management

- target the level of anxiety the patient presents with (mild to panic)
- non-pharmacological interventions
    - placing patient in a calm environment
    - encouraging rhythmic breathing and the Valsalva technique
    - offering emotional support
    - promoting an open policy for family visitation
    - allowing the patient time to overcome the episode
- pharmacological interventions
    - antihistamines
    - benzodiazepines

QUICK REVIEW QUESTION

3. A patient presents to the ED reporting a sudden onset of feeling fearful, apprehensive, and on edge. The patient is feeling mild chest pain and shortness of breath. What should the nurse ask in the assessment of this patient?

Mood Disorders and Suicidal Ideation

Characteristics

Mood disorders can include mania and/or depression. **Depression** is a mood disorder characterized by feelings of sadness and hopelessness. Patients may also report feelings of suicidality. Depression can manifest as an exacerbation of bipolar disorder or as its own disease process.

Bipolar disorder (previously called manic-depressive illness) is characterized by shifts in mood accompanied by manic behaviors or depressive behaviors. Severe episodes of either mania or depression can also result in **psychosis**, characterized by hallucinations or delusions.

Suicidal ideation is characterized by considering suicide, thoughts of attempting suicide, or planning suicide. Patients exhibiting suicidal ideation may have vague thoughts without a distinct plan, or they may have a specific plan and the means to carry it out.

Signs and Symptoms

- manic behaviors
    - feelings of elation
    - high levels of energy and increased activity
    - difficulty sleeping; may not sleep for several days
    - increased rate of speech
    - engaging in high-risk activities (e.g., excessive spending, risky sexual activity)
- depressive behaviors
    - deep or intense feelings of sadness, worry, or anxiety
    - decreased energy levels with associated decreased activity
    - sleep and appetite disturbances
    - suicidal ideation or focus on death

Treatment and Management

- screen for depression and suicidal ideation
    - Ask directly if the patient is considering suicide or has recently or in the past attempted suicide.
    - If the patient is having thoughts of suicide, do they have a concrete plan to carry it out?

- Determine the presence of risk factors such as a history of substance abuse or chronic pain.
- Assess the presence of social supports for the patient.
- interventions for patients with suicidal ideation
  - securing a contract of safety that states they will remain safe while in the hospital and in the future
  - creating a safe environment (e.g., removing dangerous items from the room)
  - establishing a 1:1 watch or line-of-sight supervision for the patient
  - having the patient evaluated by a psychiatrist before discharge
- rule out possible medical causes for depression or mania (e.g., metabolic disorders)
- medications used to treat exacerbations of bipolar disorder
  - mood stabilizers
  - atypical antipsychotics
  - antipsychotics and antidepressants (usually used long term)

QUICK REVIEW QUESTION

4. How can the nurse address patient and staff safety when a patient reports thoughts of self-harm?

HELPFUL HINT:

Never ask family members to monitor or care for patients who are agitated, delirious, violent, or suicidal. This places an undue burden on the family. They may choose to provide support, but the nurse should ensure that appropriate monitoring or restraints are in place.

Post-Traumatic Stress Disorder (PTSD)

Characteristics

Post-traumatic stress disorder (PTSD) is a psychosomatic condition triggered by a traumatic event that involved the real or potential threat of serious injury, violence, or death. The condition can take an unspecified time to present, from a month to several years. It is marked by symptoms including pain, flashbacks, debilitating anxiety, nightmares, and uncontrollable fixation on the initial event.

Patients with **post-intensive care syndrome (PICS)** experience PTSD-like symptoms after critical care, particularly if they required ventilatory support. PICS correlates with delirium and typically presents 1 – 6 months post-hospitalization.

Treatment and Management

- nursing considerations for patients with PTSD
    - providing a supportive environment
    - initiating safety precautions for patient and others
    - reviewing medications and assessing for unwanted side effects
    - providing facts and reorientation if patient is experiencing flashbacks or delirium
    - announcing self when entering the room
    - explaining care before providing to prevent startling the patient
    - maintaining routines
- measures to prevent PICS
    - limiting use of sedation
    - extubating as soon as safe
    - assessing and treating for delirium
    - encouraging family to talk with patient while the patient is under sedation
    - having patient keep a journal
    - educating patient and family on signs of PICS to monitor for

---

QUICK REVIEW QUESTION

5. The nurse is transferring a patient from ICU to progressive care. The patient had been in ICU for two weeks to treat sepsis and was intubated and sedated for several days. What should the nurse explain to the family members regarding PICS?

Substance Dependence and Abuse

ALCOHOL WITHDRAWAL

Pathophysiology

Alcohol is a CNS depressant that directly binds to gamma-aminobutyric acid (GABA) receptors and inhibits glutamate-induced excitation. Chronic alcohol use alters the sensitivity of these receptors; when alcohol use is stopped, the result is hyperactivity in the CNS. Alcohol withdrawal can be fatal.

Chronic alcohol use inhibits the absorption of nutrients, including thiamine and folic acid. Consequently, patients admitted with symptoms of alcohol withdrawal are also at risk for disorders related to vitamin deficiency, including Wernicke's encephalopathy and megaloblastic anemia.

Refractory alcohol withdrawal syndrome (RAWS) occurs when the maximum dosage of benzodiazepines is insufficient for treatment, leading to excessive sedation, respiratory depression, hyperosmolar metabolic acidosis, and an increase of morbidity and mortality.

Signs and Symptoms

- mild (6 – 24 hours after last drink)
  - tachycardia and hypertension
  - agitation and restlessness
  - tremor
  - insomnia
  - hyperactive reflexes
  - diaphoresis
  - headache
  - nausea and emesis
- severe
  - hallucinations (12 – 48 hours after last drink)
  - tonic-clonic seizures (6 – 48 hours after last drink)
  - delirium tremens (DTs) (72 – 96 hours after last drink)
    - anxiety
    - tachycardia and hypertension
    - ataxia
    - diaphoresis

Assessment

- Assess withdrawal symptoms using the Clinical Institute Withdrawal Assessment (CIWA-Ar).
  - Scores range from 0 to 67.
  - A score >20 indicates severe withdrawal symptoms.

Treatment and Management

- IV fluids
- monitor for electrolyte imbalances
- treat vitamin deficiencies and malnutrition
- benzodiazepines for agitation
- lorazepam for seizures

- treatment for RAWS: phenobarbital, propofol, and dexmedetomidine
- mechanical ventilation for patients with severe DTs or RAWS

QUICK REVIEW QUESTION

6. An ICU patient was conscious and alert 48 hours following endovascular aortic repair to an abdominal aortic aneurysm. The patient's wife expresses concern that the patient has become sweaty and confused and has been asking when he can have a drink to relax. What interventions should the nurse anticipate?

Opioid Withdrawal

Pathophysiology

Opioids are synthetically and naturally occurring substances that bind to opioid receptors in the brain, depressing the CNS. (The term "opiate" is sometimes used to refer only to naturally occurring opioids.) Chronic use of opioids increases excitability of noradrenergic neurons, and withdrawal leads to hypersensitivity of the CNS. Opioid withdrawal is rarely fatal, but death can occur, usually as a result of hemodynamic instability or electrolyte imbalances.

Signs and Symptoms

- drug craving
- nausea, vomiting, diarrhea, and abdominal cramping
- dysphoria and anxiety
- yawning
- rhinorrhea and lacrimation
- mydriasis
- piloerection
- sweating
- muscle pain and twitching
- tachycardia, tachypnea, and hypertension

Assessment

- The **Clinical Opiate Withdrawal Scale (COWS)** is an 11-item scale to help objectively assess withdrawal symptoms and ensure that patients are given the correct amount of medication.
  - □ 5 – 12: mild withdrawal
  - □ 13 – 24: moderate withdrawal

- □ 25 – 36: moderate to severe withdrawal
- □ >36: severe withdrawal

Treatment and Management

- supportive care for symptoms
  - □ benzodiazepines for anxiety, tachycardia, and hypertension
  - □ clonidine for tachycardia and hypertension
  - □ antiemetics
  - □ antidiarrheals
- possible treatments for opioid withdrawal
  - □ Immediately cease taking opioids.
  - □ Opioid replacement therapy—methadone or buprenorphine relieve symptoms without producing intoxication.
  - □ Opioid antagonists—naltrexone and naloxone block the effects of opioids.

QUICK REVIEW QUESTION

7. An opioid-naive patient in the ICU for therapeutic hypothermia treatment was mechanically ventilated for five days and received a fentanyl 0.1 mcg/kg/hr IV continuous infusion as part of the analgesia protocol. After discontinuation of the drip, the patient was treated for discomfort with hydromorphone. The patient has been extubated and opioid treatment withdrawn. What should the nurse do to monitor and prepare for opioid withdrawal in the patient?

DRUG-SEEKING BEHAVIOR
Characteristics

Drug-seeking behavior is a loose term used to describe repeated attempts by a patient to obtain a certain substance or drug. In the critical care setting, opioids and benzodiazepines are the most commonly sought-after substances, although psychotropics are also abused. Patients exhibiting drug-seeking behaviors may display the following:

- reported pain levels that do not match patient symptoms or behavior
- polypharmacy and using several different pharmacies
- requesting drugs by specific name/brand name
- requesting increases to dosing
- escalating requests for a certain drug or displaying aggression
- irritability/anger when requests for medication are denied
- refusal to consider other treatment methods

Treatment and Management

- Be empathetic with patient; avoid judgment or blame, and be cautious of labeling patient as drug-seeking.

- Perform comprehensive pain assessment using a pain assessment tool that describes the pain scale.

- Establish a functional pain goal with patient that is reasonable and realistic.

- Observe and document patterns in behavior.

- If patient requires ongoing IV analgesics and is cognitively capable, patient-controlled administration can offer improved outcomes.

- Discuss alternative or adjuvant treatments available.

QUICK REVIEW QUESTION

8. One day after a PCI for a STEMI, a patient is sitting up in bed, laughing and talking with family in the room. When the nurse enters the room to complete morning assessments, the patient's demeanor abruptly changes. Cringing, the patient complains of chronic severe lower back pain and specifically requests "Dilaudid." The nurse notes that the home medication list reports oxycodone for back pain. What should the nurse do?

Medical Nonadherence

Characteristics

There are a number of factors that can contribute to **medical nonadherence** to care plans.

- social factors
  - □ inability to afford medications or lack of insurance
  - □ lack of transportation or time
  - □ cultural norms against receiving care
- emotional or spiritual factors
  - □ depression or fear
  - □ recourse to prayer or alternative healing methods
- physical factors
  - □ immobility
  - □ inability to properly access or use medications
  - □ medication side effects
- educational factors (i.e., lack of health literacy)

Treatment and Management

- Provide supportive care that individually addresses the patient's barriers, needs, and circumstances.

- Assess for potential barriers to medical adherence when developing a care plan.

- Consult social worker for financial and supportive resources.

- Consult physician to explore alternative medications or treatments that may better meet the patient's needs.

- Maintain open communication with the patient and family over concerns.

QUICK REVIEW QUESTION

9. A patient is readmitted to the ICU with acute-on-chronic COPD exacerbation. Upon questioning, the nurse finds that the patient was not taking the medications prescribed after the last admit. The patient's spouse states there are too many pills to keep track of and they are not able to afford several of the medications. What key interventions can the nurse initiate to mitigate this nonadherence?

ANSWER KEY

1. The nurse should complete the physical assessment and discuss these findings with the physician. She should then complete the screening for child abuse and follow local policy on mandatory reporting of suspected child abuse.

2. The nurse should assess the status of the patient, including orientation, vital signs, neurovascular status of the extremities restrained, and skin integrity at the restraint points.

3. The nurse should obtain prior medical history, including cardiac and respiratory concerns, and find out if the patient has a history of anxiety reactions in the past. Medications the patient is currently taking should be reviewed. The nurse should be prepared to address any life-threatening illnesses before addressing anxiety.

4. The nurse should get a detailed accounting of the patient's plan for self-harm and determine if the patient is in possession of any objects or weapons that could cause harm to the patient or to staff. The patient's surroundings should be assessed for safety, with removal of any objects that could be used for harm. Suicide precautions should be initiated with procurement of a 1:1 safety companion assignment.

5. The nurse should educate the family on the possibility that the patient could develop symptoms of depression, labile moods, excessive fatigue, weakness, or cognitive decline in the upcoming months. The family should be encouraged to talk with the patient about their experiences in the ICU and to validate their feelings about the experience.

6. The nurse should assess the patient and take a thorough history to confirm the patient is experiencing alcohol withdrawal. The nurse should be prepared to administer benzodiazepines and assess for fluid and nutrient imbalances related to chronic alcohol use.

7. A patient who does not have prior opioid use is at risk for opioid withdrawal after more than 96 hours of opioid treatment. Screen patient for withdrawal symptoms using COWS. Anticipate orders for benzodiazepine or clonidine if patient exhibits symptoms of tachycardia, tachypnea, and hypertension.

8. After completing a thorough pain assessment, as well as setting reasonable and realistic pain goals with the patient, the nurse should review the medications and other treatments the patient used at home prior to hospitalization. A discussion with the managing physician regarding restarting the patient's home regimen rather than treating with patient's request for hydromorphone (Dilaudid) is reasonable.

9. The nurse can try to alleviate the cost of medications by working with a social worker to find assistance programs and working with the physician to find less expensive alternative medications. An interview with the patient and family may help identify other specific barriers that can be addressed. Possible interventions may include pill organizers, further education, and increased social support from family or friends.

11 MULTISYSTEM REVIEW

CCRN TEST PLAN: MULTISYSTEM

- Acid-base imbalance*
- Bariatric complications
- Comorbidity in patients with transplant history
- End-of-life care
- Healthcare-associated conditions (e.g., VAE, CAUTI, CLABSI)*
- Hypotension*
- Infectious diseases
- Life-threatening maternal/fetal complications (e.g., eclampsia, HELLP syndrome, postpartum hemorrhage, amniotic embolism)
- Multiple organ dysfunction syndrome (MODS)
- Multisystem trauma*
- Pain: acute, chronic
- Post-intensive care syndrome (PICS)*
- Sepsis
- Septic shock
- Shock states
- a. Distributive (e.g., anaphylactic, neurogenic)
- b. Hypovolemic
- Sleep disruption (including sensory overload)
- Thermoregulation
- Toxic ingestion/inhalations (e.g., drug/alcohol overdose)
- Toxin/drug exposure (including allergies)

*Topic is covered in relevant systems chapter.Bariatric Complications

- The CCRN should be prepared for acute post-op management of bariatric surgery and for delivery of pertinent dietary and lifestyle education to the patient.
- There are three types of bariatric surgical procedures intended to produce weight loss: restrictive, malabsorptive, and combination procedures.
- **Restrictive procedures** reduce the capacity of the stomach.
  - The **vertical band gastroplasty (VBG)** creates a small pouch (15 – 30 mL capacity) and is generally considered a permanent alteration.
  - The **adjustable gastric banding procedure** also creates a small pouch, which can be externally inflated and deflated to allow for flexibility in the amount of food intake.
  - The **vertical sleeve gastrectomy (SG)** surgically removes approximately 80% of the stomach, changes the organ to a sleeve shape, and permanently reduces capacity.
- **Malabsorptive procedures** limit digestion and absorption of food by altering the GI tract itself. The amount of food volume consumed is minimally affected, but the absorption of nutrients is markedly reduced. Nutritional deficits require monitoring over time.
  - The **biliopancreatic diversion with a duodenal switch (BPD)** creates an anastomosis between the stomach and the intestine.
- **Combination procedures** limit capacity and profoundly alter the absorption of nutrients.
  - The **Roux-en-Y gastric bypass (RYGB)** constructs a small gastric pouch (20 – 30 mL capacity) that has a stoma outlet to a Y-shaped section of the jejunum that has been anastomosed to the pouch.
  - This surgery allows food to bypass the lower stomach and the duodenum, decreasing digestive absorption.
- Common complications of bariatric surgery:
  - Post-op GI bleeding markedly increases morbidity and mortality and requires surgical correction.
  - Anastomotic leaks present with pain and fever. They require treatment with broad-spectrum antibiotics and possible drainage or surgical repair.
  - Stenosis is prevalent in the RYGB procedure and often requires endoscopic balloon dilation within 1 week postsurgery.
  - Kinks in the surgical sleeve (after SG) present with recurrent vomiting and inability to tolerate oral intake. This complication generally requires surgical intervention.
  - Gastroenteric or gastrobronchial fistulas are managed according to severity; they may close without intervention or require surgery.

HELPFUL HINT:

VBG is often accompanied by a cholecystectomy to reduce risk of gallstones.

- Common abdominal postsurgical emergent events such as atelectasis, pneumonia, PE, DVT, postoperative pain, and trauma from nasogastric suction are also bariatric sequelae.

- **Dumping syndrome** is a collection of symptoms that result from rapid gastric emptying; it can occur after surgery that removes or bypasses the pyloric sphincter.

  - Early dumping syndrome occurs when fluid shifts into the small bowel because of hyperosmolar stomach contents. Signs and symptoms include abdominal pain, diarrhea, tachycardia, and hypotension.

  - Late dumping syndrome (postprandial hyperinsulinemic hypoglycemia [PHH]) occurs when there is an overproduction of insulin after a high concentration of carbohydrates is delivered quickly into the intestines.

  - Dumping syndrome is managed with dietary changes. Some patients may require medication (self-administered subcutaneous Sandostatin [octreotide injection]).

  - Dumping syndrome may not occur in the critical care setting, as postoperative dietary progression may not include sufficient solids to trigger the syndrome.

QUICK REVIEW QUESTION

1. What are the anatomical changes in an RYGB and the potential adverse emergent situations in the first 3 postoperative days?

End-of-Life Care

- The implementation of high-quality **end-of-life care (EOLC)** is an important part of ICU work. The CCRN should be aware of the aspects, options, and caring responses to this event described by the 2020 AACN recommendations.

- Decision-making process:
  - The decision to withhold or withdraw life-sustaining therapy is made by the individual, with family involvement.
  - Decisions should reflect the patient's values and wishes (if possible) and are documented with input from the entire interdisciplinary team, without excluding other therapies in progress.

- Place-to-die determination:
  - The best location for an actively dying individual is usually the same single-occupancy ICU room.

- If transfer is necessary, complete information is given to the patient early, with staff support, to ease the transition.
- Discharge to home is also an option.

- Palliative care, patient comfort, and dignity:
  - Assess frequently to manage palliation of pain.
  - Both medical and nonmedical techniques should be used to maintain patient comfort.
  - Respect individual dignity and the patient's wishes for visits, spiritual support, and a nursing surrogate role (if no family is present).

- Family presence in ICU (including children's visiting practices):
  - If congruent with patient's wishes, family should be able to visit at all times.
  - Avoid unnecessary waiting outside room.
  - Provide clear, age-appropriate, and truthful explanation of dying to children before their first ICU visit.
  - When possible, provide an ICU area that children can play in.

- Preparing family and identifying their diverse needs at end-of-life event:
  - Be sensitive to cultural and personal family reactions to the active dying of a loved one.
  - Assess family needs for information and spiritual support systems.
  - Respect family dynamics during the grieving process.
  - Reassure family that the patient's pain is being managed, and frequently assess and treat emergent symptoms while giving family simple explanations.

- Determining staff presence during the active dying of individual:
  - Identify the individual's wishes.
  - If the family prefers to be alone, continue appropriate care in room without intruding on family processes.

- Family participation at end-of-life event, and after:
  - Family-centered bereavement care provides time for grieving, allows the family to participate in care of the expired patient, and continues to support families after they leave the ICU.
  - Most facilities have established policies to allow for personal mementos (e.g., locks of hair, handprints), follow-up notes, visitations, or calls, and bereavement counseling groups to reduce family suffering and PTSD responses to loss.

- Staff grieving: Debriefing honors staff grief and reduces burnout.

QUICK REVIEW QUESTION

2. What is family-centered bereavement care?

Infectious Diseases

- The CCRN exam will likely not cover signs and symptoms or management of specific infectious diseases. Instead, candidates should expect to see bacterial or viral infections appear as part of background scenarios (e.g., management of sepsis secondary to pneumonia).

- The exam may include questions about standard isolation protocols. Some general guidelines are given below.

Standard Precautions

- Assume that all patients are carrying an infectious microorganism.

- Practice hand hygiene.
  - □ Use soap and water when hands are visibly soiled.
  - □ Use antimicrobial foam or gel if hands are not visibly soiled.

- Wear gloves.
  - □ Gloves must be discarded between each patient visit.
  - □ Gloves may need to be discarded when soiled and a new pair donned.
  - □ Practice hand hygiene after removing gloves.

- Prevent needle sticks.
  - □ Immediately place used needles in puncture-resistant containers.
  - □ Recap using mechanical device or one-handed technique.

- Avoid splash and spray: wear appropriate PPE if there is a possibility of body fluids splashing or spraying.

HELPFUL HINT:

Antimicrobial foams and gels are not effective against some infectious agents, such as *C. difficile*.

Airborne Precautions

- Patient should be placed in a private room with a negative-pressure air system and the door kept closed.

- Wear N-95 respirator mask: put it on before entering the room, and keep it on until after leaving the room.

- Place N-95 or surgical mask on patient during transport.

- Examples of diseases requiring airborne precautions include chicken pox, measles, and tuberculosis. The precautions are also used for COVID-19 patients undergoing aerosol-generating procedures (e.g., intubation).

Droplet Precautions

- Place patient in a private room; the door may remain open.

- Wear appropriate PPE within 3 feet of patient.

- Wash hands with antimicrobial soap after removing gloves and mask, before leaving the patient's room.

- Place surgical mask on patient during transport.

- Examples of diseases requiring droplet precautions include influenza, pertussis, and COVID-19.

Contact Precautions

- Place the patient in a private room; the door may remain open.

- Wear gloves.
  - □ Change gloves after touching infected materials.
  - □ Remove gloves before leaving patient's room.

- Wear gown; remove before leaving patient's room.

- Use patient-dedicated equipment if possible; community equipment is to be used clean and disinfected between patients.

- During transport, keep precautions in place and notify different areas as needed.

- Examples of diseases requiring contact precautions include C. *difficile*, MRSA, and noroviruses.

QUICK REVIEW QUESTION

3. A patient is admitted to the ICU with a suspected C. *difficile* infection. What PPE should the nurse use?

Life-Threatening Maternal/ Fetal Complications

- **Preeclampsia** is a syndrome that occurs when abnormalities in the placental vasculature cause widespread arterial vasospasms. The multiple, repetitive vasospasms decrease perfusion to organs, eventually leading to tissue ischemia, microangiopathy, and end-organ dysfunction in the mother.

□ Symptoms can appear after the twentieth week of pregnancy and most commonly appear after 34 weeks. Maternal **postpartum preeclampsia** generally occurs within 6 days after childbirth but can be delayed up to 6 weeks after delivery. It can occur even if there was no evidence of preeclampsia prior to delivery.

□ Signs and symptoms: malignant hypertension, edema (despite strict bed rest), excruciating headache, vision disturbance, dyspnea, changes in LOC.

□ Diagnostic findings: proteinuria, hyperuricemia, thrombocytopenia, elevated homocysteine.

□ The reduced blood flow seen in severe preeclampsia can cause injury to multiple organs, including the liver (causing elevated liver enzymes), kidneys, (causing elevated creatinine), or myocardium (causing elevated troponin). Labs may also show hemolysis of RBCs (decreased hemoglobin, hyperbilirubinemia).

□ Sequalae: pulmonary edema (due to increased capillary permeability), abruptio placentae, intracerebral hemorrhage

□ During pregnancy, the only definitive treatment is delivery of the fetus and removal of placental tissue.

□ Postpartum preeclampsia requires anti-hypertensives, seizure prophylaxis, and anticoagulants.

□ **Eclampsia** is the onset of tonic-clonic seizures in women with preeclampsia. All patients with preeclampsia require seizure prophylaxis (magnesium sulfate [$MgSO_4$] IV pump infusion) to prevent progression to eclampsia. Recurrent seizure may be treated with amobarbital, phenytoin, or benzodiazepines.

□ Refractory hypertension is treated with labetalol or hydralazine hydrochloride.

▪ **HELLP syndrome** is currently believed to be a form of preeclampsia, although the relationship between the 2 disorders is controversial and not well understood.

□ Around 85% of women diagnosed with HELLP also present with symptoms of preeclampsia.

□ HELLP is characterized by hemolysis (H), elevated liver enzymes (EL), and low platelet count (LP).

□ Signs and symptoms: hypertension, tachycardia, dyspnea, jaundice, fatigue, RUQ pain with epigastric tenderness, dehydration.

□ HELLP severity is evaluated using the Mississippi Classification System (based on platelet count, AST/ALT levels, and LDH levels).

□ Management is focused on preventing and managing emergent complications, including DIC, pulmonary edema, PE, ARDS, MI, AKI, hepatic rupture, and infection.

HELPFUL HINT:

Be aware of how an exam question on preeclampsia is worded. Do not confuse *prepartum* preeclampsia (which requires delivery of the fetus) with *postpartum* preeclampsia (which requires ICU monitoring and management).

HELPFUL HINT:

HELLP syndrome is often mistaken for acute hepatitis, gastritis, gallbladder disease, or influenza.

- **Postpartum hemorrhage** is bleeding that occurs any time after delivery up to 12 weeks postpartum and exceeds 1,000 mL or that causes symptoms of hypovolemia.
  - □ Management: IV fluid resuscitation and blood products as needed; identify and treat underlying cause of hemorrhage.
  - □ Uterine atony: uterine massage; oxytocin 20 – 40 IU/L 0.9% NaCl IV; ergot derivatives (contraindicated for preeclampsia and hypertension); vasopressors.
  - □ Trauma: surgery to repair cause of bleed.
  - □ Retained tissue: manual removal of placental tissue.
  - □ Coagulopathy (thrombin): replace clotting factors (platelets and/or FFP).

HELPFUL HINT:

The causes of postpartum hemorrhage are known as the Four T's: tone, trauma, tissue, and thrombin.

- **Amniotic fluid embolism (AFE)** is an acute, life-threatening allergic reaction that occurs when amniotic fluid enters the maternal circulation during childbirth.
  - □ Phase 1 exhibits rapid-onset respiratory failure leading to cardiac arrest, ARDS, and multisystem organ failure.
  - □ Phase 2 (hemorrhagic phase) develops profuse bleeding (usually at the site of placental attachment, cesarean incision, and IV site) and DIC.
  - □ Treatment focuses on management of symptoms and may include massive blood transfusion protocol, hysterectomy, and management of cardiac arrest, ARDS, and multisystem organ failure.
  - □ Maternal survivors demonstrate severe neurological injury; infant survivors show cerebral palsy or limited brain function. AFE survivors and their families are at high risk for PTSD.

- **Abruptio placentae** (placental abruption) occurs when the placenta separates from the uterus after the twentieth week of gestation but before delivery. Abruption can lead to life-threatening conditions, including hemorrhage and DIC.

- In **placenta accreta**, the placenta attaches abnormally deeply into the myometrium. Because the placenta cannot detach from the uterus after delivery, placenta accreta can lead to hemorrhage and requires a hysterectomy.

QUICK REVIEW QUESTION

4. A 33-year-old prima gravida previously diagnosed with mild preeclampsia develops headache, double-vision intervals, with BP 180/101 mm Hg at 36 weeks. After a noncomplicated vaginal delivery, BP stabilizes at 145/80. Six days later, the mother presents at the ED with severe headache, overwhelming fatigue, abdominal pain, nausea, vomiting, and generalized edema. With BP of 190/110, she is transferred to ICU for management. What is the admission diagnosis, and what should the nurse anticipate for treatment?

Pain

- **Pain management** is uniquely individualized in the critical care setting, so the CCRN exam will not focus on management of individual patients. Instead, the exam will present questions that target the nurse's understanding of pain assessment and documentation.

- The goal of pain management should be timely and consistent patient responses to interventions.

- The critical care nurse should understand that pain assessment requires asking the right questions and using an appropriate and consistent pain scale (as defined by hospital policy). Pain assessment may include:
    - patient's self-reported pain (on a consistent scale)
    - a detailed interview to determine location, quality, severity, timing, and alleviating/exacerbating factors of pain
    - review of effects of previous interventions
    - use of tools such as the Behavioral Pain Scale (BPS) or Critical Care Pain Observation Tool for patients who cannot verbally communicate

- Planning for pain management is an important component of a care plan.
    - Review with patient and/or family the potential or actual discomfort levels related to the specific clinical situation.
    - Prepare patients for upcoming treatments or bedside procedures (e.g., dressing changes, line insertions or removals, treatments, transfers to testing areas) with appropriate premedication, and ensure sufficient time for premedication to take effect before initiating procedures.
    - Engage patients/family in mobility planning and implementation.

- Pain management interventions should always be properly documented.

- The pain management plan should address the side effects of analgesics (e.g., constipation, nausea, or respiratory depression related to opioid use).

HELPFUL HINT:

Sedation is NOT the correct way to treat pain and should never replace the use of appropriate analgesics.

QUICK REVIEW QUESTION

5. A 28-year-old multi-trauma patient will require, after chest wound surgical repair, intermittent prone positioning to decrease ARDS complications of prolonged ventilator therapy. The patient's wife, upset because she believes her husband is in pain during positioning, demands the nurse "give him something to stop him from hurting." What is the most appropriate pain management plan for the nurse to initiate?

Shock States

Shock is a state of circulatory failure that results in insufficient oxygenation of tissue. Shock is categorized according to the underlying cause of circulatory failure.

- **Hypovolemic shock** is the result of reduced intravascular volume.

- **Distributive shock** is the result of massive vasodilation. Types of distributive shock include anaphylactic, septic, and neurogenic shock. (Neurogenic shock is discussed in chapter 9.)

- **Cardiogenic shock** is the result of cardiac tissue damage that reduces cardiac output. (Cardiogenic shock is discussed in chapter 1.)

- **Obstructive shock** is reduced cardiac output not caused by cardiac tissue damage. Causes of obstructive shock include PE, pulmonary hypertension, cardiac tamponade, and tension pneumothorax.

Understanding the pathophysiology underlying the **three phases of shock**—no matter what the specific type/cause of shock—is the key to answering exam questions on every type of shock state.

HELPFUL HINT:

Specialty knowledge of shock trauma is not part of the CCRN exam, but CCRN candidates should know that the triad of hypothermia, acidosis, and coagulopathy in trauma patients must be stabilized to prevent irreversible damage or death.

TABLE 11.1. Phases of Shock

Phase	Pathophysiology	General Symptoms
Compensatory (early)	Activation of the sympathetic nervous system to increase/maintain blood pressure causes vasoconstriction, increased contractility of heart, and increased HR.	• restlessness, anxiety • tachycardia • tachypnea (impending respiratory alkalosis) • normal PaO_2 on ABG • pallor • oliguria • increased thirst
Progressive	Compensatory system begins to fail, and sympathetic withdrawal syndrome occurs.	• hypotension • change in LOC • increased tachycardia • decreased PaO_2 • metabolic acidosis on ABG • cool, clammy, mottled skin • nausea

Phase	Pathophysiology	General Symptoms
Refractory (late)	Severe systemic hypoperfusion leads to MODS.	• neurological: stroke, encephalopathy • cardiac: ischemia, failure • pulmonary: ARDS • renal: anuria, acute tubular necrosis • hepatic: liver failure • hematologic: DIC

HYPOVOLEMIC SHOCK

Pathophysiology

Hypovolemic shock is characterized by a profound reduction in circulating volume, leading to impaired tissue perfusion. It is the most common type of shock.

External causes of hypovolemic shock include hemorrhage, burns, GI/renal losses, or excessive diaphoresis. Hypovolemic shock can also be caused by fluid pooling in the intravascular compartment (third-spacing). Shock caused by bleeding is categorized as **hemorrhagic shock**; all other causes of hypovolemic shock are **nonhemorrhagic**.

Hemodynamic Changes

- narrowing pulse pressure (decrease in SBP, increase in DBP): cardinal sign of hypovolemic shock
- increased SVR
- decreased cardiac output
- decreased pulse pressure/low BP
- decreased CVP
- decreased PAOP

Treatment and Management

- Determine and treat cause (assessment performed concurrently with fluid resuscitation).
- Secure airway and obtain 2 large-bore IV access sites.
- Rapidly replace volume.
  - □ 0.9% NaCl or lactated Ringer's (crystalloid fluids)
  - □ Use fluid warmer if giving more than 2 L/hr

HELPFUL HINT:

During early shock, vasoconstriction occurs with activation of the **renin-angiotensin-aldosterone system (RAAS)**. **Renin** activates angiotensin I, which in turn activates **angiotensin II**, which increases systemic vascular resistance. Angiotensin II also stimulates release of **aldosterone**, which promotes Na⁺ and water retention.

HELPFUL HINT:

SVR remains high during hypovolemic state: do NOT give vasopressors.

HELPFUL HINT:

Replacing lost volume helps sustain aerobic metabolism to reduce acidosis, improves oxygen delivery/tissue uptake, decreases tachycardia, and increases renal perfusion to improve urinary output.

HELPFUL HINT:

Cold blood increases hemoglobin's affinity for oxygen and decreases tissue uptake, creates platelet dysfunction, and deforms RBCs.

- Initiate maintenance treatment when HR returns to baseline to meet target parameters:
  - MAP ≥ 65
  - CVP 6 – 10 mm Hg
  - Urine output ≥ 0.5 mL/kg/hr
- Management of hemorrhagic shock:
  - manage bleeding
  - hemorrhagic shock Class I and II (blood loss <1500 mL, BP normal): crystalloid fluids
  - hemorrhagic shock Class III and IV (blood loss >1500 mL, decreased BP): crystalloids and PRBC units
  - because PRBCs do not contain plasma or platelets, actively bleeding patients will also need FFP, cryoprecipitate, and/or platelets
  - indications for massive transfusion resuscitation: traumatic injuries; liver transplants; OB emergencies; ruptured aortic or thoracic aneurisms; Hgb <7.0 (generally transfused at higher level for MI, lactic acidosis, severe hypoxemia, or continued active bleeding)
  - ensure Hgb >7.0 and coagulation profile/platelets normalized before moving to maintenance treatment
- Blood administration risks:
  - hypothermia: use blood warmer if possible
  - hemolytic and nonhemolytic transfusion reactions (see chapter 4 for more detailed information on transfusion reactions)
  - hypocalcemia and hypomagnesemia
  - coagulopathy: requires platelets and plasma therapy
  - viral infections: transmitted from blood products

QUICK REVIEW QUESTION

6. What are the classic signs and hemodynamic changes found in hypovolemic shock?

Sepsis and Septic Shock

Pathophysiology

Sepsis, a dysregulated inflammatory response to infection, leads to organ system dysfunction. What starts as a localized response to infection leads to generalized inflammation, which in turn causes cellular damage across systems. Common organ-specific conditions seen during sepsis include:

- hypotension (due to massive vasodilation)
- pulmonary edema and ARDS
- AKI
- encephalopathy

Sepsis is a progressive process, and the guidelines for classifying its stages continue to evolve. Current Society of Critical Care Medicine guidelines define 3 stages of sepsis:

- **early sepsis:** infection + early indicators of organ dysfunction (e.g., increased RR or decreased SBP)
- **sepsis:** infection + signs of organ dysfunction
  - lung: decreased PaO_2/FiO_2 ratio
  - coagulation: decreased platelets
  - liver: increased bilirubin
  - cardiovascular: hypotension
  - brain: low GCS score
  - kidney: increased creatine
- **septic shock:** sepsis + inability to maintain adequate MAP (MAP ≥65 mm Hg and lactate 2 mmol/L)

MODS is the most severe end of the sepsis spectrum. (Note that MODS is simply a description of organ dysfunction and can have noninfectious causes.) Commonly used indicators of organ dysfunction are given below.

- **neurologic:** confusion, lethargy, disorientation, delirium, coma, seizure
- **cardiovascular:** tachycardia, dysrhythmias, elevated troponin level, hypotension requiring fluid resuscitation and vasopressor support, decreased SVR, abnormal CVP (low or high)
- **pulmonary:** tachypnea, dyspnea, hypoxemia, ARDS
- **renal:** oliguria, decreased GRF, elevated creatinine, critical-level electrolyte imbalances
- **endocrine:** hypoglycemia or hyperglycemia, adrenal insufficiency
- **hepatic:** decreased albumin, jaundice, elevated liver function tests
- **hematologic:** thrombocytopenia, coagulopathy, increased D-dimer levels
- **metabolic:** metabolic acidosis, elevated lactate levels

Older sepsis guidelines also include **systemic inflammatory response syndrome (SIRS)** as part of the sepsis continuum. SIRS is defined as 2 or more of the following:

- HR >90 bpm
- temperature 100.5°F (38.0°C) OR <96.8°F (36.0°C)

- RR >20 or PaCO$_2$ <32 (respiratory alkalosis)
- WBC >12,000 or WBC <4,000 OR a shift of bands to the left 10%

Patients with SIRS and a suspected or confirmed infection are considered to have sepsis. Noninfectious causes of SIRS include pancreatitis, burns, thromboembolism, and trauma.

Regardless of which guidelines are used, the critical care nurse should understand how sepsis may progress from infection to inflammation to organ dysfunction.

Treatment and Management

- Stat lab work:
  - 2 sets of blood cultures: 2 separate sites; obtain before initiating antibiotic therapy
  - CBC with differential, lactate levels
- Implement sepsis bundle (per facility guidelines): broad-spectrum antibiotics, IV fluids, and vasopressors as indicated.
- Identify causative agent: antibiotic/antiviral/antifungal therapy ASAP.
- IV fluid challenges:
  - initiated when lactate level 4 mmol/L
  - 30 mL/kg to start to support BP
  - IV crystalloid concentrations based on other comorbidities present
- Maintain MAP ≥65:
  - first-line vasopressor: norepinephrine infusion
  - second-line vasopressor: epinephrine infusion
  - ionotropic therapy if cardiac dysfunction: dobutamine infusion (not to exceed 20 mcg/kg/min)
  - PRBCs if Hgb <7.0
- Focused reassessment exam after initial fluid resuscitation:
  - assess tissue perfusion and volume status
  - lactate level should decrease by 10% with each fluid bolus
- SvO$_2$/ScvO$_2$ stabilized
  - SvO$_2$ 60 – 75% (target): measured with pulmonary artery catheter; mixed venous sample
  - ScvO$_2$ 70% (target): continuous monitoring (identify/use specific CVP port/line) or intermittent monitoring (CVP multiuse port/line or PICC line)
  - ScvO$_2$ = 5 – 8% higher than SvO$_2$

HELPFUL HINT:

Lactate may be considered a marker of tissue perfusion. Elevated lactate levels sustained 6 hours lead to increased mortality. Lactate 4.0 mmol/L is associated with a 28% mortality rate.

QUICK REVIEW QUESTION

7. A 69-year-old female patient with oral-medication-controlled type 2 diabetes mellitus has just completed her course of chemotherapy postmastectomy. The patient is admitted from the ED to the ICU with a temperature of 102.6°F (39.2°C), lethargy, and confusion. HR 105 bpm, BP 92/68 mm Hg, RR 22. Admission fingerstick glucose was 122 mg/dL, electrolytes and coagulation panel appeared within normal limits, lactate level was 2.4, and WBC = 14,000. What interventions should the nurse prepare for?

ANAPHYLACTIC SHOCK

Pathophysiology

Anaphylaxis is triggered when a hypersensitive reaction to an allergen (e.g., foods, medications, insect sting, latex, radiocontrast dye, blood/blood products) causes an overwhelming inflammatory response. Symptoms appear minutes to a few hours after exposure to the allergen. If untreated or ineffectively treated, anaphylaxis will progress to anaphylactic shock, refractory hypotension, and possible death.

Anaphylactic shock is characterized by massive vasodilation, resulting in fluid loss into the extravascular space, hemoconcentration, and hypovolemia. Increased pulmonary vascular resistance may lead to pulmonary edema and respiratory arrest. Dysrhythmias (especially tachycardia) are common, and patients are at risk for MI.

Signs and Symptoms

- urticaria, itching, and erythema
- pale skin
- nausea, vomiting, or diarrhea
- angioedema or tongue swelling
- laryngeal edema and difficulty swallowing
- bronchospasm and wheezing
- hypotension
- tachycardia
- alteration in LOC

Treatment and Management

- first-line treatment
  - maintain airway

HELPFUL HINT:

Epinephrine may be administered in nebulized form for laryngeal edema.

- □ 0.3 mg epinephrine 1:1,000 IM (blocks release of inflammatory mediators)
- □ glucagon 5 – 15 mcg/min infusion if patient is on beta blocker
- second-line treatment
  - □ H1 blocker: diphenhydramine (25 – 50 mg IV/IM/PO)
  - □ H2 blocker: ranitidine (50 mg IV or 150 mg PO)
  - □ steroids: prednisone (50 mg PO) OR methylprednisolone (125 mg IV)
- shock management
  - □ airway management: oxygen therapy and bronchodilators (albuterol inhaler)
  - □ volume resuscitation: IV or IO colloid infusion with volume dependent on response (1 – 3 L rapid administration not uncommon)
  - □ circulatory management (decrease afterload and preload): epinephrine infusion (2 – 8 mcg/min), dopamine infusion (5 – 20 mcg/kg/min), or norepinephrine infusion (2 – 8 mcg/min)
- Monitor for spontaneous or rebound/reemergence of anaphylaxis.

QUICK REVIEW QUESTION

8. A 33-year-old male patient is undergoing an emergent laparotomy for removal of an inflamed appendix. The circulating nurse hangs a 50 mL antibiotic IV mini bag as the incision is closed and sutured. As the still-intubated patient is being prepared for transfer to the PACU, the cardiac monitor shows SVT of 128, and the patient is markedly hypotensive. IV fluids and a dopamine drip at 8 mcg/kg/min are infusing as the patient is brought to the SICU. The receiving nurse discusses with the surgical resident a possible anaphylactic reaction. What series of initial medication orders should the critical care nurse expect for this patient?

★ Toxic Ingestion and Exposure

- During **acetaminophen (Tylenol)** overdose, toxic metabolites accumulate in the liver causing hepatotoxicity from mitochondrial dysfunction and cellular destruction.
  - □ Time and amount of drug are important considerations in acetaminophen overdose treatment. Plasma acetaminophen levels can be measured 4 – 24 hours after ingestion to predict risk of hepatotoxicity using the Rumack-Matthew nomogram.

- Gastritis symptoms usually appear within hours; symptoms of hepatotoxicity may not appear for 48 hours.

- Hepatoxicity rapidly advances to acute liver failure often complicated by encephalopathy, pulmonary edema, pancreatitis, and AKI. (See chapter 5 for detailed information on liver failure.)

- The antidote for acetaminophen overdoes is **N-acetylcysteine (Mucomyst)**; the best response occurs when it is administered within 24 hours of ingestion.

- N-acetylcysteine dosing (IV): IV 150 mg/kg over 1 hour; 50 mg/kg over next 4 hours; 100 mg/kg over next 16 hours

- N-acetylcysteine dosing (PO): 140 mg/kg loading dose; 70 mg/kg every 4 hours

- Activated charcoal may be administered within 4 hours of ingestion but is usually not well tolerated.

- **Beta blockers** block beta-adrenergic receptors in the heart (beta$_1$) and blood vessels (beta$_2$), resulting in lowered BP and HR and decreased cardiac output. They are used to treat a wide range of conditions, and most overdoses are unintentional.

  - Symptoms will vary with the beta blocker ingested, as each medication has different actions, absorption times, half-lifes, and interactions with other medications.

  - Symptoms will be seen 1 – 2 hours after ingestion and usually are most pronounced around 20 hours post-ingestion.

  - General signs and symptoms: bradycardia, hypotension, hypoglycemia, altered mental state.

  - Beta blockers with lipophilic affinity (e.g., propranolol) cross the blood-brain barrier easily and may cause seizures.

  - Beta blockers that block sodium or potassium channels (e.g., propranolol, acebutolol) can cause prolonged QRS/QTc intervals.

  - Glucagon bypasses the beta-adrenergic receptor sites affected by the beta-blocking agent and reverses the beta$_1$ blockade; it increases myocardial contractility and HR with improved AV conduction.

  - Management of symptoms may include vasopressors, MgSO$_4$ IV for prolonged QTc, sodium bicarbonate (NaHCO3) IV for widened QRS, intubation, bronchodilators for bronchospasm, gastric lavage, seizure management, insulin drip (glucose control target 100 mg/dL – 200 mg/dL)

- **Salicylate** (aspirin) overdose affects the brain's respiratory center, resulting in hyperventilation and respiratory alkalosis. The kidneys respond by producing more bicarbonate and excreting more potassium, causing metabolic acidosis.

HELPFUL HINT:

Enteric-coated pills may form a gastric **bezoar** (hard mass or concretion in the stomach) delaying absorption and excretion.

HELPFUL HINT:

The sleep aids zolpidem and zaleplon also bond to GABA/benzodiazepine receptors and are responsive to flumazenil after an overdose.

- □ Peak serum salicylate levels occur at 6 hours after ingestion (for non-enteric-coated pills).
- □ Diagnostic findings: nausea/vomiting, tinnitus, hyperventilation, hyperthermia, hypoglycemia, hypernatremia, hypokalemia
- □ Sequelae: seizure, dysrhythmias, noncardiogenic pulmonary edema, coma
- □ Management: urinary alkalinization (IV $NaHCO_3$ bolus or infusion until urine pH $\geq$ 7.5); fluid resuscitation and electrolyte replacement; hemodialysis
- □ Intubation is contraindicated unless there is respiratory failure with hypoxemia and uncontrollable acidosis. Even a temporary increase in pCO_2 rapidly increases the flow of salicylates into brain tissue, precipitating cardiovascular collapse and death.

- ■ **Benzodiazepine** overdose causes a depression of spinal reflexes and the reticular activating system by enhancing the neurotransmitter GABA.
  - □ Generally, respiratory arrest occurs with ingestion of benzodiazepines. Cardiopulmonary arrest is seen in rapid diazepam injections or when benzodiazepines are used with other depressant drugs.
  - □ Onset of symptoms are seen in 30 – 120 minutes (specific to the benzodiazepine used).
  - □ Signs and symptoms: lethargy, slurred speech, ataxia, hyporeflexia, hyporeflexia, pinpoint pupils (midline fixated and unresponsive to light), hypothermia, coma.
  - □ **Flumazenil (Romazicon)** is an antidote that competitively inhibits benzodiazepines receptors. Administer 0.2 mg IVP every 1 – 6 minutes or IV infusion 0.3 – 0.4 mg/hr.
  - □ Monitor for re-sedation after flumazenil administration: its effects often do not last as long as the drug's toxic effects.
  - □ Benzodiazepines have a very high therapeutic index, and the majority of benzodiazepine overdose cases do not require the use of an antagonist.

- ■ **Calcium channel blockers (CCBs)** restrict the flow of calcium into cells in vascular and cardiac tissues and result in vasodilation, decreased contractility, and decreased conduction velocity in the cardiac nodes. They are used to treat hypertension, vasospasms, SVT, and migraine headaches.
  - □ Dihydropyridines (nifedipine, amlodipine, felodipine, isradipine, nicardipine, nimodipine) act on vascular smooth muscle and are used to treat hypertension.
  - □ Non-dihydropyridines (diltiazem, verapamil) act on the myocardium and are used for angina and SVT.

- CCBs also reduce insulin secretion from the pancreas, causing insulin resistance and hyperglycemia, and alter glucose catabolism, ultimately increasing lactate levels.
- CCB overdose causes severe hemodynamic instability with hypotension and dysrhythmias, including sinus bradycardia, AV block, junctional rhythms, BBBs, prolonged QT, or sinus tachycardia (nifedipine only).
- Results of tissue hypoperfusion and end-organ ischemia include seizures, MI, bowel infarction, stroke, and ARDS.

TABLE 11.2. Management of CCB Overdose

Symptom Management	Reversal of Toxicity
Emergent intubation with pre-administration of atropine	Activated charcoal (within 2 hours of ingestion); whole bowel irrigation for timed-release medication
Continuous cardiac monitoring; pacing for refractory bradycardia	
IV colloids	10% calcium chloride 10 – 20 mL IV bolus; *not rapid* IVP: will cause hypotension, V-fib, AV dissociation
IV glucagon for refractory hypotension: 5 mg IV bolus, repeat bolus reconstituted in D5W (to avoid propylene glycol toxicity)	Lipid emulsion therapy (LET): high-dose IV lipid administration reverses CCB toxicity
vasopressor and/or positive inotrope to increase MAP	Hyperinsulinemic euglycemia therapy (HIET): ensure serum glucose 200 mg/dL and serum potassium ≥2.5 mEq/L
ECMO, IV catecholamine, and/or IABP for cardiogenic shock	

HELPFUL HINT:

Urinary alkalinization, hemofiltration, and hemodialysis are ineffective decontamination measures because there is large volume distribution and lipophilic affinity with CCB toxicity.

- **Opioids** depress the CNS and lower the perception of pain by stimulating dopamine release.
  - Opioid overdose can be a complication of substance abuse, unintentional or intentional overdose, or therapeutic drug error.
  - Opioid overdose causes an excessive depressive effect on the portion of the brain that regulates RR and can be fatal.
  - Signs and symptoms: opioid overdose triad (pinpoint pupils, respiratory depression, decreased LOC), hypotension, wheezing, dyspnea, nausea, vomiting, gastric aperistalsis, seizure, coma.
  - Priority is airway management and supplemental oxygen.
  - **Naloxone** is an opioid antagonist administered IV or IM; a standard dose is 0.4 mg titrated until adequate ventilation is achieved.
  - In patients who are opioid dependent, a slow dose of naloxone (0.1 – 0.4 mg every 1 – 3 minutes) is administered to prevent withdrawal symptoms.

□ Activated charcoal or whole bowel irrigation may be used if indicated.

■ **Alcohol** is a CNS depressant that directly binds to GABA receptors and inhibits glutamate-induced excitation. Chronic alcohol use alters the sensitivity of these receptors; when alcohol use is stopped, the result is hyperactivity in the CNS.

□ Alcohol withdrawal can be fatal.

□ Chronic alcohol use inhibits the absorption of nutrients, including thiamine and folic acid. Consequently, patients admitted with symptoms of alcohol withdrawal are also at risk for disorders related to vitamin deficiency, including Wernicke's encephalopathy and megaloblastic anemia.

□ Signs and symptoms: tachycardia, anxiety, irritation, tachypnea, diaphoresis, seizures.

□ Delirium tremens (DTs) may occur 72 – 96 hours after the last drink and is characterized by anxiety, hallucinations, tachycardia, hypertension, ataxia, and diaphoresis.

□ The Clinical Institute Withdrawal Assessment (CIWA) is a 10-item scale used to objectively assess withdrawal symptoms and to ensure that withdrawing patients are given the correct amount of medication.

TABLE 11.3. The CIWA of Alcohol	
Patients are given a score of 0 – 7 for each symptom, based on its severity, except orientation, which is scored as 0 – 4.	
• nausea and vomiting	
• paroxysmal sweats	
• level of anxiety	
• level of agitation	
• tremors	
• headache symptoms	
• auditory disturbances	
• visual disturbances	
• tactile disturbances	
• orientation	
< 8	No medication needed
9 – 14	Medication administration is optional
15 – 19	Administer medications ordered
>20	High risk for complications

- Pharmacological interventions for alcohol withdrawal and DTs include benzodiazepines, chlordiazepoxide (Librium), dexmedetomidine, antipsychotics (e.g., haloperidol, quetiapine), and nonbenzodiazepine anticonvulsants (e.g., phenytoin, carbamazepine, gabapentin).
- Patient will require IV fluids and electrolyte/vitamin replacement (particularly thiamine).

- **Carbon monoxide (CO)** binds to serum hemoglobin with 240 times oxygen's affinity, producing carboxyhemoglobin (CHOB) and resulting in impaired oxygen uptake by tissue. Additionally, CO can initiate an inflammatory cascade that causes delayed neurologic conditions.
  - Sources of CO include malfunctioning heaters and generators, smoke from fires, and motor vehicle exhaust. CO poisoning and cyanide poisoning often occur together.
  - Diagnostic findings: headache, malaise, dizziness, nausea, altered mental status, syncope, seizure, lactic acidosis.
  - SpO_2 pulse oximetry CANNOT screen for CO exposure, because the sensor does not differentiate between oxyhemoglobin and carboxyhemoglobin.
  - Complications: pulmonary edema, ventricular dysrhythmias, MI.
  - Management: 100% oxygen via nonrebreathing mask (high-flow oxygen) or intubation.
  - Hyperbaric oxygen therapy (HBO) initiated within 6 hours of exposure when patient has one of the following indicators: CHOB level 25% (20% in pregnant patients), loss of consciousness, severe metabolic acidosis (pH <7.1), or symptoms of end-organ ischemia (e.g., chest pain).

HELPFUL HINT:

The "cherry red" skin and lips often cited as indicative of CO poisoning are not reliable diagnostic criteria but may be included in a test scenario.

QUICK REVIEW QUESTION

9. A 58-year-old is brought to the ED after ingesting 25 enteric-coated diltiazem pills 3 hours earlier. He is administered 0.5 mg atropine and intubated. Fluid resuscitation is started with 3 L 0.9% NaCl and he receives IV calcium gluconate 60 mL bolus/10 min. After transfer to the MICU, the patient's hemodynamics are MAP 45 mm Hg, cardiac output 3.0 L/min, CI 2.0 L/min/m2, SVR 90 dynes/sec/cm5, and stroke volume variability 8%. A second 12-lead ECG shows sinus bradycardia of 53 bpm and a slightly prolonged QRS interval. What medications should the nurse anticipate administering?

ANSWER KEY

1. RYGB combines restrictive and malabsorption bariatric surgical procedures to effectively reduce the size of the stomach and to allow ingested food to bypass the lower part of the stomach and duodenum to reduce nutritional absorption. Post-op considerations include monitoring for internal bleeding at the anastomosis site; signs and symptoms of hypovolemic shock, atelectasis, pneumonia, and wound infection; pain management; and DVT prophylaxis with early ambulation.

2. Family-centered bereavement care prepares the family with information and education before the death of their loved one. It continues through the end-of-life event, with all staff demonstrating empathy and respect for the family's social, cultural, and specific grieving processes.

3. *C. difficile* requires contact protections, so the nurse should use gloves and an isolation gown.

4. The diagnosis is postpartum preeclampsia. Targeted treatment would include IV antihypertensive medications, aggressive IV seizure management, and initiation of anticoagulants, with a plan for long-term monitoring and therapy tapering after discharge.

5. The nurse should build a preemptive plan for pain management. The nurse should review the rationale for prone positioning and design a care plan that minimizes maneuvers that appear to cause the patient pain. The nurse should also determine the length of time necessary for position changes and ensure that appropriate premedications are administered. During care, the nurse needs to evaluate and document pain per hospital policies and share this information with the health care team so that consistent feedback can be given to the wife.

6. A narrowing pulse pressure (dropping SBP with increasing or maintaining DBP); decreasing BP; increased SVR; decreased cardiac output; decreased CVP (RAP); and decreased PAOP.

7. The nurse should be prepared to initiate a sepsis bundle per the hospital's protocols. This will likely include administration of broad-spectrum antibiotics and a crystalloid IV bolus fluid challenge. Vasopressors may be administered as part of the bundle if hypotension persists.

8. To stabilize the profound vasodilation response in anaphylaxis, the nurse should expect to initiate an epinephrine drip to titrate for a MAP ≥65. To counteract the histamine release in response to the antibiotic administered, the nurse would expect to give diphenhydramine 50 mg IV. Finally, methylprednisolone 125 mg IV will likely be given to reduce inflammation and potential rebound anaphylaxis.

9. The CCRN should anticipate administering a continuous calcium chloride IV infusion and should determine whether the medical team wants to repeat the 60 mL IV calcium gluconate bolus. The patient may also be administered glucagon (5 mg IV bolus followed by glucagon drip). To improve cardiac output, the nurse would anticipate starting an inotropic infusion rather than a vasopressor, because stroke volume and SVR are within normal limits. The patient may also receive IV regular insulin (1 unit/kg) as part of HIET protocols.

12 PROFESSIONAL CARING AND ETHICAL PRACTICE REVIEW

CCRN TEST PLAN: PROFESSIONAL CARING AND ETHICAL PRACTICE

- Advocacy/moral agency
- Caring practices
- Response to diversity
- Facilitation of learning
- Collaboration
- Systems thinking
- Clinical inquiry

The AACN Synergy Model

The **AACN Synergy Model** for patient care was developed in 1996 as a framework for the certification program of the American Association of Critical-Care Nurses (AACN). This patient-focused model is centered on an understanding that the characteristics of the patient/family unit inform the competencies of the nurse who delivers care.

EIGHT CORE PATIENT CHARACTERISTICS

- **Core patient characteristics** reflect the patient's biological, psychosocial, and spiritual developmental characteristics.

- Assessing patients' core characteristics enables the critical care nurse to develop an integrated, individualized plan of care with the patient/family unit.

- Core characteristics are rated from level 1 to level 5.

TABLE 12.1. Core Patient Characteristics		
Characteristic	**Description**	**Levels**
Resiliency	The ability of an individual to use coping skills and survive in the face of adversity. The relationship between resiliency and a positive patient outcome has been extensively documented.	level 1: minimally resilient level 5: highly resilient
Vulnerability	The susceptibility of patients to harm. This may include physical, psychosocial, or social vulnerability.	level 1: highly vulnerable level 5: minimally vulnerable
Stability	The ability of a patient to maintain a steady state of equilibrium. This generally refers to hemodynamic stability.	level 1: minimally stable level 5: highly stable
Complexity	The entanglement of two or more systems. Complexity requires a multifaceted assessment by the nurse.	level 1: highly complex level 5: minimally complex
Resource Availability	The number and type of resources (e.g., financial, psychological) the patient and family bring to the immediate health care situation. The nurse should be aware that a lack of resources can negatively impact a patient's recovery.	level 1: few resources level 5: many resources
Participation in Care	The extent to which the patient and family take part in care. The nurse plays a critical role in encouraging patient/family to actively participate in care.	level 1: no participation level 5: full participation
Participation in Decision-Making	The extent to which a patient/family is able to understand and make decisions regarding care. The CCRN candidate should expect exam questions that reference barriers to decision-making.	level 1: no participation level 5: full participation
Predictability	A summary of multiple factors present in the patient's condition that allow a health care provider to expect a certain trajectory. Critical pathways are tools-based scoring systems (e.g., APACHE, SOFA) used to guide care of the patient to survival of the critical illness.	level 1: not predictable level 5: highly predictable

HELPFUL HINT:

When hemodynamic measurements reflect hypoperfusion to vital organs, early recognition and rapid intervention by the nurse will prevent further destabilization, avoid multisystem organ dysfunction, and reduce morbidity/mortality.

1. A 30-year-old primigravida (37 weeks) patient is admitted preoperatively to the CVICU after a diagnosis of large dissecting thoracic aneurysm. A plan for an emergent C-section, followed by aneurysm repair, was outlined by the care team and presented to the patient and partner. The couple agreed to this plan, although this deviated significantly from their expectation of a natural childbirth. An advance directive is already on file, and the family verbalizes an understanding that the patient's partner will make medical decisions. Extended family members appear supportive and caring, and clergy related to the couple's spiritual view are present. The patient and partner both have insurance accepted by the hospital, and extended family members verbalize plans to help with the post-op care of patient and infant. The patient is being transferred to the OR as vital signs are labile.

What level would each of the core patient characteristics be?

HELPFUL HINT:

The Synergy Model requires that the nurse become an advocate for the patient to ensure equitable care.

EIGHT CORE NURSE COMPETENCY CHARACTERISTICS

- The eight **Core Nurse Competency Characteristics** reflect a continuum of knowledge, experience, skills, and attitudes.

- Each competency is rated from level 1 (competent) to level 5 (expert).

TABLE 12.2. Core Nurse Competencies		
Competency	**Level 1 Nursing Actions**	**Level 5 Nursing Actions**
Clinical judgment: clinical reasoning that incorporates clinical decision-making, critical thinking, a global grasp of the situation, and integration of nursing skills based on formal/informal experiential knowledge and evidence-based practice guidelines	• collects basic data • uses algorithms and protocols (but is uncomfortable deviating from these guidelines) • matches formal knowledge with clinical events • delegates decision-making to others; includes extraneous detail	• synthesizes/interprets complex and often conflicting patient data • makes clinical judgment based on immediate grasp of situation • uses past experience to anticipate problems • recognizes limitations

continued on next page

TABLE 12.2. Core Nurse Competencies (continued)

Competency	Level 1 Nursing Actions	Level 5 Nursing Actions
Advocacy/moral agency: representing the concerns of the patient/family and nursing staff, and acting as a moral agent to identify and help resolve ethical/clinical concerns	• works on behalf of patient • is aware of ethical issues that may occur in clinical settings • makes ethical/moral decisions based on rules	• works on behalf of patient, family, and community • advocates for patient/family regardless of personal values • suspends rules to allow the patient/family to direct moral decision-making • empowers patient/family to represent themselves
Caring practices: the application of nursing concepts like vigilance, responsiveness, engagement, and compassion to promote healing, prevent unnecessary suffering, and create a therapeutic environment	• identifies needs of patient care based on policy, procedure, and standards • manages a safe environment for patient and family • does not anticipate future needs • acknowledges end of life as a potential outcome	• insightfully recognizes/anticipates changing patient/family needs • engages fully with patient/family/community • anticipates obstacles and hazards and takes action to avoid them • promotes safety while allowing expression of grief as death/dying issues present • compassionately stands alongside patient/family transitioning through the end of life continuum
Collaboration: working with patients, families, health care colleagues, and community members to promote individual contributions to optimal and realistic patient/family goals	• is willing to be mentored, coached, or taught • is open to team members' contributions • participates in health care meetings to discuss practice issues/care activities	• reaches out to mentor others and continues self-learning by willingness to be taught • facilitates health care meetings/care delivery discussions and practice decisions • optimizes diverse resources and promotes patient/family outcomes through inclusivity

Competency	Level 1 Nursing Actions	Level 5 Nursing Actions
Systems thinking: the understanding of a body of knowledge and the tools used by nurses to manage system and environmental resources available for the patient/family and staff	• has limited strategies and outlook • sees patient/family within the specific health care unit environment • sees self as a resource • is unable to recognize negotiation as a caring tool	• develops and applies multiple strategies driven by the needs and strengths of patient/family • has a global outlook; anticipates and guides patient/family through the health care system • uses alternative resources when necessary • knows when and how to negotiate within the health care system on behalf of patient/family
Response to diversity: the ability to recognize, appreciate, and incorporate diversity into care delivery (including differences in culture, gender, lifestyle, spiritual beliefs, race, values, socioeconomics, ethnicity, and age)	• assesses aspects of cultural diversity • is guided by own belief system in provision of care • is aware of the culture of the health care environment	• anticipates and integrates cultural differences into patient/family care delivery • incorporates diverse and alternative therapies into care as presented • facilitates merging of health care culture with patient/family strengths to meet patient goals as possible
Facilitation of learning: facilitating formal and informal learning for patients, families, health care colleagues, and the community	• has limited knowledge • follows planned educational program • sees patient/family education as separate nursing care delivery task • sees patient as passive • focuses on nurse's perspective	• develops patient education programs • individualizes and incorporates health care team's educational input • evaluates patient understanding by recognizing behavioral change related to education • recognizes patient/family goals and choices • negotiates in relation to patient/family education needs

continued on next page

TABLE 12.2. Core Nurse Competencies (continued)

Competency	Level 1 Nursing Actions	Level 5 Nursing Actions
Clinical inquiry: the ongoing process of evaluating practice and creating practice change through research, experiential learning, and sharing new evidence-based practice guidelines	• follows standards and guidelines • uses evidence-based clinical changes developed by others • recognizes critical patient status changes • seeks assistance to identify needs and emergent problems	• individualizes standards, guidelines, and policies for individual or patient populations • reviews literature to acquire new knowledge • attends education/learning opportunities to address questions of practice/care delivery improvement • merges clinical judgment and clinical inquiry on the expert level

QUICK REVIEW QUESTION

2. A recently retired 68-year-old prediabetic Muslim neuro-ICU patient received tPa treatment for a left hemispheric stroke in the last 18 hours. The patient has right-sided hemiplegia and has passed a dysphagia screening. The patient is widowed, appears sad, and speaks mostly Farsi. The patient's son was out of state at a business meeting, and will not arrive until much later in the evening. The patient has refused the bacon, egg, and pancake breakfast tray. What should the nurse understand and do for this patient?

HELPFUL HINT:

Although participation in care encourages more positive outcomes, diminishes errors, and increases satisfaction with care, there are patient/family preferences or beliefs that may limit their ability or willingness to participate in care practices.

Ethical Practice Parameters
CODE OF ETHICS

■ The **American Nurses Association (ANA)** has defined a clear framework for ethical decision-making that reflects the nurse's professional responsibility to the general public, the nursing profession, and health care colleagues.

■ AACN considers the **ANA Code of Ethics for Nurses** the foundation for nursing practice. Questions on clinical competency throughout the CCRN exam will reflect this ethical practice knowledge base.

■ The CCRN candidate is expected to read and understand the Code of Ethics. The code can be viewed at the ANA's website: https://www.nursingworld.org/practice-policy/nursing-excellence/ethics/code-of-ethics-for-nurses/.

- The CCRN candidate should expect questions on the CCRN exam that address assisting patients and families through a meaningful end-of-life clinical event.
  - The ANA Code of Ethics 2015 Provision 1.4 specifically defines **The Right to Self-Determination**, which describes the patient's right to make decisions (with family) to accept, refuse, or terminate treatment.
  - The nurse should understand the moral rights of the patient and give support during the process, which includes providing information without duress, coercion, deceit, prejudice, or undue influence.

QUICK REVIEW QUESTION

3. A 58-year-old female patient who has obesity, hypertension, and DM is confirmed positive for COVID-19. She was transferred to the ICU for emergent intubation. The patient developed ARDS with an unstable hemodynamic status and acute kidney injury requiring dialysis. The nurse has been facilitating virtual visits for the patient with her daughter during the patient's stay. The daughter, who has medical power of attorney, has also been in discussion with the hospital's ICU intensivist about end-of-care decisions. During the most recent discussion, the daughter stated that she wants "everything done to save her mother." During dialysis, the patient becomes hypotensive, resulting in heart block and ACLS measures. The patient is unable to be resuscitated.

   What actions should the nurse take to help the family after the patient's death?

LEGAL AND ETHICAL PRINCIPLES

- Ethical and legal dilemmas occur daily in the critical care environment. Critical care practitioners must make decisions with speed and synthesize rapidly changing technological data, making resolving dilemmas even more challenging.

- The nurse should combine an ethical decision-making process with a systematic approach of moral examination to support the best interests of the patient.

- The nurse should be able to advocate for identifying ethical/legal issues and use the processes available to address these concerns.

- Candidates should be familiar with the following ethical principles:
  - **Autonomy** is the basic human right of freedom to self-determine a course of action that is respected and supported, without coercion, undue influence, or withholding of information by others.
  - **Beneficence** is the promotion of well-being for patients, based in the compassionate actions of doing good for others or preventing or removing harm, or actively improving another's situation.

HELPFUL HINT:

Some patient empowerment strategies may conflict with religious or cultural views that must be respected by the health care team. Expect relevant exam questions to address the referral of these situations to a facility's ethics committee.

- **Nonmaleficence** is an ethical principle that obliges a nurse to "do no harm" and/or to correct a harmful situation.
- **Veracity**, also known as "truth-telling," requires the nurse to provide information accurately and without bias to patients/family units and colleagues and within the employer-employee relationship.
- **Fidelity** is the idea that faithfulness builds a trusting relationship. It requires loyalty, fairness, truthfulness, patient advocacy, and a commitment by the nurse to keep promises.
- **Confidentiality** is a key element of the ANA Revised 2015 Position Statement on Privacy and Confidentiality,[1] which states that protection of privacy and confidentiality, including individually identifiable health information such as genetic data, is essential in the nurse-patient trust relationship.
- **Paternalism** is when health care providers make decisions they believe to be in the patient's best interests without the knowledge or consent of the patient. Nurses must work to balance patient autonomy with their adherence to other ethical values, like beneficence and nonmaleficence.
- **Justice** pertains to the fair and equitable distribution of scarce goods and resources, based on the assumption that all have equal rights. Everyone has the right to **access** to health care in the US, but health care itself is not a constitutionally mandated right. Quality of life, application of technology, and patient treatment preferences related to their personal value system must be considered in allocating resources.
- **Utilitarianism** is an ethical theory that, in the context of health care, seeks to promote the greatest achievable good based on a health care professional's actions; actions are analyzed based on positive or negative consequences, not fundamental moral principles.

QUICK REVIEW QUESTION

4. A 67-year-old woman is admitted to the ICU for multiple fractures and a closed head injury. She and her husband were hit by a car while walking across a street and the husband subsequently died from his injuries at the scene. The family and admitting physician have directed nursing staff not to tell the patient that her husband has died; however, she keeps asking the nurse if he is okay. Which ethical principles are being violated and what should the nurse do?

---

1   American Nurses Association, "Position Statement on Privacy and Confidentiality," revised June 2015, https://www.nursingworld.org/~4ad4a8/globalassets/docs/ana/position-statement-privacy-and-confidentiality.pdf.

MORAL DISTRESS

- **Moral distress** occurs when:
  - □ the nurse knows the appropriate ethical action but is unable to act on it
  - □ the nurse is required to act in a manner that violates professional and/or personal values and undermines the nurse's integrity and authenticity
- The AACN provides a framework to help nurses manage moral distress. It involves four key steps.
  - □ 1. **Identify what you are experiencing**: distinguish between moral distress, burnout, and compassion fatigue.
  - □ 2. **Assess your level of moral distress**: learn to recognize the emotional, physical, and psychological symptoms of moral distress.
  - □ 3. **Identify the causes and constraints**: determine the personal or organization constraints causing distress.
  - □ 4. **Take action**: find resources and make a plan to move forward.
- To manage the moral distress that is part of the critical care environment, nurses must feel empowered to advocate for themselves, patient/family units, and their colleagues, and to do so in a safe work environment.
- It takes **moral courage** to act in an ethical manner that reflects one's personal and professional integrity when moral principles are being compromised or undermined.
- The CCRN candidate should be prepared to see this issue of moral distress/moral courage reflected in at least one question or scenario on the exam.

HELPFUL HINT:

In March 2020, the AACN released their position statement "Moral Distress in Times of Crisis" to address moral distress during crises like the COVID-19 pandemic. It can be viewed here: https://www.aacn. org/policy-and-advocacy/aacn-position-statement-moral-distress-in-times-of-crisis

QUICK REVIEW QUESTION

5. A CCRN is asked to perform a painful procedure that the nurse feels may cause unnecessary harm to a patient with a poor prognosis. The physician determines that the particular treatment is required and is not interested in the nurse's viewpoint. What makes this situation an example of moral distress?

Ethical Decision-Making

DECISIONAL CAPACITY

- **Decisional capacity** is the ability of the patient to make informed medical decisions based on knowledge of their illness and treatment options.

- Decisional capacity is assessed using four criteria.
  - the patient's demonstrated **understanding** of the situation
  - the patient's ability to **express a choice**
  - the patient's **appreciation** of how illness or treatment options will affect them
  - the patient's ability to **reason** and understand consequences
- **Diminished decisional capacity** is common in critical care settings. Common situations that may lead to diminished decisional capacity include sedation, underlying medical conditions (e.g., hypoglycemia), and neurological injury or disease.
- If decisional capacity is determined to be diminished, a surrogate or power of attorney may be used.
- **Durable power of attorney (DPOA)** (also called medical power of attorney or health care proxy) may be appointed to make health care decisions for a patient when they do not have the capacity to do so.
  - It may be general or very specific regarding the range of decisions the surrogate can make.
  - It must be present and valid in order to be used for decisions in care.
  - If a patient is alert and competent, their medical decisions cannot be overridden by their health care proxy.

QUICK REVIEW QUESTION

6. A patient admitted to the ICU following cardiac arrest and resuscitation tells the nurse that he does not want to be resuscitated again. He also states that he is worried that his spouse, who has DPOA, will reverse this decision if he is not able to communicate. What should the nurse do?

PATIENT CONSENT

- Patient **consent** is required for treatment. In general, there are four types of consent: informed, implied, express, and involuntary.
  - **Informed consent** is used in situations where moderately invasive or high-risk procedures are going to be performed. The provider must cover key elements for informed consent to be valid (e.g., description of procedures, risks/benefits, alternatives).
  - **Implied consent** is given in situations where patients are at risk to lose life or limb, and they are unable to provide informed consent. This type of consent is only applicable during resuscitation and is no longer implied if the patient is able to give and/or express informed consent.

HELPFUL HINT:

Decisional capacity is fluid and can change based on the patient's presentation and status in the critical care setting. For example, a patient with hypoxia may regain decisional capacity after the underlying medical condition is corrected.

- **Express consent** is the assumption of consent to perform noninvasive to minimally invasive procedures. Some departments require a signature for express consent; others take verbal consent based on words or actions of patients.
- **Involuntary consent** is given when a patient is deemed not to have decisional capacity. Physicians, law enforcement officers, and psychiatrists typically enact this type of consent.

- If a pediatric patient presents for care without a legally responsible adult, the nurse must get consent for care from the legal custodian of the patient. There are some exceptions to this rule.
  - Treatment can be provided if there is immediate danger to life or limb.
  - Some states allow pediatric patients to come to the ED for care for STIs or similar issues in the absence of the legal custodian.
  - Treatment can be provided when there is high suspicion of non-accidental trauma or domestic abuse. Consent for treatment is implied until the local child services system can determine temporary legal guardianship terms.

- Patients who have intact decisional capacity have the **right to refuse any and all care**.
  - The responsibility of the nurse is to provide the patient with as much information as they can to allow the patient to make an informed decision to refuse care.
  - This also applies to surrogates or family members responsible for making care decisions.

- **Leaving against medical advice (AMA)** is when a patient requests to leave care against the advice of health care providers. If the patient chooses to do so, the physician will counsel the patient on the risks of such a departure, and then ask the patient to provide a signature acknowledging these risks.

QUICK REVIEW QUESTION

7. A diabetic patient being treated for cellulitis and wet gangrenous ulcers of the left lower extremity has been told by the multidisciplinary team that the leg below the knee must be amputated. The patient vehemently disagrees and refuses to undergo an amputation. The patient has been educated about the risks and benefits and is advised of the immediate risk of sepsis, losing her leg above the knee, and possibly death. How should the nurse proceed?

_____

ADVANCE DIRECTIVES

- **Advance directives** are written statements of individuals' wishes with regard to medical treatment decisions such as resuscitation, intubation, and other interventions. They are made to ensure that the wishes of the individual are carried out in the event the person is unable to express those wishes at the time of care.

- Advance directives must be documented, valid, and up to date before they can be honored in the clinical setting. In order to honor an advance directive, the physician must see the paperwork, validate the paperwork, and place an order that indicates the advance directive status of the patient.

- Advance directives generally dictate the level of lifesaving measures to be taken in certain circumstances.

    - **Do not resuscitate (DNR)** typically indicates that no resuscitation measures (e.g., CPR, defibrillation) should be taken.

    - **Do not intubate (DNI)** indicates that the patient does not wish to be intubated if the need presents.

    - **Allow natural death (AND)** indicates the patient does not want any intervention that may sustain life or prevent a natural progression to death.

- Any combination of DNR, DNI, and AND may be requested, as can other directives present in the documentation if applicable to the patient's circumstance.

- DNR, DNI, and AND all allow for palliative care and comfort measures.

- **Living wills** allow an individual to state which treatments they would like in the event they are unable to express such at the time of illness. They are used in situations such as a patient having a terminal illness or being in a vegetative state.

- In the absence of legal documentation to guide decision-making, a multidisciplinary approach should be taken to inform patients and families of treatment options.

HELPFUL HINT:

Advance directives may also address organ donation and specify which organs a patient is choosing to donate and/or specific recipients

QUICK REVIEW QUESTION

8. An 85-year-old patient arrives at the ED for nausea and dizziness. Soon after arrival, the patient becomes unresponsive and requires CPR. The patient's daughter states the patient does not wish to be resuscitated. What should the nurse do next?

FAMILY PRESENCE

- Family presence in critical care settings, particularly during procedures or resuscitation, is a complex and controversial topic.

- Generally, family presence, even during invasive procedure and resuscitation, is recommended.

- Evidence shows that family members assert that it is their preference and right to be present for these efforts, especially in the case of pediatric care.

- Family members should be invited to be present if appropriate and their presence should be governed by local policy and guidelines for consistency and provision of boundaries.

- If a family member is behaving inappropriately or interfering with care, they should not be present.
  - Aggressive or interfering family members may be taken to a separate, private area to deescalate.
  - Security may be needed if family members are violent or pose a danger to patients or staff.

- The critical care nurse should make every effort available (within hospital policies) to ensure that patients and their families have the time they need together.

HELPFUL HINT:

Family members may find their experience in the critical care unit difficult, and a staff member should be assigned to be available to discuss what is occurring. A chaplain or other community support staff may also be requested.

QUICK REVIEW QUESTION

9. A nurse is caring for a 68-year-old patient in a COVID-19 unit that does not allow visitation. Security has detained the patient's son at the entrance to the unit. The man is calm, but he tells the nurse that he knows his mother is dying and will not leave without seeing her. What actions should the nurse take?

PAIN MANAGEMENT

- **Pain management** in critical care is a complex and controversial issue in the context of the current opioid crisis facing the United States.

- Both non-pharmacological and pharmacological approaches to pain should be considered.
  - Non-pharmacological interventions include repositioning the patient, keeping the patient relaxed or distracted, and applying ice, heat, or massage.
  - Pharmacological interventions include acetaminophen, NSAIDs, opioids, muscle relaxants, and local anesthetics.

- Nurses manage expectations for pain relief with patients.

HELPFUL HINT:

It is a common myth that some patients feel less pain. Medication should never be withheld from a patient based on the patient's race, age, religion, gender identity, or cognitive ability.

- Pain assessment is a numerical score as well as a subjective description of the nature of pain from a patient's perspective.
- Measurement of pain should occur as frequently as every measurement of vital signs, or more frequently if indicated.
- Patients may have unrealistic expectations of pain management and will need education on the subject. Establishing a goal for pain with the patient may help mitigate this issue.

QUICK REVIEW QUESTION

10. The nurse is taking care of a 63-year-old patient admitted with septic pneumonia. The patient is refusing any pain medication aside from PO acetaminophen. The nurse observes that the patient is guarding and cringing when coughing and suggests that the patient may get more relief from a different type of pain medication. The patient states that their sibling died of an opioid overdose and that they will never take any opioids. What should the nurse do?

Communication and Teaching
COMPONENTS OF COMMUNICATION

- **Therapeutic communication** is a set of communication techniques that address the physical, mental, and emotional well-being of patients.

TABLE 12.3. Dos and Don'ts of Patient Communication

Do...	Don't...
• make eye contact with the patient • introduce yourself and use the patient's name • speak directly to the patient when possible • ask open-ended questions • speak slowly and clearly • show empathy for the patient • be silent when appropriate to allow the patient time to think and process emotions	• use medical jargon • threaten or intimidate the patient • lie or provide false hope • interrupt the patient • show frustration or anger • make judgmental statements

- A variety of techniques are used for therapeutic communication.
  - **Active listening** includes facing the client, being attentive to what they are saying, and maintaining eye contact if culturally appropriate.

- □ **Sharing observations** may open the conversation up to how the patient is feeling.
- □ **Empathy,** or trying to understand and accurately perceive the patient's feelings and experiences, can make the patient more comfortable.
- □ **Using touch,** such as a gentle hand on the shoulder or arm, when appropriate or welcome, can offer comfort.
- □ **Silence** allows the patient a moment to absorb or process information given.
- □ **Summarizing and paraphrasing** information back to a patient helps ensure or confirm understanding.
- □ **Asking relevant questions** that pertain to the situation helps the nurse gather information for decision-making.
- ■ Communication includes both verbal and nonverbal components.
  - □ **Verbal communication** is the use of language to convey information. Characteristics of verbal communication include tone, volume, and word choice.
  - □ **Nonverbal communication** includes behavior, gestures, posture, and other non-language elements of communication that transmit information or meaning.

QUICK REVIEW QUESTION

11. A patient admitted for monitoring post-MI has just been emergently intubated. The spouse enters the room and begins to cry and aggressively accuse the nurse of providing poor care. The nurse tells the spouse, "Your behavior is disrupting the patient's recovery. I need you to calm down and come with me to the conference room."

Why is the nurse's response inappropriate, and what would a better response be?

_____

BARRIERS TO COMMUNICATION

- ■ Certain **barriers** can prevent effective communication between the nurse and patient. Such barriers include language differences, sensory impairments, cognitive impairments, time constraints, and personality conflicts.

- ■ **Language barriers** can occur when a nurse does not speak the patient's primary language or speaks it as a second language.
  - □ The organization should provide professional interpretation services for the patient when necessary.
  - □ It is not appropriate for staff to act as interpreters.

☐ If waiting for translation services would prevent the patient from receiving needed care, the nurse should use nonverbal communication (such as gestures) with the patient.

■ **Sensory impairments** include hearing or vision loss as a result of heredity, disease, or injury.

☐ Patients with sensory impairments should be offered interpretation services when needed.

☐ Whenever possible, the nurse should ask the patient what their preferred method of communication is.

■ **Cognitive impairments** can often result from trauma or injury, particularly stroke. In these cases patients may not be able to speak due to motor impairments, or they many have neurological impairments that prevent them from processing communication.

☐ The nurse should determine the method of communication that works best for the patient.

☐ The nurse should be aware of changes in a patient's cognitive status.

■ **Time constraints** are common in all care settings and can be the result of understaffing, high-acuity patient loads, or unanticipated emergencies. When the nurse is speaking with patients and their families under time constraints, the nurse should share this issue with the patient.

QUICK REVIEW QUESTION

12. A patient is admitted to the critical care unit following an ischemic stroke. The patient's first language is Spanish, but they understand some English. The nurse assigned to perform the admission assessment does not speak any Spanish. What should the nurse do?

EDUCATION PLANS

■ The critical care nurse should understand how to develop and implement a **patient education plan** tailored to the learning needs of each patient.

■ **Procedural education** should be included if a patient is going to or already has undergone a procedure that they will have to recover from. Such education should include details about the procedure, what the patient can expect after the procedure, and the responsibilities of the patient in their own care after the procedure.

■ **Risk factor modification** should be included when a patient needs to make lifestyle changes to promote healthy outcomes, such as quitting smoking or following a restricted diet.

- **Disease management** education should focus on the patient's role in managing a chronic condition. Topics may include the disease process, monitoring and management of disease symptoms, medication administration, and management of medication side effects.

- **Health promotion** education includes ways that patients can prevent deterioration in their health, including diet, exercise, and managing stress.

QUICK REVIEW QUESTION

13. The nurse is providing patient education after a patient returns from a PTA procedure. The patient appears anxious. What should the nurse include in the teaching plan?

CONDITIONS FOR LEARNING

- Adult learners have several distinct traits that critical care nurses should consider while developing patient education plans.
    - Adult learners are **independent** and **self-directed**. Nurses should actively engage them in the learning process and encourage them to help develop their health plans.
    - Adult learners are **results-oriented** and **practical**. Nurses should give them information that they can apply immediately.
    - Adult learners may be **resistant to change** and will require justification for new behaviors.
    - Adult learners may **learn more slowly** than younger learners. However, they may be more skilled at integrating new knowledge with previous experience.

- Psychologist Benjamin Bloom described three domains of learning.
    - The **cognitive domain** includes collecting, synthesizing, and applying knowledge.
    - The **affective domain** involves emotions and attitudes, including the ability to be aware of emotions and to respond to them.
    - The **psychomotor** domain relates to motor skills, including the ability to perform complex skills and create new movement patterns.

- Patient education plans should address all three learning domains. For example, a patient who is learning about smoking cessation may need to be taught about the negative health impacts of smoking (cognitive domain), how to manage negative emotions related to quitting (affective domain), and how to correctly apply a nicotine patch (psychomotor domain).

HELPFUL HINT:

The "knowledge, skills, and attitude" discussed in nursing education align with the three learning domains: **knowledge** is cognitive learning, **skills** are psychomotor learning, and **attitude** is affective learning.

- The critical care nurse should assess patients' source of **motivation** in the context of managing their health in order to better educate, encourage, and advocate for them.
  - **Intrinsic motivation** is the desire to achieve a goal, seek challenges, or complete a task that is driven by enjoyment and personal satisfaction (e.g., exercising because it is enjoyable).
  - **Extrinsic motivation** is the desire to accomplish a goal that is driven by external rewards or punishment (e.g., exercising to prevent cardiac-vascular disease).

HELPFUL HINT:

Patient health literacy improves as patients become more involved in their own care.

- Patients' **readiness to learn** can be shaped by many factors, including openness to new information, emotional response to illness (e.g., denial, anxiety), religious and cultural beliefs, and social support systems.
- The nurse must assess the **functional status** of a patient before developing an education plan for that patient. Doing so ensures that the plan aligns with the patient's abilities and capacity to learn.
- **Health literacy** is the degree to which an individual has the ability to obtain, process, and understand basic health information needed to make personal health decisions. Interventions for patients with low health literacy include:
  - asking patients questions to assess their current knowledge
  - using plain language and short sentences
  - limiting important points to three or fewer
  - using teach-backs to confirm the patient's understanding
  - using visual materials such as videos or models
  - discussing issues in terms of short time spans (<10 years)
  - being consistent when discussing numeric values (e.g., units, risk, dosage)
  - simplifying procedures and regimens as much as possible

QUICK REVIEW QUESTION

14. A nurse is teaching a patient how to take their own blood pressure. While the patient is trying to apply the cuff, the nurse asks the patient to state their target BP range. The patient becomes visibly frustrated and claims to not know. How can the nurse's teaching style meet this patient's needs?

_____

ANSWER KEY

1. The patient shows level 1 in Vulnerability, Stability, Complexity, and Predictability, and level 5 in Resiliency, Resource Availability, Participation in Care, and Participation in Decision-making.

2. If the patient follows a halal diet, then he would not be able to eat from his breakfast tray (which includes bacon). The patient is also experiencing barriers to communication, including a limited English-speaking ability, and is likely overwhelmed navigating his condition without any family or spiritual support. The nurse can address this patient's needs by using dietary, chaplain, and translator services to promote nutritional intake, address the patient's significant spiritual distress, and help the patient communicate with health care providers.

3. The nurse should be fully engaged with the daughter and create a compassionate, supportive, therapeutic environment. The nurse should provide comfort and an opportunity for the daughter to share her emotions/concerns surrounding her parent's death. During the process, the nurse should respect the daughter's grieving practices. The nurse should describe the postmortem care procedures to the family in a sensitive manner and give the daughter an opportunity to see the patient again. Offering CISM or grief support services to the family is also appropriate.

4. The ethical principle of veracity is being violated. The patient is requesting the truth and it is being withheld. The physician is also practicing paternalism by making decisions without involving the patient. The nurse should consult the ethics committee of the facility to review the situation.

5. When the nurse is required to act in a manner that violates their professional and/or personal values, it undermines their integrity and authenticity, creating an internal locus of moral distress. The recognition that challenging the institutional hierarchy also creates risk to the nurse is an external source of moral distress.

6. The patient is correct that the DPOA may override his decision should he become incapacitated. To prevent this from happening, the patient should be encouraged to have a conversation with his spouse and physician to clarify his wishes. He should also be encouraged to complete the necessary legal forms (e.g., DNR) to ensure that he is not resuscitated again.

7. The nurse can explore the reasons the patient does not want to amputate, further educate on the risks of noncompliance, and assist with answering any questions that the patient may have. If there is a reason to doubt that the patient is competent, a psychiatric consult may be ordered to verify intact decisional capacity. Otherwise, the patient is within her rights to refuse care and the nurse should adopt a supportive role.

8. Continue to resuscitate the patient, and ask the daughter to procure the DNR paperwork, if it is available. Explain that the ED team cannot act on the request until it has been verified as a valid, legal document.

9. The nurse should express empathy for the patient's grief but explain that the hospital visitation policies currently do not allow any visitors to enter the COVID-19 unit. The nurse should offer alternatives to the son that meet the hospital's policies, such as virtual visits. Depending on local policies, the nurse may go through the proper channels to inquire about a compassionate exception to allow for visitation.

10. The nurse should explain to the patient that proper use of opioids in the acute care setting does not increase the chance of addiction. If the patient continues to refuse opioids, the nurse may try other modalities of nonmedicinal pain relief such as repositioning, heat, ice, and distraction. The nurse should discuss the patient's refusal of ordered meds with physician and, if there are no contraindications, request an NSAID.

11. The nurse is not creating a supportive and therapeutic environment aligned with caring practices. The nurse's words place blame for the patient's condition on the spouse. Telling the spouse to calm down invalidates their emotions. The nurse should empathize with the patient's family member and attempt to deescalate the conflict. For example, the nurse could say, "I understand that you are upset. Would you like to come to the conference room with me to discuss the situation?"

12. The nurse should arrange for an interpreter to be present during the admission assessment to communicate information between the patient and the care team. The nurse should not try to communicate with the patient in a language other than Spanish.

13. To reduce the patient's anxiety, the nurse should explain that the health care team is monitoring the patient after the procedure. The nurse could say something like, "We will be checking your vital signs and heart rhythm frequently to assess for any changes." The nurse should not give the patient false reassurance or provide results of the procedure.

14. Psychomotor skills require concentration. When the nurse asked the patient about a BP target while the patient was trying to apply the cuff, the nurse disturbed the patient's focus on this skill. The nurse should help the patient learn to apply the cuff, and once that skill has been mastered, the nurse can ask questions from the cognitive domain.

13 PRACTICE TEST ONE

1. A labetalol IV infusion is started on a patient who was admitted with BP 230/108 and is being continuously monitored. After 1 hour, the patient reports dizziness and a headache. The nurse rechecks the BP and finds it is 120/62. What is the priority intervention for this patient?

   A) Continue to monitor.

   B) Notify physician that therapy is effective.

   C) Decrease rate of drip per titration orders.

   D) Complete an NIH stroke scale assessment.

2. The priority nursing intervention for a patient in pulseless electrical activity is to

   A) administer 1 mg epinephrine IV.

   B) begin high-quality CPR.

   C) prepare to defibrillate the patient.

   D) open the patient's airway.

3. A patient with a GI bleed has a critical HgB value of 4.5 g/dL, and a massive transfusion protocol is initiated. During the blood transfusion, the patient develops crackles in their lung bases and dyspnea. What transfusion reaction is likely occurring?

   A) allergic reaction

   B) febrile nonhemolytic reaction

   C) transfusion-associated circulatory overload

   D) acute hemolytic reaction

4. What classification of medication should be used cautiously in the presence of decreased glomerular filtration rate?

   A) NSAIDs

   B) ACE inhibitors

   C) statins

   D) loop diuretics

5. A 55-year-old female injured in a car accident is in the ICU being treated for a pelvic ring fracture. An hour after bathing and repositioning, the patient's vital signs are as follows: BP 96/54, HR 127, O_2 sat 96%, and RR 24. The patient is diaphoretic and reports pain in the lower back. What is the priority intervention for the nurse?

   A) Administer analgesics.

   B) Reposition patient.

   C) Increase IV fluids because patient is having a vagal response.

   D) Call physician for a pelvic CT order.

6. A patient admitted for difficulty with breathing is found to have unilateral infiltrates in the bases of the right mid and lower lobes. How should this patient be positioned?

A) on their left side

B) on their right side

C) prone

D) semi-Fowler's

7. After a cardiac catheterization, the cardiologist's report reveals that the patient's pulmonary artery pressure is 35 mm Hg, with right ventricular hypertrophy. What other findings would indicate that this condition is decompensating?

A) left ventricular hypertrophy

B) normal cardiac output

C) increased right atrial pressure

D) decreased pulmonary artery pressure

8. A 19-year-old male diagnosed with viral meningitis is being treated in the ICU for elevated ICP. The nurse notes an increase in urine output, from 30 mL/hr to 550 mL/hr. What lab values would support a diagnosis of SIADH versus diabetes insipidus?

A) serum Na+ of 115

B) urine osmolality 280 mOsm/kg

C) urine specific gravity 1.003

D) elevated HgB and Hct

9. A patient is comatose and has been intubated and sedated to reduce encephalopathy after a drug overdose 3 days ago. What factor would prevent confirmation of brain death?

A) all sedation, opioids, analgesics, intoxicants, and poisons cleared from system

B) absence of acid-base, endocrine, or electrolyte dysfunction

C) core temperature 31.9°C

D) BP sustained at 110/80 with norepinephrine bitartrate titratable IV infusion

10. A family member requests to speak to the charge nurse about the care of her 98-year-old mother. She states that her mother had been in several abusive relationships when younger and is apprehensive about having male nurses and caregivers. How can the charge nurse alleviate patient safety concerns?

A) Explain that resources and staffing is short; there is no way to assign certain caregivers.

B) Rearrange patient assignments so that only females are providing care, if possible.

C) Purposefully assign male caregivers so that the patient can get used to it.

D) Accompany male caregivers in, and provide an introduction at the beginning of the shift.

11. A 39-year-old morbidly obese patient is recovering from bariatric surgery. The patient was slightly hypertensive at 150/99 in the hour after returning to the unit from PACU. The nurse checks the patient again in 30 minutes and finds that the patient is diaphoretic and difficult to arouse. The vital signs are as follows:
BP 92/65
HR 120
RR 15
O_2 sat 98% on 2 L
What action should the nurse immediately take?

A) Position the patient Trendelenburg and notify physician.

B) Increase IV fluid rate.

C) Recheck vitals in 15 minutes since the MAP is within normal limits.

D) Place a cold cloth on the patient's head since they appear overheated.

12. An 18-year-old female, postpartum 1 day, is being monitored for preeclampsia in the ICU. What clinical sign would indicate the patient is progressing to HELLP syndrome?

A) icteric sclera

B) urine output of 200 mL/hr

C) troponins < 0.012

D) PLT 320,000/mL

13. A 32-year-old patient is admitted after a heroin overdose. The patient has been administered naloxone and is regaining consciousness. The patient becomes extremely agitated and is making indirect threats. What deescalation technique should be attempted first?

A) Allow patient to freely move around room and halls.

B) Place patient in seclusion.

C) With assistance from security, place patient in restraints.

D) Use firm, but calm verbal redirection.

14. A 43-year-old female with multiple sclerosis is admitted to the ICU after surgical complications for a scheduled hip surgery. The patient was unable to be postsurgically extubated. While repositioning the patient, the nurse notes that the patient's arms are stiff and contracted. What medication would the nurse request from the physician?

A) gabapentin

B) amitriptyline

C) baclofen

D) fentanyl

15. A patient is being monitored in the CCU with a Swan-Ganz catheter. Assessment reveals the patient is short of breath, and fine crackles are auscultated. The patient tells the nurse that they are coughing up pink-tinged sputum. The nurse inflates the balloon and receives a pulmonary capillary wedge pressure result of 28 mm Hg. What condition should the nurse suspect?

A) mitral valve regurgitation

B) cardiogenic shock

C) acute respiratory edema

D) hypotension

16. A nurse is admitting a patient for left lower extremity cellulitis with antibiotic treatment. While auscultating the lungs, the nurse notes crackles in the bases. The patient's family member states that the patient's "smoker's cough" has been worse than usual. What should the nurse do after completing the assessment?

A) Document findings.

B) Initiate antibiotic as ordered.

C) Encourage cough and deep breathing.

D) Obtain sputum sample.

17. A patient with an acute deep vein thromboembolism in the left lower extremity has been treated with catheter-directed thrombolytics for 24 hours. The patient has a history of recurrent GI bleeds with aspirin and clopidogrel. What intervention will likely be ordered to prevent pulmonary embolism?

A) angiogram

B) low-molecular-weight heparin

C) thrombectomy

D) IVC filter

18. A systolic heart murmur is noted in a patient exhibiting dyspnea and angina. The patient says that they have had a syncopal episode before being brought to the ED. The nurse identifies +3 pitting edema in the lower extremities. What should the patient be asked regarding their health history?

A) recent viral infection

B) childhood rheumatic fever

C) suicide risk

D) fall risk

19. A patient with severe abdominal cramping has no bowel sounds. What signs and symptoms would support a diagnosis of bowel infarction?

A) abdominal distension, jaundice, and altered mental status

B) pH 7.44, serum amylase 200 U/L, and WBC 18,000/mL

C) hematochezia, diarrhea, and LDH 300

D) McBurney's point, intractable abdominal pain, and WBC 12,000/mL

20. A patient with myasthenia gravis is admitted to the ICU with increasing muscular weakness, cramping, and diarrhea. The patients states that she mixed up her medication and took six 180 mg tablets of pyridostigmine that morning. What medication should the nurse expect to administer?

A) atropine

B) labetalol

C) IV immunoglobulin

D) insulin

21. A patient is scheduled to have a bone marrow biopsy at the bedside. The patient requests pain medication to be given for the procedure. How should the nurse address this request?

A) Notify the patient that this is not a painful procedure and medication is not required.

B) Administer the medication 15 minutes before the procedure starts.

C) When the physician is administering lidocaine to the area, administer the medication.

D) Wait to see if the patient needs the medication, and administer it if the patient appears to be in pain.

22. After stabilizing a patient brought in emergently with dyspnea that quickly escalated to respiratory failure requiring intubation and mechanical ventilation, the nurse asks the family if anyone knows what the patient's wishes are and if the patient had a durable power of attorney assigned. The family members are in shock and say that they don't know. What action would protect patient autonomy?

A) Assure family that it does not matter at this point.

B) Review hospital records to check if patient has submitted a living will.

C) Assign the responsibility to the most competent-seeming family member.

D) Enter order for patient to be full code.

23. A facility is going through the Magnet process and is offering a program that will pay for the study guide and exam fees for certification for nurses in the ICU and Med/Surg. What developmental reason should a nurse attempt to seek certification in their area of specialty?

A) to prove that the nurse is smarter than colleagues

B) to certify clinical skills competence

C) to be a part of the hospital's quota of certified nurses

D) to promote personal growth and increase knowledge base in one's specialty

24. A nurse is reviewing a patient's medications on admission. Which medication is NOT of concern when considering fall risk?

A) valproic acid

B) diazepam

C) terazosin

D) cholecalciferol

25. During dialysis, a patient suddenly reports a headache and blurred vision and cannot remember the day. What are they likely experiencing?

A) hypotension

B) cerebral edema

C) onset of migraine

D) dementia

26. Which of the following complications should be monitored in a patient with hyperosmolar hyperglycemic state?

A) metabolic acidosis and hypotension

B) pulmonary embolism, hypokalemia, and fluid deficit

C) coma, pleural effusion, and tachycardia

D) fluid overload, increased ICP, and infection

27. A 72-year-old male patient is confirmed with ischemic stroke by a CT scan. The symptoms began approximately 4 hours ago. There is no history of diabetes or stroke. Which of the following would be a contraindication for alteplase therapy?

A) time window

B) NIH stroke scale score of 30

C) patient took aspirin this morning

D) BP 175/95

28. A patient is admitted to the ED with chest pain. A 12-lead ECG is performed, with ST elevations noted in leads II, III, and aVF. The nurse should prepare to administer

A) nitrates.

B) diuretics.

C) morphine.

D) IV fluids.

29. A nurse reviews the 12-lead ECG on a patient 2 days after right ventricular infarction. The patient's ECG reads normal sinus rhythm with a first-degree heart block. Which result would the nurse expect to see on the ECG?

A) a PR interval > 0.20 and consistent throughout the ECG

B) a PR interval that will lengthen, lengthen, and drop a QRS

C) 2 P waves for every QRS

D) no correlation between the P waves and QRSs

30. A patient arrives at the ICU from the ED with a non-rebreathing mask delivering 15 L/min with an O_2 sat of 94%. The patient is resting comfortably and reports no current discomfort. ABG values are as follows:

pH 7.56

pO_2 89 mm Hg

pCO_2 65 mm Hg

HCO_3 24 mEq/L

Which condition noted in the patient's history would require immediate intervention by the nurse?

A) asthma

B) COPD

C) respiratory fibrosis

D) respiratory hypertension

31. A patient is being treated for an acute occlusion of the superficial femoral artery. Which of the following indicates that the patient is at an optimal level of anticoagulation therapy?

A) aPTT 94 seconds

B) fibrinogen ≤ 150 mg/dL

C) PLT 45,000/mL

D) elevated D-dimer

32. A patient admitted for treatment of a DVT of the calf complains of dyspnea and chest pain. The nurse should first

A) administer oxygen at 2 L/min PRN.

B) place patient in a semi-Fowler's position.

C) prepare patient for diagnostic tests.

D) obtain vital signs.

33. A 34-year-old patient is recovering from bilateral PEs after a pelvic fracture during a ski accident. During this stay, the patient was intubated for 3 days. The patient is being readied for discharge after a total of 10 days in the facility. What potential post-ICU complication should the patient be educated about?

A) need for supplemental O_2 because of being vented

B) ICU-related PTSD

C) dysphagia

D) paying hospital bills without insurance

34. A sentinel event is identified and reported to the charge nurse. After entering the physician's verbal order into the MAR, the dayshift nurse failed to communicate to the oncoming shift that an amiodarone drip was ordered to be discontinued. The medication ran through the night, and at 0300, the patient experienced a hypotensive event that required administration of a vasopressor. What action would be beneficial in a systems-thinking solution?

A) Require all IV drips to be reviewed by the house supervisor.

B) Require all IV drips to be cosigned when initiated.

C) Reassign both nurses to medical/surgical units where they will not encounter vasoactive drips.

D) Require bedside reporting to verify IV infusions with MAR orders.

35. A patient in the ED with chronic pain is requesting more IV pain medication for reported 10/10 pain. The physician will not give any more medication. How should the nurse approach this patient?

A) Inform the patient that it is the physician's decision.

B) Discuss chronic pain relief and realistic expectations with the patient.

C) Ignore the patient's pain complaint.

D) Discuss drug-seeking concerns with the patient.

36. A patient is sedated with fentanyl and midazolam for a lumbar puncture at the beside. The nurse is evaluating the patient 2 hours after the procedure and finds that the patient is lethargic and has pinpoint pupils. What action should be taken?

A) administration of naloxone

B) administration of flumazenil

C) sternal rub to stimulate patient

D) raising head of bed and letting patient wake up on their own

37. A 43-year-old knife wound victim with significant blood loss is transferred to the ICU. The ED nurse notes that a CT has verified that the knife did not puncture any organs. An IV was started in the ED, and the patient received about 300 mL of NS. The patient is now lethargic and having a difficult time answering questions. What intervention should the nurse immediately initiate after checking vitals?

A) Start a vasopressor to treat the patient's hypotension.

B) Initiate fluid protocol for hemorrhagic shock.

C) Continue to monitor.

D) Call security to ensure the patient has no weapons in their belongings.

38. A patient is arriving via EMS with possible ST elevation, and a STEMI code is activated. A subsequent ECG shows elevation in all leads except for aVR and V1. Which of the following medications should be used cautiously?

A) NS bolus

B) nitroglycerin

C) atropine

D) epinephrine

39. Which laboratory finding indicates that a 62-year-old male patient is at risk for ventricular dysrhythmia?

A) magnesium 0.8 mEq/L

B) potassium 4.2 mmol/L

C) creatinine 1.3 mg/dL

D) total calcium 2.8 mmol/L

40. A patient with AIDS has been admitted to the ICU for complications related to pneumonia. What would the nurse expect the ordering provider to initiate immediately?

A) sulfamethoxazole/trimethoprim

B) fluid bolus

C) supplementary nutrition

D) inhaled steroid nebulizer treatment

41. Along with an infection, which of the following conditions would indicate that the patient has sepsis?

    A) PLT 220,000/mL

    B) GCS 10

    C) creatinine 1.6 mg/dL

    D) bilirubin 4.0 mg/dL

42. The nurse is reviewing the history of a patient with heart failure. Which of the following coexisting health problems will cause an increase in the patient's afterload?

    A) diabetes

    B) endocrine disorders

    C) hypertension

    D) Marfan syndrome

43. During assessment, a patient has new-onset confusion, blurred vision, and slurred speech. Their vital signs are within normal limits. What initial assessment would be best for this patient?

    A) NIH stroke scale assessment

    B) ECG

    C) CT scan of head

    D) blood glucose levels

44. Several hours after an emergent percutaneous cholecystectomy, a patient's family reports that the patient is having new, severe pain. An assessment of the patient reveals a firm, distended abdomen and high-pitched bowel sounds, with patient rating the pain as 8/10. What is the nurse's first priority?

    A) Insert nasogastric tube and start low, intermittent suction.

    B) Administer simethicone and continue to monitor.

    C) Administer morphine PRN and reassess in 20 minutes.

    D) Send patient for CT scan.

45. A patient presents to the ED with chest pain, dyspnea, and diaphoresis. The nurse finds a narrow-complex tachycardia with these vital signs: HR 210, BP 70/42, and RR 18. Which priority intervention should the nurse anticipate?

    A) Administer adenosine 6 mg IV.

    B) Defibrillate at 200 J.

    C) Administer amiodarone 300 mg IV.

    D) Prepare for synchronized cardioversion.

46. What comorbidity requires cautious monitoring of the patient when they are being administered desmopressin?

    A) heart failure

    B) psoriasis

    C) rheumatoid arthritis

    D) hypothyroidism

47. A new mother is 3 days postpartum and is being treated in the ICU for postpartum hemorrhage. The nurse notes that the patient is very tearful and despondent during conversation. The patient confides that she is feeling incredibly sad and is having disturbing thoughts about her child. What is the best intervention by the nurse?

    A) Call a rapid response.

    B) Immediately leave to inform the attending physician.

    C) Ask the client if she has thoughts of harming herself or her child.

    D) Assure the patient that these feelings are normal and will pass in time.

48. A Hispanic patient recovering from PE is weaning off BiPAP. She is concerned that she has not been taking the herbs prescribed by her curandero. How can the nurse incorporate the patient's preferences into her current health regimen?

    A) Tell the patient that she should not take medications not prescribed by a medical doctor.

B) Find out what herbs the patient was using, and discuss continuation with the physician.

C) Call the curandero, and tell them to stop giving the patient any herbal preparations.

D) Tell the patient that those herbs are already in the medications she is receiving in the hospital.

49. A patient with suspected occlusion of the left anterior descending artery develops cardiogenic shock. The patient has received a 1000 mL fluid bolus and is on a dobutamine drip. Hemodynamics are measured via a Swan-Ganz catheter, and the cardiac output results are 2 mL/min. The patient's BP has decreased to 89/42. What would be the expected next action?

A) Titrate dobutamine up, to increase cardiac output.

B) Administer another fluid bolus.

C) Start a norepinephrine drip.

D) Begin an esmolol drip.

50. Which type of MI causes ST elevation in leads V1 – V6?

A) lateral

B) right ventricular

C) anterior

D) inferior

51. The nurse is preparing to suction a patient with a tracheostomy tube. The patient has had thick secretions that are hard to suction out. What action is NOT appropriate for this patient?

A) Oxygenate with 100% O_2 for 30 seconds before suctioning.

B) Use a sterile suction catheter.

C) Apply continuous suction for ≤ 15 seconds with each pass.

D) Increase suction to 250 mm Hg.

52. A patient who has tested positive for COVID-19 is being transferred from a step-down unit to the ICU for increasing lethargy, dyspnea, and hypoxemia. A V/Q test returns indicating right-to-left shunting. The blood gas levels return at PaO_2 of 61 mm Hg and $PaCO_2$ of 45 mm Hg. The patient is on a 3 L high-flow nasal cannula. What immediate action is required by the nurse?

A) Administer an albuterol breathing treatment.

B) Increase the high-flow nasal cannula to 4 L.

C) Call respiratory, and prepare patient for intubation.

D) Notify the physician that the patient's condition is responding to treatment.

53. Which diagnosis does the ECG in the exhibit support?

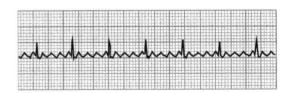

A) atrial flutter

B) atrial fibrillation

C) torsades de pointes

D) ventricular fibrillation

54. The nurse is reviewing the labs of a newly admitted patient. Which of the following findings would be the most critical?

A) ALT 33 units/L

B) BNP 760 pg/mL

C) WBC 10,450/mL

D) direct bilirubin 0.2 mg/dL

55. A patient has started receiving bolus enteral feedings through an NG tube. The patient begins coughing, and rhonchi are heard on auscultation. The feeding is immediately stopped, and a chest X-ray obtained. The feeding tube is positioned correctly, and the cause is attributed to reflux. What interventions would prevent this from happening in the future?

A) bolus feeding at a faster rate

B) keeping the head of bed at > 15 degrees

C) requesting change from bolus feed to continuous

D) keeping patient NPO

56. What diagnostic finding is indicative of DKA?

A) blood glucose level 175 mg/dL

B) metabolic alkalosis

C) presence of serum ketones

D) decrease in serum potassium

57. Before providing patient care, the nurse sees two care assistants whispering outside the patient's room. One of the aides admits to telling the other to make sure to double glove because the patient has AIDS. What is the best response by the nurse?

A) Agree that this would offer more protection.

B) Reproach the aides for discussing a patient in the hallway.

C) Educate both care assistants on the importance of using standard precautions, and explain that no other precautions are needed to keep both staff and patient safe.

D) Notify the manager that the care assistants were breaking HIPAA rules.

58. A patient and the patient's spouse are feeling overwhelmed while the nurse is teaching them how to take care of and flush a new cholecystectomy drain. What is the best method to ensure they will be able to complete the tasks once the patient is discharged?

A) Use the teach-back method.

B) Give instructional pamphlet to take home.

C) Evaluate their learning preferences and needs.

D) Tell them not to worry and that home care will do it.

59. A patient is diagnosed with idiopathic thrombocytopenic purpura and has undergone treatment with IV immunoglobulin and corticosteroids. After being sent home several weeks ago, the patient is now readmitted with epistaxis, generalized purpura, and PLT 26,000/µL. What should the nurse prepare the patient for?

A) platelet transfusion

B) emergent splenectomy

C) antibiotics

D) arterial line for monitoring

60. The treatment that a patient is undergoing for HIV includes the antidepressant imipramine. The patient is admitted to the MICU with anorexia, abdominal pain, weight loss, hypotension, fatigue, confusion without hypoglycemia, electrolyte abnormalities, and hyperpigmentation of the skin. Which of the following is the most likely diagnosis?

A) adrenal insufficiency

B) myxedema

C) SIADH

D) Crohn's disease

61. A patient arrives at the ED extremely agitated and anxious. The patient has a history of anxiety disorder and visits the ED several times a year. Which medication should the nurse expect to administer to the patient?

A) haloperidol

B) phenytoin

C) lorazepam

D) chlordiazepoxide

62. A patient is recovering after a Roux-en-Y gastric bypass, and the nurse is preparing the discharge instructions to review with the patient and family. What post-op complication related to this type of bypass surgery may require a further procedure after discharge?

    A) stenosis

    B) gallstones

    C) post-op GI bleeding

    D) anastomotic leak

63. A patient has esophageal varices secondary to portal hypertension and has been medically treated for an upper GI bleed. Vital signs are as follows:
    BP 115/82
    HR 48
    RR 16
    temp 38.7°C
    The patient is alert and oriented. The nurse is about to administer the patient's morning medications. What order should the nurse question?

    A) octreotide 50 mg 4 times per day

    B) nadolol 40 mg 2 times per day

    C) lansoprazole 40 mg 1 time per day

    D) loratadine 10 mg 1 time per day

64. Which of the following medications would be contraindicated for a patient with mesenteric ischemia?

    A) heparin

    B) digitalis

    C) metoprolol

    D) cephalexin

65. A patient is admitted to the ICU for peritonitis secondary to an infection around the peritoneal dialysis catheter. The patient's vital signs are as follows:
    BP 83/52
    HR 120
    RR 18
    temp 39.3°C

What is the most likely method of dialyzing to be ordered for this patient?

    A) peritoneal dialysis with new catheter at different site

    B) intermittent hemodialysis

    C) delay dialysis until peritonitis is treated

    D) continuous renal replacement therapy

66. After a craniotomy to repair an arteriovenous malformation, a patient experiences rhinorrhea. What test may be performed to definitively determine if the fluid is CSF?

    A) halo test

    B) glucose oxidase

    C) beta-2-transferrin

    D) CT scan

67. An 84-year-old female patient with a Foley catheter was admitted from an adult care facility. Antibiotics were initiated for a probable UTI. The patient was very agitated and restless for the first 2 days. On the third day, the patient's assessment reveals a flat affect and listlessness. What is the most likely cause for the change in the patient's behavior?

    A) The patient has adjusted to the new settings.

    B) The patient is experiencing hypoactive delirium.

    C) The patient is not getting enough sleep.

    D) The delirium has subsided.

68. A patient has an HR of 112 and is diaphoretic. A finger-stick blood glucose result is 43 mg/dL. What is the most appropriate intervention?

    A) Check the serum blood glucose level.

    B) Have patient drink 4 oz of orange juice.

    C) Administer 15 g of glucose gel sublingually.

    D) Administer 0.5 ampule of D50 via IV push.

69. A 50-year-old patient is scheduled for a percutaneous alcohol ablation of the intraventricular septum to decrease the size of the septal wall. Which type of cardiomyopathy does this patient most likely have?

    A) idiopathic dilated cardiomyopathy

    B) restrictive cardiomyopathy

    C) ischemic dilated cardiomyopathy

    D) hypertrophic cardiomyopathy

70. Which of the following clinical signs is NOT seen in an inferior wall MI?

    A) ST elevation in leads II, III, and aVF

    B) ST depression in leads I and aVL

    C) AV heart blocks requiring temporary pacing

    D) tachycardia

71. Which of the following medications is contraindicated in the treatment of heart failure with reduced ejection fraction?

    A) hydralazine and isosorbide dinitrate

    B) lisinopril

    C) carvedilol

    D) nifedipine

72. A 36-year-old male in a motorcycle accident is admitted to the ICU after being intubated in the field. During assessment, the nurse notes pink secretions suctioned from the orotracheal tube and crepitus around the neck and upper torso. BP is 101/63 with titratable norepinephrine bitartrate at 4 mcg/min IV infusion. HR is 105, and temperature is 36.2°C. The patient appears to be resting comfortably with a dexmedetomidine infusion. Which of these findings should be immediately reported to the physician?

    A) BP

    B) HR

    C) temperature

    D) crepitus

73. Which of the following ABG results should the nurse expect for a patient with acute respiratory distress syndrome in respiratory acidosis?

	pH	PCO$_2$	HCO$_3$
A)	7.47	32	24
B)	7.33	46	24
C)	7.30	40	20
D)	7.36	38	26

74. A patient with a history of cirrhosis has arrived at the ED with a new onset of confusion. The patient's skin is jaundiced. Labs are as follows:
    ammonia 130 mcg/dL
    ALT 98 units/L
    blood glucose 128 mg/dL
    The nurse should prepare to administer

    A) lactulose.

    B) bisacodyl.

    C) mesalamine.

    D) insulin 2 units.

75. A hemodialysis patient is admitted with a potassium level of 7. What would the nurse expect to see on this patient's ECG?

    A) shortened PR interval

    B) ST elevation

    C) tall, peaked T waves

    D) extra P waves

76. A patient is being closely monitored after a fall. The nurse notices a slight increase in ICP. The nurse should intervene by

    A) increasing oxygen flow.

    B) elevating the head of the bed to 90 degrees.

    C) turning and repositioning the patient on their side.

    D) suctioning the patient at least hourly.

77. The nurse learns that the patient is a member of the local Native American tribe. The nurse recently attended an event celebrating Native American culture and learned about smudging. What is the best way to incorporate the patient's beliefs into care?

A) Call the local tribe to request a visit from the spiritual leader.

B) Notify the patient that they can smudge in the room if the door is closed.

C) Bring aromatherapy supplies into the room as a substitute for smudging.

D) Ask the patient if they have any cultural preferences for their care.

78. What signs would indicate that a patient with a subarachnoid hematoma is responding to treatment and that ICP is reducing?

A) The P2 waveform is taller than the P1.

B) The patient's temperature has increased by 2°C.

C) Hunt and Hess assessment has been reduced to 2.

D) Patient has increased rhinorrhea.

79. A patient becomes nauseated after receiving chemotherapy. The nurse has already administered 2 doses of ondansetron, and the patient is allergic to prochlorperazine. The patient requests aromatherapy to help with nausea. The patient is sharing a room with another patient who has severe allergies. What can the nurse do to incorporate the patient's request into care?

A) Have a discussion with the patient about medications being more effective than home remedies.

B) Tell the patient it is against hospital policy, even though there is no policy prohibiting alternative therapy.

C) Allow patient to use oils and scents, and hope that the other patient is not affected.

D) Try to obtain a private room for the patient so that they may use their aromatherapies.

80. A patient's ECG shows torsades de pointes, and $MgSO_4$ is ordered stat. The nursing priority is to

A) monitor the patient for bradycardia and respiratory depression.

B) prepare the patient for synchronized cardioversion.

C) monitor the patient for tachycardia and hyperventilation.

D) prepare the patient for Swan-Ganz catheter.

81. A patient has undergone surgery to remove a supratentorial intradural tumor. The patient's urine osmolality decreases to 265 mOsm/kg. What medication is likely to be the cause?

A) beta blockers

B) intraoperative NS 0.9% bolus

C) phenytoin

D) albuterol

82. A patient is being assessed for adequate abdominal perfusion pressure. The patient's MAP is 65 mm Hg, and IAP measured via intravesical pressure is 14 mm Hg. What should the nurse's next step be?

A) Increase IV fluids.

B) Raise the head of the bed to 90 degrees.

C) Continue to monitor.

D) Notify the physician.

83. A patient is brought to the ED in supraventricular tachycardia (SVT) with an HR of 220. EMS has administered 6 mg of adenosine, but the patient remains in SVT. What medication should the nurse anticipate administering to the patient next?

A) 12 mg adenosine IV

B) 1 mg epinephrine IV

C) 300 mg amiodarone IV

D) 0.5 atropine IV

84. Which of the following chest X-ray readings is consistent with acute respiratory distress syndrome?

   A) bilateral, diffuse white infiltrates without cardiomegaly

   B) bilateral, diffuse infiltrates with cardiomegaly

   C) tapering vascular shadows with hyperlucency and right ventricular enlargement

   D) prominent hilar vascular shadows with left ventricular enlargement

85. Which of the following increases a patient's risk of Fournier gangrene?

   A) well-controlled diabetes

   B) dapagliflozin 10 mg 1 time per day

   C) nystatin powder

   D) straight catheter use at home

86. A nurse is assessing a patient in traction for a complicated fracture of the scapula after a water-skiing collision. The nurse notes maroon petechiae on the upper chest extending to the axilla. What should the nurse suspect?

   A) side effect from enoxaparin injections

   B) contusions from the accident

   C) fat emboli

   D) compartment syndrome

87. A 64-year-old female is brought into the ED by her family for new-onset slurring of words, confusion, and unilateral weakness. The triage nurse activates the facility's stroke protocols. Which of the following assessments should the nurse expect to perform before the patient is taken for a CT scan?

   A) stat ECG

   B) lumbar puncture

   C) blood glucose test

   D) urinalysis

88. The nurse notices that a food tray being removed from a patient's room is mostly untouched. The nurse goes in to ask the patient if they are experiencing nausea. The patient answers that they are avoiding gluten and cannot eat what is being served. Reviewing the patient's chart, the nurse does not find a diagnosis of celiac disease. What should the nurse do to make sure that the patient is getting enough to eat?

   A) Tell the patient to have family bring in food that is gluten-free.

   B) While serving the next meal, assure patient that all items are gluten-free even if they contain wheat products.

   C) Notify the physician that the diet needs to be modified to be gluten-free.

   D) Call dietary for guidance, and provide the patient with a menu that identifies food choices that are gluten-free.

89. A nurse is concerned with the increasing rate of pressure ulcers seen on the unit in the past six months. What action would demonstrate that the nurse is performing at the highest level of competency in clinical judgment?

   A) asking a charge nurse for help when encountering a difficult patient situation

   B) identifying and defining the issue, then designing an evidence-based practice project for improvement

   C) continuing to practice because that is the way it has always been done on this unit

   D) notifying the manager about the issue, and hoping that it is fixed

90. Three hours ago, a patient underwent a left heart catheterization with intervention to the right coronary artery. The access site was via the right radial artery, and the radial band was removed 1 hour ago. What sign should the nurse be concerned with?

   A) BP 105/62

   B) HR 52

   C) right digit capillary refill > 3 sec

   D) lower back pain

91. The nurse is caring for a patient who presents to the ED with the following ABG results:
pH 7.32
$PaCO_2$ 47 mm Hg
HCO_3 24 mEq/L
PaO_2 91 mm Hg
The nurse should expect the patient to present with

A) chest pain.

B) nausea and vomiting.

C) deep, rapid respirations.

D) hypoventilation with hypoxia.

92. A patient with a traumatic brain injury has the following labs:
Na^+ 110
serum osmolality 235 mOsm/kg
urinary specific gravity 1.045
What treatment may be ordered for this patient?

A) hypertonic fluid bolus

B) torsemide

C) insulin

D) beclomethasone

93. A patient with crackles in bases, dyspnea, and fluid overload is admitted to the ICU for treatment of acute pulmonary edema. The physician orders aminophylline. What additional order should the nurse ensure is completed for this patient?

A) acetaminophen 500 – 1000 mg PRN TID

B) D5 fluid bolus 500 mL

C) furosemide 40 mg IV push

D) telemetry monitoring

94. Five days after percutaneous coronary intervention for MI, a patient develops a new, high-pitched, holosystolic, harsh murmur found at the cardiac apex and widely radiating. A nurse should suspect

A) papillary muscle rupture.

B) post-MI aortic stenosis.

C) ventricular septal defect.

D) pulmonary embolism.

95. A patient is admitted for an acute asthmatic attack leading to respiratory failure. The patient was stabilized with breathing treatments and O_2 delivery through a high-flow nasal cannula at 30 L/min. After 2 hours, the nurse responds to the call light. The patient has become dyspneic, tachycardic, and extremely anxious. Blood gases are drawn, with these results: PaO_2 46 mm Hg and $PaCO_2$ 62 mm Hg. What intervention would the nurse anticipate from the physician?

A) increase O_2 of high-flow nasal cannula to 35 L/min

B) BiPAP

C) albuterol nebulizer treatment

D) 0.5 – 2 mg morphine IV push for air hunger

96. A patient arrives in the ICU with family at the bedside. The patient speaks only Vietnamese, but the family speaks English and Vietnamese fluently. Although the nurse sets up the video translator service, it is not functioning, and the images and sound are unclear. What can the nurse do to ensure that the patient understands and participates in their care?

A) Have the family act as translators, and notify the charge nurse.

B) Draw pictures for the patient, demonstrating care.

C) Continue to use a facility-approved video translation service.

D) Attempt to troubleshoot with IT over the phone.

97. A nurse new to a facility is unsure about the facility's NPO sedation rules. How can the nurse ensure that the appropriate guidelines are being met while caring for a patient who will be having a lung biopsy tomorrow?

A) Search online for evidence-based practice on NPO before sedation.

B) Refer to the facility's policies and procedures.

C) Call the surgeon to ask their preference.

D) Hold all intake after midnight.

98. A 79-year-old patient is admitted to the neuro-ICU after an ischemic stroke. The patient received TNKase 2 days ago and is still in bleeding precautions. The patient has made significant improvements and is sitting up in bed, eating a soft diet with the assistance of family. The nurse walks by the room and notices that a family member is passing several pills to the patient. What action should the nurse take?

A) Call security to seize the medications and escort the family out.

B) Stop the patient from taking the pills, and seek more information about what they are.

C) Stop the patient from taking the pills, and berate the family for doing such a dangerous act.

D) Assume they are vitamins, and go to the next patient.

99. A patient is admitted to the ICU after an abdominal aortic aneurysm repair that resulted in blood loss of 2000 mL. After surgery, HgB is 6.2 g/dL. The patient's history includes congestive heart failure and the placement of a cardiac stent within the past year. Crystalloid fluids have been administered, and the patient's BP is 80/52. The physician orders 4 units of PRBCs to be transfused immediately. What other orders would the nurse expect?

A) stat HgB

B) transfusion of FFP and PLT

C) furosemide

D) norepinephrine

100. A patient has died after 33 days in the neuro-trauma ICU. What is the best way for the staff to cope with this loss?

A) Increase workload so there is no time to dwell on the experience.

B) Apologize to the family.

C) Refer to a counselor a week after the patient's death.

D) Take time to debrief and share feelings regarding the loss.

101. When caring for a patient with esophageal varices, the nurse should first prepare to administer

A) phenytoin.

B) octreotide.

C) levofloxacin.

D) pantoprazole.

102. A patient is admitted with severe gastroenteritis and fluid loss due to excessive vomiting and diarrhea. CBC results are as follows: WBC 14,000 /mL, HgB 15 g/dL, Hct 53%, and sodium 152 mmol/L. What symptom would be expected?

A) bradycardia

B) hyporeflexia

C) hyperreflexia

D) ICP 20 mm Hg

103. The nurse is reviewing the labs of a patient with renal failure and notes a serum potassium level of 7.2 mEq/L. The nurse should prepare to administer which of the following medications to protect cardiac status?

A) aspirin

B) insulin

C) calcium gluconate

D) digoxin

104. An 18-year-old patient with a crush injury to the right lower extremity develops increased pain at the site. The nurse assesses the pressure bandage and finds that the patient can no longer move the toes and that capillary refill is 6 seconds. What is the priority intervention?

A) Remove dressing.

B) Elevate extremity.

C) Increase IV fluids.

D) Notify the physician, and ask for an increased range for analgesic therapy.

105. The nurse is caring for a patient after transsphenoidal craniotomy. What potential complication would be indicated by fluid balance overload?

A) cardiac dysrhythmias

B) CSF rhinorrhea

C) diabetes insipidus

D) SIADH

106. Which of the following should NOT be done when suctioning the endotracheal tube of a patient with TBI?

A) keeping each pass < 10 seconds

B) 100% oxygenation before and after each suction

C) deeper suction to remove more secretions with fewer passes

D) limit suction passes to 2 times

107. A patient's IV site has infiltrated with dopamine. The nurse stopped the infusion, aspirated the infusing medication until blood was returned, and flushed the catheter per hospital protocol. What intervention would be best to preserve skin integrity?

A) Request an order for a PICC line to infuse dopamine through.

B) Administer NSAIDs.

C) Apply a cold compress to site.

D) Contact physician for hyaluronidase injection.

108. A nurse is freshly off orientation and is caring for a vented patient. The patient suddenly desaturates in oxygen levels to 85%. What action shows that the nurse is progressing in the competency of clinical judgment?

A) immediately calls respiratory for assistance

B) texts the preceptors for advice

C) suctions the patient, repositions them, and then evaluates O_2 sats for improvement

D) calls a rapid response

109. A patient displaying distended neck veins, hypotension, and muffled heart sounds after receiving a penetrating chest trauma from a gunshot injury is most likely experiencing the development of

A) aortic injury.

B) tension pneumothorax.

C) cardiac tamponade.

D) hemothorax.

110. Which definition best describes a hospital facility's ethics committee function?

A) an end-of-life guidance and support group composed of community clergy and hospital health care teams

B) a group of physicians and administrators who develop policies to address legal issues related to advance directive statements

C) a multidisciplinary consulting group that addresses conflicts between doctors, patients, and their families

D) a multidisciplinary team of resource persons for patients, families, health care clinicians, and other members of the facility

111. To clinically evaluate for salicylate consumption, when should the nurse draw salicylate levels?

A) immediately

B) 3 hours after symptoms of overdose first occur

C) 6 hours after ingestion

D) within 24 hours

112. A patient on the ventilator in the ED begins to decompensate. The O$_2$ sat is decreasing, and the patient is becoming more anxious. There is a noted shift in the location of the patient's trachea. What does the nurse suspect?

A) ventilator equipment failure

B) endotracheal tube obstruction

C) tension pneumothorax

D) too much positive end-expiratory pressure

113. A 52-year-old patient undergoes emergency surgery for a ruptured appendix with possible peritonitis. During surgery, the patient received 3 L NaCl IV and 2 units PRBCs, and broad-spectrum IV antibiotics were initiated. The patient was stable before extubation and transfer to the SICU. Five hours later, the patient developed respiratory distress and bilateral rales on auscultation. A stat ABG shows the following:
pH 7.48
PaO$_2$ 56 mm Hg
PaCO$_2$ 38 mm Hg
HCO$_3$ 21 mEq/L
The patient is placed on high-flow 100% oxygen, without improvement, and a chest X-ray shows bilateral pulmonary opacities. The nurse should suspect

A) acute post-extubation laryngeal edema.

B) acute exacerbation of bronchial asthma.

C) pulmonary edema.

D) pneumonia.

114. A patient who had a stroke 3 days ago has failed a swallow study. An NG tube has been inserted and verified via auscultating an air bolus. What action would next be appropriate?

A) Flush the tube with 30 – 60 mL of water.

B) Infuse fiber-fortified tube feeding formula per order.

C) Verify placement with an X-ray.

D) Crush and administer scheduled medication per orders.

115. Which of the following is the recommended intervention for a stage 2 pressure ulcer?

A) lessening pressure to area and monitoring

B) skin grafting

C) moist dressings

D) debridement

116. The nurse is caring for a patient who says he wants to take his own life. The patient has a detailed, concrete plan. The nurse places the patient on suicide precautions, which include a 24-hour sitter. The patient becomes angry and refuses the sitter. Which action is the most appropriate?

A) Place the patient in soft wrist restraints.

B) Have security sit outside the patient's door.

C) Assign a sitter despite the patient's refusal.

D) Allow the patient to leave AMA.

117. The rhythm shown in the figure is exhibited by a patient complaining of "heart pounding" and dyspnea.

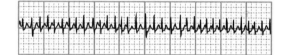

The telemetry monitoring tech notified the bedside nurse of the rhythm change and the rapidly increasing ventricular response rate. Which of the following drugs should the nurse anticipate administering?

A) lidocaine

B) amiodarone

C) epinephrine

D) digoxin

118. Which of the following drugs would be contraindicated for a patient with low systemic vascular resistance?

A) vasopressin

B) dopamine

C) nitroprusside

D) norepinephrine

119. A mechanically ventilated patient with bilateral pneumonia has sudden-onset anxiety and begins to cough up thick tracheal secretions. Cardiac monitor show sinus tachycardia 118, BP 148/82, RR 32, and a drop in O_2 sat to 88%. Which of the following is an appropriate initial intervention?

A) Administer 100% O_2 manual ventilation via ambu-bag to endotracheal tube.

B) Suction the endotracheal tube using an in-line closed suction system.

C) Discuss FiO_2 adjustment with the respiratory therapist and pulmonologist.

D) Increase IV sedation infusion to manage patient's anxiety.

120. A patient with new-onset diabetes after long-term steroid therapy is concerned about adhering to a new diet and insulin therapy. What referral would best meet the patient's health education needs?

A) follow-up appointment with primary care provider

B) psychiatric consult

C) diabetes educator

D) no referral (patient does not meet criteria for a consult)

121. A physician orders a stat medication for a patient, but in light of the patient's condition, the nurse does not understand why it is being administered. The nurse has looked up the medication in the drug book and still is puzzled. What action should the nurse take before administering the medication?

A) Call the physician to clarify the order.

B) Administer the medication as this is a trusted physician.

C) Do not give it, and mark "Patient not available" in the medication administration record.

D) Tell the charge nurse that the patient is refusing to take it.

122. A 23-year-old female with a history of status asthmaticus is a direct admit to the ICU with severe shortness of breath despite use of her rescue inhaler. Auscultation of her lung fields reveals minimal air movement. She is immediately intubated, and mechanical ventilation is initiated with the following settings:
FiO_2 = 60%
tidal volume = 400ml
positive end-expiratory pressure = 12
respiratory rate = 18
Repeat ABGs after 60 minutes show the following:
PaO_2 = 76
$PaCO_2$ = 60
SpO_2 = 93%
pH = 7.10
Which of the following interventions should the nurse anticipate to improve the patient's respiratory acidosis and hypercapnia?

A) Decrease the tidal volume.

B) Decrease the FiO_2.

C) Increase the RR.

D) Increase the inspiratory time.

123. A patient is admitted to the ICU for management of pancreatitis. During the admission assessment, which complication should the nurse should carefully assess for?

A) atelectasis

B) high blood glucose

C) light sensitivity

D) low urine output

124. Which post-MI complication is characterized by chest pain, ST elevation in all the upright leads, and an auscultated friction rub?

A) ruptured papillary muscle

B) pericarditis

C) re-infarction

D) extension of the original MI

125. What is the most important determinant of adequate coronary artery blood flow to ensure myocardial tissue perfusion?

A) supraventricular tachycardia

B) HR

C) preload

D) afterload

126. When blood glucose levels fall below normal levels, what organ is triggered to release a hormone to restore normal glucose levels?

A) liver

B) pancreas

C) adrenal medulla

D) medulla oblongata

127. A nurse responds to the call light of a patient who had a fall from a ladder. The chart notes an injury at T5. The patient is diaphoretic and has marked erythema in the upper half of the body. The tele monitor alarm signals that the patient's HR is 45. What other symptoms would support autonomic dysreflexia?

A) profound erythema across patient's body

B) tachycardia and severe headache

C) severe headache and cold, clammy lower extremities

D) hypotension > 20 mm Hg drop from baseline BP

128. A 70-year-old patient with a history of Marfan syndrome required an open-reduction internal-fixation of the left femur from a high-velocity motor vehicle crash. Six hours post-op, the patient has become hypertensive and has an acute onset of severe, tearing pain in the abdomen and back; the pain radiates downward. A nurse should suspect

A) pulmonary embolism.

B) cardiac tamponade.

C) aortic dissection.

D) acute coronary syndrome.

129. A patient with a history of COPD is admitted to the ED with dyspnea. ABGs are drawn with the following results:
pH 7.30
PO_2 87 mm Hg
PCO_2 52 mm Hg
HCO_3 28 mEq/L
Which of the following orders should the nurse verify?

A) Administer high-flow oxygen at 15 L.

B) Administer nebulized albuterol treatment.

C) Administer IV fluids.

D) Administer prednisone dose pack.

130. After receiving treatment for sepsis, what is the most likely reason the patient would develop acute kidney injury?

A) septic-induced hypovolemia

B) fluid overload from NS bolus

C) nephrotoxic antibiotics

D) underlying kidney disease that was not previously detected

131. A patient admits to having "3 – 4 servings of hard liquor" each night. What symptoms should be monitored in the first 6 hours?

A) delirium tremens

B) Wernicke encephalopathy

C) agitation and restlessness

D) hyperosmolar metabolic acidosis

132. A 36-year-old female with right upper quadrant pain, jaundice, and fatigue is being worked up for possible acute hepatitis. The patient is 30 days postpartum. What other condition should be ruled out, and what tool would be used to evaluate the patient?

A) HELLP syndrome; Mississippi Classification System

B) pre-eclampsia; NIH stroke scale

C) postpartum hemorrhage; Glasgow Coma Scale

D) abruptio placentae; Edinburgh Depression Scale

133. A peripheral nerve stimulator is being used to titrate an IV neuromuscular blocking agent dose to maintain an 80% blockade on a patient with no evidence of anasarca. Which of the following sites and corresponding responses should the nurse use to monitor muscle response?

A) ulnar nerve, 2 twitches of the thumb

B) facial nerve, 6 twitches of the eyebrow

C) posterior tibial nerve, 4 twitches of the great toe

D) facial nerve, 0 twitches

134. A nurse has read a new article in a nursing journal that would be of benefit to the neurosurgical unit. What is the best way to share this evidence-based practice with colleagues?

A) Email the article to the manager.

B) Tell a few close coworkers about the article.

C) Wait until the next staff meeting next month to bring it up.

D) Bring in the article and post it in the break room.

135. The nurse is reviewing the discharge instructions with a patient and family. The patient will be continuing to take 2 new medications at home that were started during this hospitalization. The patient asks how much the new medications cost. Which of the following responses advocates for the patient?

A) Tell the patient to contact their insurance company once they get home.

B) Call pharmacy for a free sample.

C) Remind the patient that the medication is needed to prevent rehospitalization.

D) Call pharmacy on patient's behalf for cost, and find out if there are less expensive generic options.

136. A transgender patient is comatose and vented in the ICU with a primary diagnosis of DKA. The patient's family wants the care team to call the patient by the birth name of "Angela," but the patient's chart indicates that the patient uses he/him pronouns and prefers to be called "John." What is the appropriate response by the nurse to recognize the patient's gender identity?

A) Educate the family that the patient has previously stated the preference of being called "John."

B) Call the patient "Angela" while the family is in the room.

C) Use the patient's legal name, which is still Angela, since it would be against policy to use another name.

D) Tell the patient's family that they should be more sensitive and supportive of the patient's choices.

137. A 78-year-old patient with increasing dementia is admitted to the ICU after a family member found her unconscious with an empty bottle of metoprolol. The nurse prints out a telemetry strip and measures the QT to be 500 ms. What medication would be expected to be ordered based on this clinical finding, and why?

A) atropine for bradycardia

B) $MgSO_4$ to prevent torsades de pointes

C) insulin drip for glucose control

D) glucagon to improve atrioventricular conduction

138. A brain death evaluation is being completed on a patient 4 days after discontinuation of therapeutic hypothermia. What action does NOT occur during this test?

A) preoxygenation for 10 minutes with O_2 sat readings of 100%

B) vent settings reduced to 10 breaths per minute and a positive end-expiratory pressure of 5 cm H_2O

C) test aborted if systolic BP decreases to < 100 without vasopressors

D) delivery of 100% O_2 at 6 L/min flow

139. A patient is admitted to the ICU after being struck by a vehicle while crossing a road. The patient has bruising around the eyes and at the base of the skull. When transferring the patient from the cart to a bed, what important action must be taken?

A) log roll

B) seizure precautions

C) monitoring for dysrhythmias

D) hyperventilate before and after movement

Use the following case to answer questions 140 and 141.

A 42-year-old female patient is admitted to the ICU for a malignant pleural effusion related to metastatic breast cancer. A total of 2.9 L of fluid is rapidly evacuated through the left thoracostomy. The patient describes pleuritic chest pain and begins to cough vigorously and uncontrollably. The chest X-ray shows fluffy infiltrates and unilateral haziness.

140. The nurse should suspect

A) hemothorax.

B) re-expansion pulmonary edema.

C) tension pneumothorax.

D) heart failure.

141. Which of the following is the most appropriate immediate intervention for this scenario?

A) Administer IV fluid resuscitation.

B) Intubate, and mechanically ventilate with low VT and high respiratory rate settings.

C) Perform needle decompression of chest.

D) Stop pleural fluid evacuation, and administer supplemental oxygen.

142. Grey Turner's sign in a patient with blunt abdominal trauma most likely indicates which one of the following?

A) retroperitoneal bleed

B) cholelithiasis

C) liver failure

D) hypoxemia

143. A patient 4 weeks after a small bowel resection is admitted to the ICU with a high-output enterocutaneous fistula. The nursing priority is to

A) administer antibiotics.

B) preserve and protect the skin.

C) apply a wound VAC to the area.

D) provide quiet time for relaxation.

144. A patient comes to the ED with complaints of nausea and vomiting for 3 days. The ECG reading is shown in the exhibit.

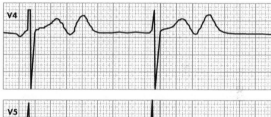
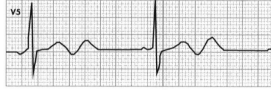

The nurse should suspect

A) hyperkalemia.

B) hypokalemia.

C) hypercalcemia.

D) hypocalcemia.

145. A college student is admitted to the ICU with new-onset confusion, severe headache, pyrexia, and nuchal rigidity. The physician is performing a lumbar puncture at the bedside, and the nurse is preparing to collect the fluid in tubes to send to the lab. The CSF appears clear. What diagnosis is the physician attempting to rule out?

A) bacterial meningitis

B) influenza B

C) viral meningitis

D) bacterial brain abscess

146. The nurse is caring for a patient who has dementia and who has pulled out 3 peripheral IVs. Which intervention should the nurse use to manage this patient?

A) Place the patient in restraints or mitts.

B) Tell the family that they need to stay with the patient.

C) Replace the IV, and wrap it in gauze to hide it from view.

D) Tell the patient that if they pull out another IV, the nurse will have to use a PICC line.

147. During the compensatory phase of shock, a patient's vital signs is as follows: BP 105/64, HR 113, O_2 sat 92%, RR 16. What other signs would be expected during this phase?

A) decreased level of consciousness

B) urine output < 30 mL/hr

C) cool, mottled skin

D) nausea

148. A 67-year-old cancer patient is in the ICU after developing pneumonia secondary to neutropenia after chemotherapy. The patient has discussed her wishes with her physician and has decided that she does not want to pursue any more treatment. She has signed documentation to change her status from Full Code to Do Not Resuscitate. Her daughter speaks privately to the primary nurse, saying she wants the status changed back and that her mother is just giving up. What intervention is most appropriate to maintain the daughter's trust?

A) Allow time for the daughter to express her feelings.

B) Tell the daughter that it is her mother's choice.

C) Call the physician to speak with the daughter.

D) Say nothing, and continue with another patient's care.

149. The nurse is taking care of a 32-year-old who has been admitted for renal failure due to extensive heroin use. The nurse is angry that this patient continues to be readmitted to the hospital and is exhibiting drug-seeking behavior. What should the first action of the nurse be?

A) Provide analgesia PRN as requested by the patient.

B) Notify physician of drug-seeking behavior.

C) Tell the charge nurse that she needs to switch assignments.

D) Assess own values to remove personal bias from care provided.

150. A patient with a history of atrial fibrillation is admitted to the ICU for a persistent HR of > 140. The patient is not in distress, and other vital signs are stable. The physician orders adenosine. What is the expected result of this medication?

A) slow rate to verify underlying rhythm

B) chemical cardioversion

C) antidysrhythmic effect

D) anticoagulation

1. **C)** Treatment for hypertensive crisis should aim to decrease the BP by less than 25% within the first 2 hours. Decreasing more within this time frame can lead to poor cerebral perfusion, as evidenced by the dizziness and headache in this patient. The IV infusion should be reduced per titratable parameters, and the physician notified. It would not be appropriate to continue therapy at the current rate as severe hypotension may result. An NIH stroke scale assessment is appropriate for patients during hypertensive crisis, but this is not the priority intervention at this time.

    Objective: Cardiovascular

    Subobjective: Hypertensive crisis

2. **B)** The priority intervention for a patient in pulseless electrical activity (PEA) is to immediately begin high-quality CPR. Epinephrine is appropriate for PEA but is not the priority intervention. A patient in PEA should not be defibrillated, as it is a nonshockable rhythm. Opening the patient's airway is not a priority.

    Objective: Cardiovascular

    Subobjective: Dysrhythmias

3. **C)** The patient is exhibiting signs of transfusion-associated circulatory overload, with symptoms of congestive heart failure or pulmonary edema.

    Objective: Hematology and immunology

    Subobjective: Transfusion reactions

4. **B)** ACE inhibitors may worsen acute tubular necrosis, which is the most common intrarenal damage seen in the ICU.

    Objective: Renal and genitourinary

    Subobjective: Acute kidney injury

5. **D)** This patient is at elevated risk for hemorrhage. A vessel may have been perforated when the patient was repositioned, and this should be ruled out via CT exam. As the patient had been repositioned a while ago, a vagal response to the repositioning is unlikely. The patient should be moved as little as possible to prevent destabilizing the fracture.

    Objective: Musculoskeletal

    Subobjective: Fractures

6. **A)** Since this patient has disease on the right side, they should be positioned with the "good" lung down (on their left side).

    Objective: Respiratory

    Subobjective: Acute respiratory infection

7. **C)** The elevated pulmonary artery pressure indicates that the patient has been diagnosed with pulmonary arterial hypertension (PAH). If the patient is experiencing right-sided heart failure, the condition has transitioned to decompensated. Increased right atrial pressure also indicates decompensated PAH. Left ventricular hypertrophy is not an indication of worsening PAH. Normal cardiac output indicates that the condition is compensated. Decreased pulmonary artery pressure would indicate that treatment is improving the patient's condition.

    Objective: Respiratory

    Subobjective: Pulmonary hypertension

8. **A)** Both diabetes insipidus and syndrome of inappropriate antidiuretic hormone secretion (SIADH) are the result of inappropriate excretion of ADH, resulting in a sodium/fluid imbalance. In SIADH, ADH is elevated, causing water retention. This would be reflected in a decrease in serum sodium (< 120 mEq/L), because the sodium would be diluted. All the other values indicate a fluid deficit.

    Objective: Endocrine

    Subobjective: SIADH

9. **C)** The patient must have a core temperature above 32°C if they are to be evaluated and declared brain dead. All the other responses meet the conditions required for a brain-death evaluation that is not distorted by potentially influencing factors.

    Objective: Neurological

    Subobjective: Brain death

10. **B)** If at all possible, the charge nurse should attempt to assign per patient preference. Patients and family members should never be told that staffing is short. Purposefully assigning male caregivers will promote distrust of nursing staff and the facility. If it is not possible to assign a female caregiver, response D would be the next-best solution.

    Objective: Professional caring and ethical practice

    Subobjective: Advocacy/moral agency

11. **A)** Postoperative hemorrhage is a risk after bariatric surgery. The decrease in BP by > 30 systolically is clinically significant even though the MAP is > 60, as is the decrease in cognitive status. The Trendelenburg position will promote perfusion to the brain while the nurse then contacts the physician. Fluids should not be increased without a physician's order. The patient's diaphoresis is unlikely to be caused by overheating, and a cold cloth will not treat this potential medical emergency.

Objective: Multisystem

Subobjective: Bariatric complications

12. **A)** HELLP is characterized by hemolysis, elevated liver enzymes, and a low platelet count. Hepatic failure and hemolysis lead to elevated bilirubin levels. This presents as jaundice, which would cause the yellowing of the sclera noted in this scenario. The other options are all within normal limits and would not indicate organ failure.

Objective: Multisystem

Subobjective: Life-threatening maternal/fetal complications

13. **D)** Firm, calm verbal redirection with limit setting should be attempted before placing a patient in seclusion or restraints. For the safety of other patients, the patient should not be allowed to roam hallways.

Objective: Behavioral and psychological

Subobjective: Aggression

14. **C)** The patient is likely experiencing muscle spasticity secondary to multiple sclerosis. Baclofen is a muscle relaxer that is common for treatment of this condition. The nurse would expect baclofen to be ordered in conjunction with an IV pain medication, such as morphine. Gabapentin and amitriptyline are commonly used to treat pain but are not utilized for acute pain. Fentanyl is a strong opioid and would not be a first-choice medication for treating spasticity or pain.

Objective: Neurological

Subobjective: Neuromuscular disorders

15. **C)** Pulmonary capillary wedge pressure (PCWP) is an indirect measure of the left atrial pressures. Along with the other symptoms presented, acute pulmonary edema should be suspected with severely elevated PCWP or pulmonary artery occlusion pressure (PAOP). In cardiogenic shock, the PAOP may be normal to > 15 mm Hg. Hypotension will often show a normal or lower PAOP because the heart is inefficiently pumping blood to the pulmonary system.

The PAOP will be elevated with mitral valve stenosis, not regurgitation.

Objective: Cardiovascular

Subobjective: Acute pulmonary edema

16. **D)** The respiratory findings are suspect for community-acquired pneumonia (CAP). The physician should be notified, an order for a culture and screen obtained, and the sputum sample collected and sent to lab before starting antibiotic treatment. It is important to screen for and identify CAP on incoming patients to prevent delays in patient treatment. The other answers are all appropriate once the sample is sent to the lab.

Objective: Respiratory

Subobjective: Acute respiratory infection

17. **D)** An IVC filter—a small, umbrella-shaped device with metal spines—is deployed within the inferior vena cava and catches emboli before they reach the lungs; the device prevents pulmonary embolism. The patient's history of recurrent GI bleeds is a relative contraindication for anticoagulant use. An angiogram and a thrombectomy are interventions to identify and treat thromboembolism.

Objective: Cardiovascular

Subobjective: Acute peripheral vascular insufficiency

18. **B)** The patient's symptoms along with the heart murmur are associated with mitral valve disease. This condition would be supported by a history of rheumatic fever, which can damage the heart valves. The damage can lead to heart failure, but the condition usually appears 15 years or more after the initial infection. A viral infection could precipitate pericarditis. All patients should be screened for suicide and fall risks.

Objective: Cardiovascular

Subobjective: Structural heart defects

19. **C)** Jaundice is a sign of liver failure. Metabolic acidosis, not alkalosis, is usually seen with bowel infarctions. McBurney's point is a sign of appendicitis. Hematochezia, diarrhea, and an elevated LDH (low-density lipoprotein) are all signs or symptoms of bowel infarctions.

Objective: Gastrointestinal

Subobjective: Bowel infarction, obstruction, perforation

20. **A)** The patient is in cholinergic crisis due to acetylcholinesterase inhibitor overdose. Atropine is effective in addressing the muscarinic effects of excessive acetylcholine by occupying the receptor

sites and reducing the nicotinic effects such as muscle flaccidity and respiratory failure. IV immunoglobulin is used as supportive care for myasthenia gravis but is not usually administered for cholinergic crisis. Labetalol and insulin are not used to directly treat cholinergic crisis or myasthenia gravis.

Objective: Neurological

Subobjective: Neuromuscular disorders

21. **B)** A bone marrow biopsy can be extremely painful, and the patient's request should be honored. Providing the pain medication before the procedure allows sufficient time for the medication to take effect. The pain medication will likely not have relieving effects if given only at the start of the procedure. It would not be appropriate to withhold pain medication and administer it only if the nurse deems it necessary.

Objective: Multisystem

Subobjective: Pain

22. **B)** To protect patient's rights, the nurse should verify that the patient has not already filed a durable power of attorney or living will with medical records during a previous visit. If there are no records on file, it would be appropriate for the nurse to request that the physician discuss the options with family. The physician should enter an order for the patient to be full code after this discussion. Answers A and C are not clinically sound and do not promote autonomy.

Objective: Professional caring and ethical practice

Subobjective: Advocacy/moral agency

23. **D)** Certification is an excellent way for a nurse to promote personal growth, advocate for the nursing profession, and increase knowledge in the nurse's specialty. Passing the exam does not prove that the nurse is any smarter. The exam does not evaluate clinical skills; it is knowledge based. Fulfilling a quota for the facility does not provide the nurse development or enrichment.

Objective: Professional caring and ethical practice

Subobjective: Clinical inquiry

24. **D)** Valproic acid is used to treat seizures, diazepam is a benzodiazepine, and terazosin is a vasodilator. These all have associated risks related to falls. Cholecalciferol is a vitamin D_3 supplement.

Objective: Musculoskeletal

Subobjective: Functional issues

25. **B)** Cerebral edema may occur during dialysis. This may also be referred to as dialysis equilibrium syndrome.

Objective: Renal and genitourinary

Subobjective: Manage patients requiring renal therapeutic interventions

26. **B)** Patients with hyperosmolar hyperglycemic state (HHS) are at higher risk for microemboli leading to PE, shifts in serum potassium, and fluid deficits. Metabolic acidosis is associated with DKA. Pleural effusion is not a complication of HHS. Fluid deficit is a primary symptom; fluid overload is not typical.

Objective: Endocrine

Subobjective: Hyperosmolar hyperglycemic state (HHS)

27. **B)** A contraindication for alteplase therapy in this scenario is the NIH stroke scale score of > 25. For eligible patients, the time frame may be increased to 4.5 hours. Although the BP is elevated and should be managed, it is less than the threshold of 185/110. Aspirin is not a contraindication and would be administered again > 24 hours after alteplase is given.

Objective: Neurological

Subobjective: Stroke (ischemic)

28. **D)** The symptoms indicate right-sided MI, so IV fluids are the priority treatment for this patient. When treating patients with right ventricular infarction, nitrates, diuretics, and morphine are to be avoided because of their pre-load-reducing effects.

Objective: Cardiovascular

Subobjective: Acute coronary syndrome

29. **A)** First-degree heart block is associated with an elongated PR interval that is consistent and uniform throughout the reading. An inconsistent lengthening that drops a QRS is associated with a second-degree type I heart block. Two P waves for every QRS may indicate atrial malfunction. No correlation between the P and QRS waves is indicative of a third-degree heart block.

Objective: Cardiovascular

Subobjective: Myocardial conduction system abnormalities

30. **B)** The pO_2 level is elevated for a patient who has COPD. This can decrease their hypoxic drive and lead to an increased retention of CO_2. The nurse should collaborate with respiratory therapy to decrease the O_2 and continue to monitor the ABGs. For this patient population, the pO_2 should be kept around 60 mm Hg, and the O_2 sat at 88 – 94% to reduce the risk of hypercapnia. The other conditions are typically not associated with chronic hypercapnia that would lead to this concern.

31. **A)** An aPTT of 94 seconds indicates that heparin therapy is within the optimal range for preventing blood clot formation. Fibrinogen levels that are ≤ 150 mg/dL and PLT levels < 60,000/μL indicate that the patient is at a higher risk for bleeding issues. D-dimer is a test used to evaluate risk for thrombus or embolus; an elevated result indicates a higher probability of developing an occlusion.

    Objective: Cardiovascular

    Subobjective: Acute peripheral vascular insufficiency

32. **B)** The patient is experiencing symptoms of a PE and should first be placed in a semi-Fowler's position to clear the airway. Vital signs should then be obtained to compare with established baseline data, followed by administration of oxygen as ordered. Finally, the patient should be prepared for diagnostic tests such as blood gases, ventilation-perfusion lung scan, and pulmonary angiography.

    Objective: Respiratory

    Subobjective: Acute pulmonary embolus

33. **B)** Approximately 10% of patients develop post-ICU PTSD, including night sweats, flashbacks, and anxiety issues. The patient should be educated about, and provided resources to address, PTSD.

    Objective: Professional caring and ethical practice

    Subobjective: Caring practices

34. **D)** Systems thinking employs strategies such as root-cause analysis. Analysis would reveal that this situation could happen to any nurse and that it occurred because the nurses did not review the drips of this patient together. Requiring a bedside report that reviews the IV infusions with the MAR (medication administration record) would help prevent this breakdown. Having a house supervisor review all IV drips would be time-consuming and infringe on that role's responsibilities. Requiring all IV drip orders to be cosigned by a nurse might also be time-consuming and could be helpful in initiating a drip but would not have prevented the drip from continuing to run.

    Objective: Professional caring and ethical practice

    Subobjective: Systems thinking

35. **B)** Having a frank, professional conversation about chronic pain relief is the nurse's priority. The nurse should not immediately assume the patient is drug-seeking; nor should the nurse ignore the patient's pain complaint.

Objective: Professional issues

Subobjective: Patient (pain management and procedural sedation)

36. **B)** The administration of sedation has put this patient at risk for oversedation. The cause is most likely the midazolam, a benzodiazepine, because the onset of symptoms is 30 – 120 minutes after administration. Because the symptoms indicate a medical emergency, the reversal drug flumazenil must be administered. Sternal rub is also appropriate, but not the priority.

    Objective: Multisystem

    Subobjective: Toxic ingestion/exposure

37. **B)** Undifferentiated trauma patients should initially be treated for hemorrhagic shock until proven otherwise. As the patient only received a small bolus in the ED, fluid resuscitation per protocol should be started immediately. Once the patient has received sufficient fluids, the BP should be evaluated, and, if necessary, vasopressors started. The patient requires an intervention, so simply continuing to monitor would not be appropriate in this case. Security should be notified of the patient, and the belongings searched, but this action does not take precedence over treating the patient.

    Objective: Multisystem

    Subobjective: Multisystem trauma

38. **B)** ST elevation in all leads except aVR and V1 is indicative of cardiac tamponade. This causes pressure that prevents venous return and decreases BP, which may cause ischemia. Nitroglycerin should be avoided or used under physician direction and close monitoring. Both an NS bolus and epinephrine are appropriate to improve volume status and to stabilize hemodynamics, as needed. Atropine is not contraindicated and would be appropriate if needed to treat bradycardia; however, cardiac tamponade is usually associated with tachycardia.

    Objective: Cardiovascular

    Subobjective: Cardiac tamponade

39. **A)** Abnormalities in magnesium levels may put the patient at risk for ventricular dysrhythmia. A hypomagnesemia level of 0.8 mEq/L would be of concern (normal range is 1.5 – 2.5 mEq/L). The other values are within normal ranges.

    Objective: Cardiovascular

    Subobjective: Dysrhythmias

40. **A)** The first line of treatment for a patient with AIDS and an opportunistic infection is antibiotics. The other

treatments may be a part of the plan of care, but antibiotics would be initiated first.

Objective: Hematology and immunology

Subobjective: Immune deficiencies

41. D) A normal bilirubin is between 0.3 and 1.2 mg/dL. A level of 4.0 mg/dL indicates liver damage and could be used alongside an infection to diagnose sepsis. The other lab levels listed are all within normal limits.

Objective: Multisystem

Subobjective: Septic shock

42. C) A history of hypertension will cause an increase in afterload. Diabetes will cause complications with microvascular disease, leading to poor cardiac function. Endocrine disorders will cause an increase in cardiac workload. Marfan syndrome causes the cardiac muscle to stretch and weaken.

Objective: Cardiovascular

Subobjective: Heart failure

43. D) The nurse should begin with assessing the patient's blood glucose levels and treat accordingly. While confusion, blurred vision, and slurred speech are symptoms of a stroke, an ECG and NIH stroke scale assessment would be reasonable tests to order if the blood glucose levels were within normal range. A CT scan may be ordered, depending on further assessment.

Objective: Endocrine

Subobjective: Hypoglycemia (acute)

44. D) Because of the sudden nature and intensity of the pain, a stat CT scan would rule out possible perforation or volvulus. The other interventions would be reasonable after perforation or volvulus is ruled out.

Objective: Gastrointestinal

Subobjective: Bowel infarction, obstruction, perforation

45. D) With a BP of 70/42, the patient is experiencing unstable supraventricular tachycardia (SVT) and therefore requires immediate synchronized cardioversion. Defibrillation is not indicated, because the patient is awake and has an organized heart rhythm. Adenosine can be used in patients with stable SVT, but this patient is not stable. Amiodarone is not indicated for patients in unstable SVT.

Objective: Cardiovascular emergencies

Subobjective: Dysrhythmias

46. A) Vasopressin and desmopressin may cause cardiac, cerebral, and mesenteric artery vasospasm. In a patient with heart failure, vasospasm may affect cardiac perfusion and inhibit the pumping function; therefore, cardiac monitoring is indicated.

Objective: Endocrine

Subobjective: Diabetes insipidus

47. C) Before assuming that the patient is thinking of harming herself or her child, the nurse must collaborate with the patient to address these signs of postpartum depression. The patient is not in immediate danger, and the patient should not be stigmatized for confiding in the nurse. The patient should not be left alone without the nurse's determining any suicidal tendencies. The physician may be contacted later. The patient's feelings should not be dismissed, and the nurse has the opportunity to educate the patient on the symptoms of postpartum depression and provide resources for help.

Objective: Professional caring and ethical practice

Subobjective: Collaboration

48. B) The safety and efficacy of the herbs should be explored, and the herbs incorporated into the patient's care, if possible. Curanderos are an important part of some Hispanic and Indigenous cultures. Telling the patient to stop the use of these herbs or warning the curandero to stop treatment may cause distrust of Western medicine. Directly lying to the patient should never be a considered an appropriate response.

Objective: Professional caring and ethical practice

Subobjective: Response to diversity

49. C) If the cardiac output is not improving, a second vasopressor (such as norepinephrine) is typically initiated. Dobutamine is an inotropic but may also cause systemic vasodilation. The patient has already received a fluid bolus, and the pressure remains low. The dobutamine drip would not be increased, given the increasing hypotension, and may be ordered to discontinue. Esmolol is a beta blocker and is contraindicated with cardiogenic shock.

Objective: Cardiovascular

Subobjective: Cardiogenic shock

50. C) ST elevation in leads V1 – V4 indicates a primarily anterior infarction. Accompanying elevation in leads V5 – V6 suggests some lateral involvement as well. Lateral STEMI will have elevation in leads I, aVL, V5, or V6. Right ventricular (inferior) infarction elicits elevation in leads II, III, and aVF.

Objective: Cardiovascular

51. **D)** Suction should be kept at the lowest possible pressure, usually between 800 and 120 mm Hg, and < 200 mm Hg if necessary. Catheters should not be reused, and a sterile suction catheter should be used with each suction session. Oxygenating the patient before and after suctioning prevents hypoxia. Continuous, not intermittent suction, is best practice, and passes should be limited to ≤ 15 seconds to prevent a vagal response.

    Objective: Respiratory

    Subobjective: Tracheostomy

52. **C)** COVID-19 can cause fluid to build up in the alveoli, resulting in shunting. PaO_2 will continue to decrease as shunting increases, while $PaCO_2$ remains stable. The patient's PaO_2 levels indicate hypoxemia. This emergent condition requires positive airway pressure and intubation and ventilatory support. Increasing O_2 delivery will not improve PaO_2, because the issue is a deficit of gas exchange related to the pulmonary edema.

    Objective: Respiratory

    Subobjective: ARDS

53. **A)** In atrial flutter, there are no discernible P waves, and a distinct sawtooth wave pattern is present. The atrial rate is regular, and the PR interval is not measurable. In atrial fibrillation, the rhythm would be very irregular with coarse, asynchronous waves. Torsades de pointes, or "twisting of the points," is characterized by QRS complexes that twist around the baseline and is a form of polymorphic ventricular tachycardia. It may resolve spontaneously or progress to ventricular fibrillation, which is emergent: the ventricles are unable to pump any blood, because of disorganized electrical activity. Untreated, ventricular fibrillation quickly leads to cardiac arrest.

    Objective: Cardiovascular

    Subobjective: Dysrhythmias

54. **B)** BNP, or B-type natriuretic peptide, is a hormone released by the heart in response to pressure changes within the heart. This measurement is used to gauge the severity of congestive heart failure. A normal range in a patient with heart failure is 0 – 100 pg/mL. A BNP of 760 pg/mL indicates severe heart failure. ALT (alanine aminotransferase) tests liver enzymes. The normal range of ALT is 7 – 56 units per liter, so a value of 33 units/L is within normal limits. WBC count normally ranges from 4,500 to 11,000/μL, so a value of 10,450 is within normal limits. Direct bilirubin is a by-product of RBC breakdown. Normal lab values for direct bilirubin range from 0 to 0.3 mg/dL, so a value of 0.2 mg/dL falls within normal limits.

    Objective: Cardiovascular

    Subobjective: Heart failure

55. **C)** The bolus increases the probability of aspiration due to the noted reflux; delivering the bolus faster would worsen the reflux. The head of the bed should be kept at > 30 degrees during feedings unless otherwise contraindicated. Delivering the enteral nutrition at a slower rate would help prevent reflux and is an appropriate intervention. Because the patient requires nutrition, a restriction of caloric intake could worsen outcomes.

    Objective: Respiratory

    Subobjective: Aspiration

56. **C)** The presence of ketones is a highly reliable indicator of DKA. The patient would have a blood glucose level > 250 mg/dL, metabolic acidosis, and an increase in serum potassium.

    Objective: Endocrine

    Subobjective: Diabetic ketoacidosis

57. **C)** The best action for the nurse would be to treat this as a teaching moment and provide the care assistants with the information needed to keep themselves safe and to decrease the stigma surrounding this diagnosis. Double gloving offers no more protection during standard patient care than does single gloving. Reproaching the staff may cause a lack of trust and a breakdown of relationships. Since both aides were participating in the care of the patient and were not speaking loud enough to be heard by others, HIPAA laws were not violated.

    Objective: Professional caring and ethical practice

    Subobjective: Caring practices

58. **C)** Effective teaching must start with evaluating the learner's preferences and needs. Choices A and B are both appropriate if they align with the information gathered from the evaluation of the patient's and spouse's learning styles. The patient and spouse may not always have home care available and should know and feel comfortable with the basic care and management of the drain.

    Objective: Professional caring and ethical practice

    Subobjective: Facilitation of learning

59. **A)** Although the patient may need a splenectomy in the future, the nurse must now stabilize the patient by correcting platelet levels. Antibiotics are not indicated

to treat idiopathic thrombocytopenic purpura, and an arterial line is contraindicated because of the bleed risk.

Objective: Hematology and immunology

Subobjective: Coagulopathies

60. **A)** Adrenal insufficiency, a serious pathologic condition found in critically ill patients, is caused by the decreased production of cortisol, aldosterone, and androgen. Imipramine is an inhibitor of glucocorticoid production and may lead to adrenal insufficiency. Myxedema is a deficiency of thyroxine and is also known as advanced hypothyroidism. SIADH, caused by an inappropriate and excessive release of ADH from the posterior pituitary gland, alters the equilibrium of water in the body. Crohn's disease is a regional, chronic, nonspecific inflammatory disease of the bowel.

Objective: Endocrine

Subobjective: Adrenal insufficiency

61. **C)** Lorazepam is a short-acting antianxiety medication used to treat patients with a high level of anxiety. Haloperidol is an antipsychotic used to treat schizophrenia, and phenytoin is an antiseizure medication; neither would be ordered for anxiety. Chlordiazepoxide is a medium- to long-acting benzodiazepine that would take several hours to have a full effect.

Objective: Behavioral

Subobjective: Anxiety

62. **A)** Stenosis is seen specifically with Roux-en-Y gastric bypass (RYGB) and requires endoscopic balloon dilation. Stenosis is usually seen within the first week post-op. Because gallstones are a common complication with vertical band gastroplasty, the gallbladder is often prophylactically removed during the bypass procedure. The risk for post-op bleeding is highest in the immediate post-op period, not after discharge, and would require emergent surgical correction. Anastomotic leaks are a risk with all bypass procedures and are not specific to RYGB.

Objective: Multisystem

Subobjective: Bariatric complications

63. **B)** Nadolol is a beta blocker, and this patient is already bradycardic. Consultation with the physician is required before administration. While loratadine is not utilized to treat esophageal varices, there is no contraindication to administering this medication. The other medications and dosages are all appropriate.

Objective: Gastrointestinal

Subobjective: Hepatic failure/coma

64. **B)** Vasoconstrictors like digitalis are contraindicated with mesenteric and colonic ischemia because they may further decrease blood flow to the bowel. The other options are all part of the medical management of bowel infarctions.

Objective: Gastrointestinal

Subobjective: Bowel infarction, obstruction, perforation

65. **D)** The patient will still require dialysis, but dialysis via the peritoneal route is contraindicated with the presence of infection. The patient's vital signs are not stable enough to handle the fluid shifts of intermittent hemodialysis. Continuous renal replacement therapy is appropriate for hemodynamically unstable patients in the ICU setting.

Objective: Renal and genitourinary

Subobjective: Manage patients requiring renal therapeutic interventions

66. **C)** The gold standard for identifying a fluid as CSF is either the beta-2-transferrin or the beta-trace-protein lab test. The halo test is subjective; it requires interpretation of the presence of a halo appearance on a piece of gauze. The glucose oxidase test may give false positives for patients with diabetes. A CT scan will show where a leak is occurring and would be appropriate if the fluid is determined to be CSF.

Objective: Neurological

Subobjective: Neurosurgery

67. **B)** There are 2 types of delirium: hypoactive and hyperactive. Patients experiencing delirium may have one set of symptoms or the other set, or they may have a mix of both. The patient may need more rest, but lack of rest is not the most likely cause of the flat affect. Moreover, this complacency should not be confused with adjusting.

Objective: Neurological

Subobjective: Delirium

68. **D)** This is a critical blood glucose level. There is no time to wait for a serum blood glucose result. The patient is at high risk for seizures at this low of a glucose level, and oral intake would therefore not be safe. The patient should be administered an 0.5 ampule of D50 (dextrose 50% solution) via IV.

Objective: Endocrine

Subobjective: Hypoglycemia (acute)

69. **D)** Alcohol septal ablations are used to treat left ventricle outflow obstruction caused by hypertrophic

cardiomyopathy. This treatment is not indicated for other cardiomyopathies.

Objective: Cardiovascular

Subobjective: Cardiomyopathies

70. **D)** The AV (atrioventricular) node's arterial supply is from the conus off the right coronary artery. Occlusion interrupts the normal conduction pattern, resulting in the bradycardia and AV heart blocks that are most commonly seen in a right-sided (inferior wall) infarction. The ECG changes listed are also associated with inferior wall MIs.

Objective: Cardiovascular

Subobjective: Acute coronary syndrome

71. **D)** First-generation calcium channel blockers such as nifedipine are contraindicated in the treatment of heart failure with reduced ejection fraction (HFrEF) because they reduce contractility. ACE inhibitors such as lisinopril are the first-line treatment of HFrEF. Hydralazine, a selective arteriole dilator, and isosorbide dinitrate, a nitrate that is a selective venous dilator, are used together to create an effect similar to ACE inhibitors when patients are unable to tolerate an ACE inhibitor. Beta blockers, such as carvedilol, are prescribed to patients with HFrEF to prevent progression of the disease.

Objective: Cardiovascular

Subobjective: Heart failure

72. **D)** Crepitus is an abnormal finding caused by an air leak into the subcutaneous tissue and must be reported to the physician immediately. Because the patient was intubated in the field and has signs of crepitus and hemoptysis, the patient should be evaluated for tracheal perforation. Although the BP is on the lower side, the titratable norepinephrine bitartrate drip is not at max level and may be increased. The HR is high but would most likely decrease if the BP were raised. The patient's temperature is within normal limits.

Objective: Respiratory

Subobjective: Thoracic trauma

73. **B)** A pH of 7.33 with an increased PCO_2 and normal HCO_3 indicates respiratory acidosis. Option A indicates respiratory alkalosis. Option C indicates metabolic acidosis. Option D indicates a normal ABG.

Objective: Respiratory emergencies

Subobjective: Interpret blood gas results

74. **A)** The patient's ammonia level and ALT are elevated, which is expected with cirrhosis. Lactulose is given to lower ammonia levels in patients with cirrhosis. Bisacodyl is a laxative and is not indicated for this patient. Mesalamine is an anti-inflammatory given for ulcerative colitis. The patient's blood glucose is not elevated enough to require 2 units of insulin.

Objective: Gastrointestinal

Subobjective: Hepatic failure/coma

75. **C)** Tall, peaked T waves are a classic sign of hyperkalemia. Other indicators of hyperkalemia include ST depression, prolonged PR intervals, and absent P waves.

Objective: Renal and genitourinary

Subobjective: Life-threatening electrolyte imbalances

76. **A)** Increasing ICP requires nursing intervention; the nurse should increase the rate of oxygen because hypoxia can worsen ICP. Elevating the head of the bed, repositioning the patient, and suctioning the patient are not recommended interventions for patients experiencing (or at risk for) ICP because these interventions can actually increase the pressure.

Objective: Neurological

Subobjective: Increased intracranial pressure

77. **D)** Calling the local spiritual leader without the patient's request or permission may be violating HIPAA laws. Answers B and C indicate that the nurse is making cultural assumptions about the patient. Before assuming that the patient may wish to participate in certain cultural practices, the nurse should ask the patient if there are any cultural preferences that would affect their care.

Objective: Professional caring and ethical practice

Subobjective: Response to diversity

78. **C)** The Hunt and Hess grading scale evaluates severity of symptoms caused by a subarachnoid hemorrhage. The lower the value, the less symptomatic the patient is, indicating that ICP would be reducing and the patient improving. When measuring ICP waveforms, the P1 wave would normally be highest. For every 1°C a patient's temperature increases, there is an increase in ICP. Rhinorrhea is a sign of elevated ICP, which causes CSF drainage.

Objective: Neurological

Subobjective: Increased intracranial pressure

79. **D)** Even though it may not be possible, the nurse should attempt to find a private room so that the patient could use aromatherapy. If the nurse dismisses the purposefulness of a patient's alternative therapies, the nurse is imposing their own belief system onto

the patient. The other patient's health should never be jeopardized. Most health care facilities allow alternative therapies in conjunction with conventional medicine. The patient should never be told something that is not true.

Objective: Professional caring and ethical practice

Subobjective: Response to diversity

80. **A)** Magnesium sulfate ($MgSO_4$) is a CNS depressant and can cause marked bradycardia and respiratory depression. The nursing priority is to monitor the patient's vital signs for CNS depression after this drug is administered. Tachycardia and hyperventilation are not side effects of $MgSO_4$. A Swan-Ganz catheter and synchronized cardioversion are not indicated.

Objective: Cardiovascular

Subobjective: Dysrhythmias

81. **C)** The low urine osmolality is indicative of diabetes insipidus. Phenytoin, used postoperatively to prevent surgically induced seizures, may cause drug-induced diabetes insipidus by making the kidneys unresponsive to the action of ADH.

Objective: Endocrine

Subobjective: Diabetes insipidus

82. **D)** The equation for abdominal perfusion pressure (APP) is MAP – IAP (intra-abdominal pressure). An adequate APP is 60 mm Hg or greater. This patient's APP is 51 mm Hg, which is insufficient for adequate perfusion. The physician should be notified for orders such as increasing IV fluids. Raising the head of the bed and continuing to monitor do not address this specific issue.

Objective: Gastrointestinal

Subobjective: Abdominal compartment syndrome

83. **A)** The drug of choice for supraventricular tachycardia (SVT) is adenosine. The first dose of 6 mg has already been given, so the next appropriate dose would be 12 mg. The other options are not the next appropriate intervention for a patient in SVT.

Objective: Cardiovascular

Subobjective: Dysrhythmias

84. **A)** The typical chest radiography for a patient with acute respiratory distress syndrome (ARDS) is bilateral, diffuse white infiltrates without cardiomegaly. Options C and D show results for abnormal heart tissue but not for lung tissue and give no information about infiltrates.

Objective: Respiratory emergencies

Subobjective: ARDS

85. **B)** Dapagliflozin, an SGLT2 inhibitor used to manage diabetes, does have the rare risk of causing Fournier gangrene. Poorly controlled diabetes is a risk factor for infection and possible gangrene. Nystatin powder, used to treat integumentary yeast infections, does not increase the risk of Fournier gangrene. Long-term indwelling catheters, not straight catheters, may also contribute to the development of necrotizing fasciitis conditions such as Fournier gangrene.

Objective: Integumentary

Subobjective: Necrotizing fasciitis

86. **C)** Petechiae in this region are a cardinal sign of a fat embolism, which is a risk after a fracture of the scapula and long bones. Petechiae related to subcutaneous enoxaparin would appear on the lower abdomen at the injection site. Contusions would appear as mottled blue and purple bruising. Petechiae are not a sign of compartment syndrome.

Objective: Musculoskeletal

Subobjective: Fractures

87. **C)** Severe hypoglycemia can mimic stroke signs; a finger-stick blood glucose test would quickly rule out hypoglycemia without delaying the CT scan. A lumbar puncture may be done if the CT scan is inconclusive and if a hemorrhagic stroke is suspected. The patient is not exhibiting chest pain or signs of MI, an ECG is not necessary. A urine specimen may be difficult to collect at this time because of the patient's condition and may be postponed until after the CT scan.

Objective: Neurological

Subobjective: Stroke (ischemic)

88. **D)** Giving the patient a menu of choices available for various dietary preferences allows the patient to order a meal without waiting for the physician to put in a new dietary order. The physician should be notified of the dietary preference during rounds that day and should clarify if the patient has celiac disease or is gluten intolerant so that this condition may be added to the chart.

If the patient is still unsatisfied by the food selection, suggesting that the family bring in some food choices may be appropriate. It is never appropriate to lie to a patient, and misleading statements about gluten content may cause serious health issues if the patient does indeed have celiac disease.

Objective: Professional caring and ethical practice

Subobjective: Response to diversity

89. **B)** Level 5 in clinical judgment involves synthesizing and interpreting complex patient data. Taking the initiative to design a project embraces autonomy and contributes to the practice of nursing. The other responses are at the lowest level of clinical practice and involve gathering basic data to identify an issue, but they do not act on that information autonomously.

Objective: Professional caring and ethical practice

Subobjective: Clinical judgment

90. **C)** The HR and BP are within normal limits, and the scenario does not indicate that the patient is having any distress related to cardiac output. With interventions on the right coronary arteries, the patient may have refractory bradycardia. Because the access site was through the right radial artery, the back pain is highly unlikely to be due to a retroperitoneal bleed; nor is the patient having any signs of hemorrhage. With the radial band now off, the capillary refill to the right hand should have returned to normal. In this situation, neurovascular insufficiency is of concern, and the physician should be notified of this finding.

Objective: Cardiovascular

Subobjective: Acute peripheral vascular insufficiency

91. **D)** These ABGs indicate acute respiratory acidosis. Common signs of respiratory acidosis include hypoventilation with hypoxia, disorientation, and dizziness. Untreated respiratory acidosis can progress to ventricular fibrillation, hypotension, seizures, and coma. Deep, rapid respirations and nausea and vomiting are signs of metabolic acidosis. Chest pain is not a symptom of respiratory acidosis.

Objective: Respiratory

Subobjective: Interpret blood gas results

92. **B)** The patient's labs history and labs suggest syndrome of inappropriate antidiuretic hormone secretion (SIADH). Torsemide is used off label to decrease ADH secretion and promote diuresis. Hypertonic fluids may be an appropriate treatment but should be used to slowly correct Na^+ imbalances to decrease the risk of permanent neurological damage. Insulin and beclomethasone are not used primarily to treat SIADH.

Objective: Endocrine

Subobjective: SIADH

93. **D)** Because aminophylline may cause tachydysrhythmias, the patient's hemodynamic and cardiac rhythms should be monitored closely for sudden changes. Acetaminophen may be indicated to promote patient comfort but is not a priority. A fluid bolus is contraindicated in the case of fluid overload. The patient may require furosemide, but this is related to the disease process and not associated with the aminophylline order.

Objective: Cardiovascular

Subobjective: Acute pulmonary edema

94. **A)** This heart sound at the cardiac apex is specific to mitral or tricuspid regurg, which would be caused by a papillary muscle rupture. Aortic stenosis would be heard as a harsh systolic murmur over the right second intercostal space, with radiation to the right neck. A pleuritic rub may be auscultated in the presence of pulmonary embolism.

Objective: Cardiovascular

Subobjective: Cardiac/vascular catheterization

95. **B)** BiPAP is the appropriate choice to improve gas exchange and decrease the patient's respiratory work. The patient is in type 3 respiratory failure, a mix of hypoxemia and hypercapnia. Merely increasing the O_2 concentration will not help with hypercapnia. And because the PaO_2 labs show that the patient is already severely hypoxemic, and 35 L/min is at the maximum delivery rate for the high-flow nasal cannula, increasing the O_2 would be insufficient for type 3 respiratory failure. A breathing treatment has been provided already within the past 2 hours, so albuterol nebulizer treatment is unlikely to provide any improvement at this point. Morphine may help alleviate air hunger, but the sedation may also decrease respiratory depth and worsen hypercapnia.

Objective: Respiratory

Subobjective: Acute respiratory failure

96. **A)** The patient's care should not be delayed because of translational or technology issues. The charge nurse should be notified that the system is not working so that IT can work on the problem. Drawing pictures and continuing to use the malfunctioning system may increase the risk of misunderstanding. Attempting to troubleshoot over the phone delays patient care. The nurse should continue the care that the patient needs at this time with the family's assistance in explaining what is occurring. The family should not be used to translate information needed for informed consent if the patient is still capable of making their own decisions.

Objective: Professional caring and ethical practice

Subobjective: Response to diversity

97. **B)** NPO guidelines vary slightly depending on the resource. To ensure best practice within the facility,

the nurse should refer to the facility's policy and procedures for guidance. Searching online for evidence-based practice may bring up resources that are not valid or that contradict the facility's standards. It would not be appropriate to call the surgeon for this matter. Deciding to simply hold all intake after midnight would also not be appropriate if the surgery was scheduled later in the afternoon or if the patient has diabetes.

Objective: Professional caring and ethical practice

Subobjective: Clinical inquiry

98. B) The immediate action should be to prevent the patient from taking the pills and to find out what they are and if the patient has already taken any. The patient's family should then be educated about the importance of not giving any medications or supplements to the patient while the person is in the hospital. Calling security or berating the family will not help ensure patient safety or educate the family on why this is a safety risk. Even vitamins may be contraindicated with certain medications, and several herbal supplements may increase bleed risk.

Objective: Professional caring and ethical practice

Subobjective: Clinical judgment

99. B) As the patient may still be actively bleeding from the continued hypotension despite fluid resuscitation, clotting factors such as FFP and platelets should be administered with the PRBCs. HgB should be redrawn after blood has been transfused. After the patient has stabilized, furosemide should be considered, to prevent fluid overload and pulmonary edema due to congestive heart failure. Norepinephrine is a vasopressor and should not be administered until the patient's hypovolemic state has been stabilized.

Objective: Multisystem

Subobjective: Shock states

100. D) Debriefing should occur shortly after the causative event. Doing so has been shown to prevent staff burnout. Apologizing to the family assigns blame to the staff. Increasing workload after a traumatic event will further increase the risk for burnout.

Objective: Multisystem

Subobjective: End-of-life care

101. B) Esophageal varices can lead to death via hemorrhage. Octreotide is a vasoconstrictor used to control bleeding before an endoscopy. Phenytoin is an anticonvulsant, levofloxacin is an antibiotic, and

pantoprazole is a proton pump inhibitor; none of these are indicated at this time.

Objective: Gastrointestinal

Subobjective: Acute GI hemorrhage

102. C) The patient is hypernatremic. Hyperreflexia is seen with hypernatremia and may be elicited. Tachycardia is seen with both hyper- and hyponatremia. Hyporeflexia and increased ICP are typical of hyponatremia.

Objective: Renal and genitourinary

Subobjective: Life-threatening electrolyte imbalances

103. C) Calcium gluconate is administered to the patient with hyperkalemia for cardiac and neuromuscular protection. Aspirin is used for acute coronary syndrome but would not be a first-line drug for this condition. Insulin may be given to lower potassium levels but does not protect cardiac status. Digoxin is an antidysrhythmic and is not indicated for hyperkalemia.

Objective: Renal and genitourinary

Subobjective: Life-threatening electrolyte imbalances

104. A) The priority is to prevent tissue ischemia. The pressure dressing may be too tight, or the patient could be developing compartment syndrome. Once the dressing is removed, the nurse must reassess circulatory status. Elevating the extremity is contradicted with compartment syndrome. It would be appropriate to increase IV fluids if the urine output decreased to < 30 mL/hr. The nurse should first assess the patient for the cause of increased pain before administering higher doses of analgesics.

Objective: Musculoskeletal

Subobjective: Compartment syndrome

105. D) Syndrome of inappropriate antidiuretic hormone (SIADH) is a condition where the body makes too much ADH, causing the kidneys to retain too much fluid. Cardiac dysrhythmias are not typical with craniotomies. They may occur as a side effect of anesthesia but typically are not accompanied by fluid retention. CSF rhinorrhea is caused by a CSF leak. Diabetes insipidus would cause polyuria and fluid balance deficit.

Objective: Neurological

Subobjective: Neurosurgery

106. C) Suctioning deeply can induce coughing and overstimulate the patient. The other options are all appropriate for this patient.

Objective: Neurological

Subobjective: Traumatic brain injury

107. A) A PICC line should be placed to continue the dopamine infusion at a different site and to prevent a reoccurrence of infiltration. NSAIDs may be given for pain, but they will not preserve skin integrity. A cold compress may cause further damage by keeping the vesicant in a localized area. Hyaluronidase may be used for parenteral nutrition or calcium chloride infiltrations but is contraindicated with vasoconstrictive medications such as dopamine.

Objective: Integumentary

Subobjective: IV infiltration

108. C) In option C, the nurse is demonstrating clinical competence in using nursing judgment to intervene before delegating a decision. The other options delegate decision making to others. Texting a preceptor for advice without intervening on the patient's behalf would put the patient at risk for serious complications.

Objective: Professional caring and ethical practice

Subobjective: Clinical judgment

109. C) Cardiac tamponade occurs from accumulation of blood in the pericardial sac, decreasing cardiac output. Tension pneumothorax presents with absent or diminished breath sounds, dyspnea, and tachypnea. Aortic injury presents with profound hypotension and a loud systolic murmur. Hemothorax occurs when blood collects in the pleural cavity, causing tachypnea, dyspnea, and dullness upon percussion.

Objective: Cardiovascular

Subobjective: Cardiac trauma

110. D) An ethics committee addresses and provides guidance to any member with an ethics inquiry within the committee's jurisdiction. The committee may be represented by numerous individuals who have a vested interest in providing solutions and support in the facility. The committee is not limited to personal or legal conflicts.

Objective: Professional caring and ethical practice

Subobjective: Advocacy/moral agency

111. C) Labs should be drawn at 6 hours after ingestion, because peak serum levels will occur at this time. The nurse can then base treatment on the severity of the overdose.

Objective: Multisystem

Subobjective: Toxic ingestion/exposure

112. C) Tracheal deviation and decompensation are key characteristics of tension pneumothorax. The nurse should check the ventilator for malfunction and the endotracheal tube for obstruction, but the tracheal shift must be immediately addressed. Too much positive end-expiratory pressure will not cause tracheal shift.

Objective: Respiratory

Subobjective: Pleural space abnormalities

113. C) In this scenario, fluid overload in surgery forced fluid into the alveoli from circulatory burden. This noncardiogenic-based pulmonary edema was evident by both bilateral rales and the lack of PaO_2 improvement on high-flow oxygen. There is no mention of stridor, a classic indication of laryngeal edema post-extubation, and deterioration to respiratory distress in asthma would be distinguished by a silent chest, rather than rales. Diminished air flow/air movement is indicated by the marked reduction of breath sounds over all fields in asthma, whereas rales indicate a collection of fluid in lung tissues or pleural spaces. While pneumonia and pulmonary edema have similar diagnostic qualities, the sudden onset after fluid resuscitation points toward a noninfectious process.

Objective: Respiratory

Subobjective: Noncardiogenic pulmonary edema

114. C) Best practice is to always verify NG tube placement with an X-ray before first use. The other actions are appropriate once placement is verified.

Objective: Gastrointestinal

Subobjective: Intervene to address barriers to nutritional /fluid adequacy

115. C) Stage 2 pressure ulcers are treated with moist dressings such as petroleum-impregnated gauze.

Objective: Integumentary

Subobjective: Pressure injury

116. C) The nurse should assign a sitter because the patient's safety is more important than his right to refuse care. Placing the patient in restraints does not guarantee his safety and may escalate the situation. If the patient manages to get out of the restraints, he might hang himself with the restraints. Having security sit outside the door does not provide direct observation of the patient and uses up a limited resource of the facility. Allowing the patient to leave against medical advice (AMA) leaves the nurse and the facility vulnerable to legal action if the patient hurts himself or dies by suicide after leaving.

Objective: Behavioral and psychosocial

Subobjective: Suicidal ideation and/or behaviors

117. B) Amiodarone has been shown to control the ventricular rate in atrial fibrillation with rapid ventricular response and may assist in a spontaneous conversion to sinus rhythm. Lidocaine, epinephrine, and digoxin are not used to correct atrial fibrillation.

Objective: Cardiovascular

Subobjective: Dysrhythmias

118. C) Nitroprusside is a vasodilator that lowers systemic vascular resistance; it is not appropriate for patients with low systemic vascular resistance. Vasopressin, dopamine, and norepinephrine are vasoconstrictors that increase systemic vascular resistance.

Objective: Cardiovascular

Subobjective: Hemodynamic monitoring

119. B) Removal of the copious secretions causing mechanical obstruction of the patient's endotracheal tube airway is the first priority in this scenario. An in-line closed suction system is an effective and sterile intervention that is immediately available. Manual ventilation will not clear the clogged endotracheal tube or improve oxygenation but will waste time and increase distress for the patient. There is no need to increase IV sedation, because in this example, anxiety is a reasonable response to airway obstruction and a drop in O_2 sat. Increasing sedation is counterproductive to weaning protocols, which are designed to prevent weakening of a patient's breathing musculature while they are intubated. The health care team will continuously discuss management of FiO_2 (fraction of inspired oxygen), but this acute event requires simple, immediate nursing intervention.

Objective: Respiratory

Subobjective: Therapeutic interventions related to mechanical ventilation

120. C) The patient should have a consultation with a diabetes educator before being discharged. Because a follow-up appointment with the primary care provider might not be scheduled immediately, the patient should feel well educated before discharge. A psychiatric consult is not indicated, as the patient's concern is not a mental health disorder related to food, and the new-onset diabetes is a medical condition that requires education. The statement that the patient does not meet criteria is false.

Objective: Professional caring and ethical practice

Subobjective: Facilitation of learning

121. A) Many medications are ordered for off-label use; however, the nurse should verify that this is the correct medication and dosage. Administering a medication without knowing what it is for is reckless and could jeopardize the patient's condition. Options C and D suggest that the nurse make a false statement; the nurse should not attempt to lie to bypass responsibilities. These actions could jeopardize the nurse's career and license.

Objective: Professional caring and ethical practice

Subobjective: Clinical inquiry

122. C) Increasing the minute ventilation (MV = tidal volume [V_T] x RR) would improve both hypercapnia and respiratory acidosis. Increasing either V_T or RR would increase MV, decrease PCO_2 (treating hypercapnia), and help return the pH to normal range (as the acidosis resolves). An increase in V_T is limited by lung size (respiratory mechanics) and would potentially cause lung injury if plateau pressures were raised aggressively; decreasing the V_T will NOT help this patient. Decreasing the FiO_2 is unwarranted, and manipulating it only affects oxygenation, not ventilation. Increasing the ventilator RR will achieve the desired CO_2 reduction and improve acidosis. Increasing the RR is limited by the expiratory time (increasing the RR will reduce expiratory time), and if expiratory time is set too "short," the patient will show evidence of auto-positive end-expiratory pressure.

Objective: Respiratory

Subobjective: Manage patients requiring mechanical ventilation

123. A) Atelectasis and other respiratory problems are common in patients with acute pancreatitis. The nurse should thoroughly assess lung sounds and note any adventitious or diminished breath sounds, look for signs of orthopnea or dyspnea, and monitor O_2 sat levels. High blood glucose, light sensitivity, and low urine output are not complications of pancreatitis.

Objective: Gastrointestinal emergencies

Subobjective: Pancreatitis

124. B) Pericarditis will cause global elevation in upright ECG leads. A ruptured papillary muscle causing valve prolapse or regurg does not produce specific ECG changes and may be heard as a murmur. Re-infarction or extension of initial MI will show specific ECG changes, depending on the location of the infarction, and may be accompanied by a crushing-chest feeling, jaw or back pain, and diaphoresis.

Objective: Cardiovascular

Subobjective: Acute coronary syndrome

125. B) Coronary artery perfusion occurs during diastole, and the length of time the heart is in diastole directly affects coronary artery perfusion. HR is the determinant of blood flow to the coronary arteries: elevated HR reduces the amount of time in diastole, thus reducing the amount of coronary artery perfusion by decreasing both the volume of blood flow and the time for perfusion to occur.

Objective: Cardiovascular

Subobjective: Hemodynamic monitoring

126. C) The adrenal medulla releases epinephrine to stimulate the sympathetic nervous system to achieve homeostasis of blood glucose levels.

Objective: Endocrine

Subobjective: Hypoglycemia (acute)

127. C) Autonomic dysreflexia is the result of overstimulation of the autonomic nervous system for spinal cord injuries above the T6 level. The condition causes flushing and diaphoresis above the injury and cold, clammy skin below the level of injury. Answer C supports this diagnosis. Hypertension and bradycardia are also classic signs.

Objective: Neurological

Subobjective: Acute spinal cord injuries

128. C) The patient has 2 predisposing conditions for the diagnosis of aortic dissection: Marfan syndrome and blunt chest trauma (from the car crash). Patients with aortic dissection typically present with sudden onset of severe, tearing chest pain. Pulmonary embolism would elicit symptoms such as dyspnea, a feeling of impending doom, and chest pain. Cardiac tamponade presents with muffled heart tones, jugular venous distention (JVD), and hypotension. Acute coronary syndrome exhibits crushing chest pain radiating to the left arm and jaw, as well as ST elevation on an ECG.

Objective: Cardiovascular

Subobjective: Aortic dissection

129. A) The patient with COPD should start out with low-flow oxygen delivery. Too much oxygen can decrease the hypoxic drive and cause respiratory arrest. The other interventions are appropriate in the treatment of a patient with COPD exacerbation.

Objective: Respiratory emergencies

Subobjective: Chronic conditions

130. A) The hypovolemic shock experienced during sepsis has a high potential to cause acute kidney injury.

Objective: Renal and genitourinary

Subobjective: Acute kidney injury

131. C) Agitation and restlessness are most common during the first 6 hours after the last drink, and symptoms are generally mild. Delirium tremens and metabolic changes are more likely to occur 72 – 96 hours after the last drink. With Wernicke encephalopathy, the changes in the brain occur slowly over a long period of alcoholism.

Objective: Behavioral and psychosocial

Subobjective: Substance use disorders

132. A) Right upper quadrant pain is often attributed to acute hepatitis, gastritis, or gallbladder disease. But because the patient has recently delivered, this sign, along with signs of hepatic failure, should prompt screening for HELLP syndrome via the Mississippi Classification System. NIH stroke scale assessment is used to evaluate for stroke symptoms. The Glasgow Coma Scale assesses for level of consciousness, and the Edinburgh Depression Scale assesses for postpartum depression.

Objective: Multisystem

Subobjective: Life-threatening maternal/fetal complications

133. A) The testing location of choice is the ulnar nerve, and 2 twitches at any site indicate an 80% blockade. If anasarca is grossly present, the secondary choice of stimulation is the facial nerve. However, 0 twitches indicates a need to troubleshoot electrode placement, retest, and if the response is the same, the nurse must immediately reduce the neuromuscular blocking agent dose (perhaps by as much as 50%). Testing should be repeated every 15 – 30 minutes per hospital protocol/policy until at least 2 twitches are obtained.

Objective: Respiratory

Subobjective: Manage patients requiring mechanical ventilation

134. D) Posting the article in a high-traffic area would be the most effective way to share new knowledge with colleagues. Mailing the article to the manager does not ensure that it will be distributed to the intended audience. As the nurse believes the information will benefit the entire unit, the article should be shared with the unit, rather than just a few select colleagues. Sharing the article now would give colleagues an opportunity to review the article before bringing it up at the next staff meeting so that everyone will be aware of the information.

Objective: Professional caring and ethical practice

Subobjective: Collaboration; clinical inquiry

135. D) When advocating for the patient, the nurse should act to provide a solution. Finding out the cost and less expensive alternatives before the patient's discharge enables the patient to ask the physician for a generic or alternative medication that is more affordable before the patient learns that they cannot pay for it. Telling the patient to call after they are home does not answer their question about the cost and does not give the patient alternatives before discharge. Free samples offer only a short-term solution.

Objective: Professional caring and ethical practice

Subobjective: Advocacy/moral agency

136. A) The patient's declared preference for being called "John" should be respected, and the family should be made aware of the patient's wishes. Calling the patient a different name to appease family is disrespectful to his wishes. Studies have shown that vented, sedated patients often remember conversations and events. While the legal name should still be used as the patient identifier for safety purposes, nicknames or preferred names are acceptable while providing care. The nurse should not pass judgment on the patient's family, but to prevent confusion, the family should be made aware of previous conversations or statements by the patient.

Objective: Professional caring and ethical practice

Subobjective: Response to diversity

137. B) A QT > 470 ms in females is considered prolonged. This places that patient at an increased risk for torsades de pointes. Magnesium sulfate (MgSO4) is utilized in patients with prolonged QT to decrease this risk. The patient may have a prolonged QT without being bradycardic. Insulin and glucagon are both used in the treatment of beta-blocker overdose but are not given specifically for QT prolongation.

Objective: Multisystem

Subobjective: Toxic ingestion/exposure

138. C) Options A, B, and D are all appropriate actions defined by standard brain death evaluations. The evaluation should not be aborted unless the systolic BP decreases to < 90 despite increasing vasopressor dosage.

Objective: Neurological

Subobjective: Brain death

139. D) Battle sign and raccoon eyes indicate that this is a basilar skull fracture, and spinal cord injuries are frequently concurrent. The patient should be log-rolled during transfer to prevent cord injury. The patient should be placed in seizure precautions after being moved to bed. Critical care monitoring is essential for this patient but is not directly related to the patient transfer. Hyperventilation should take place before and after suctioning a patient with a TBI, not with movement.

Objective: Neurological

Subobjective: Traumatic brain injury

140. B) A pleural effusion is excess fluid that has collected in the pleural space. The CCRN candidate is aware that a pleural effusion should be evacuated slowly, with intermittent clamping and that no greater than 1000 – 1500 mL should be removed, to prevent re-expansion pulmonary edema. Removal of a large amount of fluid increases the negative intrapleural pressure and leads to lung collapse when the lung is unable to re-expand sufficiently to fill the thoracic space.

Objective: Respiratory

Subobjective: Pleural effusions

141. D) Immediate stoppage of further evacuation of pleural fluid and giving supplemental oxygen is the most appropriate intervention for this emergent re-expansion pulmonary edema crisis. If patient's condition continues to deteriorate, noninvasive positive-pressure ventilation or intubation with positive-pressure mechanical ventilation may be required. Unless the patient is hypotensive, fluids should not be administered, as the excess fluid would return to the thoracic space. Since the issue is not ventilatory, intubation is unnecessary. Needle decompression is also unnecessary and may worsen this condition.

Objective: Respiratory

Subobjective: Pleural effusions

142. A) Signs and symptoms of retroperitoneal bleed include hypotension, bradycardia, Grey Turner's sign (ecchymosis along flanks), and abdominal or flank pain.

Objective: Gastrointestinal

Subobjective: Acute abdominal trauma

143. B) The nursing priority for patients with fistulas is preserving and protecting the skin. Antibiotics may be given but are not the first priority. Wound VACs (vacuum-assisted closures) should not be used simply to manage drainage or in patients with increased bleeding risk. Providing a quiet environment is important, but skin integrity is the first priority with this patient.

Objective: Gastrointestinal

Subobjective: GI surgeries

144. B) The patient has had nausea and vomiting; the vomiting can cause hypokalemia. A U wave can be noted on an ECG or a cardiac monitor. Hyperkalemia would show peaked T waves. Hypercalcemia may produce a shortened QT interval, and hypocalcemia may show QT prolongation.

Objective: Renal and genitourinary

Subobjective: Life-threatening electrolyte imbalances

145. C) As the patient is a college student and has the symptoms of meningitis, the viral type would be more likely. The clear appearance of the fluid also supports this diagnosis. Bacterial meningitis is less common, and the CSF would appear cloudy. Influenza B is not tested via CFS. While a brain abscess does exhibit similar symptoms, a CT scan or an MRI would be used to rule out.

Objective: Neurological

Subobjective: Neurological infectious disease

146. C) Many patients with dementia pull out an IV because they see it as something unusual attached to their body. Placing the IV in an inconspicuous place, such as where it can be covered by the gown or wrapped up in gauze, prevents the patient from pulling it out, because the patient cannot see it. Restraints should not be the first-line intervention for this patient; this intervention may increase confusion and agitation. Family members can help watch the patient and prevent them from removing the IV, but many patients have no family close by who can stay with them around the clock. Threatening the patient with a more invasive procedure should never be used as a means of obtaining cooperation.

Objective: Neurological

Subobjective: Dementia

147. B) Oliguria (decrease in urine output) is a compensatory mechanism to prevent volume loss associated with this phase of shock. The patient would be more likely to be anxious, not lethargic. The patient would also be extremely thirsty. Nausea and cool, mottled skin are signs of progressive phases.

Objective: Multisystem

Subobjective: Shock states

148. A) The daughter should be allowed time to express her feelings and vent. The nurse has an opportunity to answer questions that the daughter may have and to provide a bridge to encourage further discussion with the patient. Although the daughter may have further questions for the physician, the nurse should not automatically pass along that responsibility.

Objective: Professional caring and ethical practice

Subobjective: Advocacy/moral agency

149. D) The nurse should first recognize any personal bias that may be a barrier in providing care to this patient. The nurse should assess the patient's pain and symptoms before notifying the physician about drug-seeking behavior. Anger at a patient's choices is not an appropriate cause for having a different nurse assigned to the patient.

Objective: Professional caring and ethical practice

Subobjective: Advocacy/moral agency

150. A) Because the patient has a history of atrial fibrillation, the fast rhythm is probably due to this condition, but it may not be easily distinguishable from supraventricular tachycardia, because of the rate. Adenosine would be administered to slow the rate and identify the underlying rhythm before further treatment. The patient is stable, and immediate cardioversion is not indicated. Moreover, adenosine will not cardiovert an atrial fibrillation or atrial flutter. Calcium channel blockers, cardiac glycoside, or beta blockers—not adenosine—would be ordered to treat dysrhythmias. Adenosine has no blood-thinning attributes.

Objective: Cardiovascular

Subobjective: Dysrhythmias

14 PRACTICE TEST TWO

1. A patient was diagnosed with pulmonary hypertension after a right heart catheterization revealed a pulmonary artery pressure of 35 mm Hg. The patient is being treated in the ICU for right-sided heart failure. What signs would indicate that the patient is transitioning to compensated pulmonary hypertension?

   A) increased right atrial pressure and decreased cardiac output

   B) increased right atrial pressure and increased right ventricular hypertrophy

   C) decreased pulmonary artery pressure and right-sided heart failure

   D) normal cardiac output and right atrial pressure with right ventricular hypertrophy

2. A patient in the ED is diagnosed with a right ventricular infarction with hypotension. The nurse should prepare to administer which of the following to treat the hypotension?

   A) NS fluid boluses 1 – 2 L

   B) dopamine at 10 mg/kg/min

   C) D5W fluid boluses titrate 3 L

   D) furosemide drip at 20 mg/hr

3. A patient is suspected of experiencing HELLP syndrome. What additional clinical signs would support this diagnosis?

   A) bradycardia, hypertension, and dyspnea

   B) left upper quadrant pain, fluid volume overload, and tachycardia

   C) hypotension, dyspnea, and fatigue

   D) right upper quadrant pain, hypertension, and dehydration

4. Which of the following statements about intra-aortic balloon pumps is NOT true?

   A) improves blood flow to the coronary arteries

   B) decreases afterload and decreases cardiac output

   C) requires concurrent anticoagulation therapy

   D) contraindicated for aortic regurgitation

5. A nurse responds to the telemetry alarm in a patient's room and finds that the intubated and mechanically ventilated patient has become agitated, is not responding to name as previously, and is fighting the vent. What monitoring values would indicate type 2 respiratory failure in this patient?

   A) PaO_2 48 mm Hg

   B) $PaCO_2$ 35 mm Hg

   C) O_2 sat 88%

   D) $PETCO_2$ 50 mm Hg

6.   A patient is admitted for severe dyspnea, lethargy, and chest pain rated at 7/10. An echocardiogram finds the patient has severe aortic stenosis, and a transcatheter aortic valve repair (TAVR) is scheduled. With a history that includes stomach ulcers with GI bleeding requiring intervention, the patient is very concerned about taking any blood thinners. The patient states that they cannot take full-strength aspirin. What alternative medication would likely be ordered after TAVR placement?

A) prasugrel

B) tirofiban hydrochloride

C) clopidogrel

D) enoxaparin

7.   Five days after total hip arthroplasty, a patient's lab values show a platelet count of 38,000/μL. What medication should be reviewed and discontinued immediately?

A) levofloxacin

B) aspirin

C) ketorolac

D) heparin

8.   An IV site that is infusing vancomycin is assessed by a nurse. The skin around the site is found to be reddened and swollen, and the patient says the area is itchy. What is the likely cause?

A) allergic reaction

B) phlebitis

C) extravasation

D) thrombosis

9.   A comatose patient with encephalopathy scores a 7 on the GCS. In completing the neuro assessment for the patient, the nurse sees that there has been no significant change in the patient's condition. What assessment should be questioned if it were noted as present in the patient's chart?

A) asterixis

B) PERRLA

C) decorticate posturing

D) tremor

10.   Five days after vertical sleeve gastrectomy surgery, a patient is started on a soft diet. Each time after eating or drinking, the patient has emesis of the majority of the intake. What diet would be expected to be ordered after the physician is notified of these symptoms?

A) smaller, more frequent meals

B) full diet

C) NPO until further notice

D) liquid-only diet

11.   One day after mitral valve replacement, a nurse is encouraging the patient to participate in physical therapy. The patient says that they are too tired and sore to walk today. The patient has been refusing pain treatment, aside from acetaminophen, because of fear of opioid addiction. What would be the best intervention from the nurse to promote mobility?

A)   Allow the patient to rest and try again tomorrow.

B)   Make the patient walk even if they are in pain.

C)   Create a multimodal pain relief plan that patient is agreeable to.

D)   Administer a dose of ibuprofen.

12.   A patient has been diagnosed with brain cancer that has progressed to the point that surgery was deemed too risky. The physician told the patient that symptoms are likely to worsen in the next 3 months and will probably be debilitative. The patient has no family in the area and says that they are not close to any friends. The nurse notes that the patient is tearful and seems depressed. What consult would be appropriate for this patient?

A) hospice

B) second opinion from another oncologist

C) home care

D) psychiatric

13. After precepting a nurse for three months, the orientee is now off orientation and has a full patient assignment. When walking by a patient's room, the former preceptor notices that the newer nurse is struggling to zero the arterial line. How should the former preceptor assist?

A) Continue walking; the new nurse needs to figure it out at some point.

B) Ask if assistance is needed and answer any questions.

C) Print out instructions and leave on the newer nurse's station for next time.

D) Go in the room and do it for the newer nurse.

14. A patient was admitted with bipolar disorder after an attempted suicide by wrist cutting. The patient has been treated for blood loss, was started on mood stabilizers, and is exhibiting an improved outlook on life. They state that they are better and want to be discharged. What is the best course of action?

A) Allow the patient to leave, to promote patient autonomy.

B) Allow the patient to leave as long as they are with a family member or friend.

C) Call psychiatrist to request an evaluation before discharge.

D) Place patient in restraints to prevent elopement.

15. A patient with an NG tube has residuals of 200 mL, 250 mL, and 300 mL, respectively, with each 4-hour assessment. What medication would the nurse anticipate would be ordered?

A) omeprazole

B) sodium polystyrene sulfonate

C) metolazone

D) metoclopramide

16. A patient being treated for DKA has a blood glucose level of 430 mg/dL and an order for continuous IV insulin. What lab must be checked before IV insulin is administered?

A) WBC

B) potassium

C) sodium

D) INR

17. An 18-year-old patient arrives in the ED after a fall from a building. The patient is guarding the left side and states pain is 7/10 in the thoracic region. The vitals are as follows:
BP 124/82
HR 99
RR 22
O_2 sat 98% on RA
What is the priority nursing intervention?

A) Auscultate lung sounds.

B) Provide pain medication as ordered.

C) Reposition to improve breathing.

D) Continue to document admission history.

18. A nurse is caring for a patient with a congestive heart failure exacerbation. The patient is experiencing dyspnea with an O_2 sat of 84% on room air. Which of the following priority treatments would the nurse expect to perform?

A) providing the patient with positive airway pressure

B) administering a calcium channel blocker

C) laying the patient flat to facilitate oxygenation

D) preparing for chest tube placement

19. A 30-year-old patient with a known history of cocaine use is admitted after a 10-minute episode of chest tightness and dyspnea after a family argument. Symptoms have resolved by time of arrival. A cardiology consult is initiated, and a 12-lead ECG shows ST depression in the precordial leads. A nurse should suspect

A) mitral valve prolapse.

B) posterior wall MI.

C) anxiety disorder.

D) pulmonary embolism.

20. The nurse is getting a report on a 45-year-old male, Jacob P., from the previous shift. The patient arrived at the unit less than 1 hour ago, and the outgoing nurse admits to being behind in the admission process but had checked in on the patient to ensure that they were stable. That nurse tells the oncoming nurse that the patient is "a bit strange. You'll see," then leaves. The nurse enters the patient room and sees the patient is wearing a long wig and lipstick. How should the nurse address the patient?

A) The nurse should always refer to the patient by the name listed on the chart.

B) Request that the patient remove the wig and makeup.

C) Just ask the patient their birthdate and don't address patient by a name.

D) Verify name and birth date on wristband, and ask how the patient would prefer to be addressed.

21. A patient is admitted to the ICU for dyspnea and hypoxia related to exacerbation of asthma. The nurse is going through the home medications and finds that the patient is taking a supplemental turmeric powder that is not in the pharmacy's formulary. The patient brought their own medications in and asks if they can just take their own. What is the priority action by the nurse?

A) Consult with physician and pharmacy to allow patient to take supplemental medication not on formulary.

B) Allow patient to take their own supplements, since they are OTC.

C) Remove patient's medications from room and give to security.

D) Notify pharmacy that patient will be taking their own meds to reduce costs.

22. A patient being treated for postpartum preeclampsia has progressed to eclampsia. A magnesium sulfate ($MgSO_4$) drip has been running for 6 hours, and the patient continues to have seizure activity. What additional medication would likely be ordered?

A) labetalol

B) hydralazine hydrochloride

C) phenytoin IV push over 1 minute

D) benzodiazepines

23. After a recent upper respiratory infection, a 56-year-old male is given supportive care in the ICU for symptoms including unsteady gait, new-onset weakness in the lower extremities that started distally and has progressed to below the waist, and diminished reflexes. Vital signs are as follows:
BP 168/72
HR 46
O_2 sat 90% on 4 L high-flow nasal cannula
Temp 39.3°C
What neuromuscular disorder is the likely cause of these symptoms?

A) cerebral palsy

B) myasthenia gravis

C) muscular dystrophy

D) Guillain-Barré syndrome

24. Which of the following is NOT a treatment in the management of cerebral vasospasm?

A) hyponatremia

B) hypervolemia

C) hemodilution

D) hypertension

25. A patient who is on anticoagulant therapy has an unwitnessed fall while walking to the bathroom without nonslip footwear. After assessing the patient and gaining assistance to move the patient back to the bed, what should the nurse do next?

A) Complete incident report per hospital protocol.

B) Notify the family of the patient's fall.

C) Notify the physician, and prepare patient for a head CT scan.

D) Continue to monitor the patient for neurological symptoms.

26. A patient with *C. diff* is experiencing skin breakdown, and the nurse is considering a fecal management device to prevent further discomfort to the patient. What conditions would prevent this device from being used on this patient?

A) anticoagulant therapy

B) urinary tract infection

C) colectomy 9 months ago

D) presence of hemorrhoids

27. The nurse is caring for a patient receiving total parenteral nutrition. During the assessment, the nurse notes an absence of breath sounds on the right side, where the central catheter is placed. Which of the following does the nurse suspect is responsible for this abnormal assessment finding?

A) air embolism

B) fluid overload

C) pneumothorax

D) refeeding syndrome

28. A comatose, vented patient is on strict I&O measurements. Assessment reveals the patient's temperature is 35.8°C, HR is 122, and urine is dark and cloudy. The physician orders a broad-spectrum antibiotic. How should the nurse proceed?

A) Administer the antibiotic as ordered.

B) Consult the physician for a culture before administering the antibiotic.

C) Check the patient's allergies before giving the antibiotic.

D) Screen the patient for sepsis.

29. A patient is being treated for rapidly evolving DIC. Which of the following lab values would the nurse expect?

A) increased hemoglobin

B) decreased D-dimer

C) increased platelets

D) decreased fibrinogen

30. An 89-year-old male with acute-on-chronic congestive heart failure is in the ICU. An echocardiogram showed significant hypertrophy with an ejection fraction of 15%. There have been multiple attempts at extubation with no success. The spouse who is the documented durable power of attorney has decided to withdraw supportive care after discussion with the physician about the patient's expected quality of life. Family arrives and a daughter becomes verbally confrontational with the spouse. What should the nurse do first?

A) Notify the physician to talk with family.

B) Demand that the daughter leave the room.

C) Call security.

D) Proceed with the withdrawal process while other family deals with the daughter.

31. After ingesting a bottle of aspirin and being brought into the ED, a patient is in the ICU with seizure activity and is in atrial fibrillation. What intervention would likely be avoided unless the patient is experiencing extreme respiratory distress?

A) potassium replacement

B) mechanical ventilation

C) fluid resuscitation

D) D50 to treat blood glucose < 40 mg/dL

32. An 89-year-old female is being treated for pneumonia secondary to influenza B infection. Broad-spectrum antibiotic therapy was started yesterday after sputum cultures were sent to lab. The patient's temperature remains elevated despite antipyretics, and a chest X-ray reveals significant opacity in the left lower lobe. What intervention may be considered to treat this patient?

    A) positioning on left side

    B) thoracentesis with culture of collected fluid

    C) diuretics

    D) infusion of albumin

33. A total of 3 mg of atropine has been administered incrementally for a patient with an HR of 38. After the last dose, the HR is palpable at 42, BP is 83/45, and O_2 sat is 96% on 3 L nasal cannula. The patient is diaphoretic and nauseous before having a syncopal episode. What intervention would be appropriate?

    A) Begin a phenylephrine infusion.

    B) Administer 1 mg of atropine.

    C) Begin transcutaneous pacing.

    D) Administer 1 mg of epinephrine IV push.

34. Which of the following lab values should the nurse expect to order for a patient receiving IV heparin therapy for a pulmonary embolism?

    A) hematocrit

    B) HDL and LDL

    C) PT and PTT

    D) troponin level

35. A 42-year-old male patient is admitted to the CCU with an initial diagnosis of acute coronary syndrome with MI ruled out. Patient history includes the use of sildenafil within the last 3 hours and one 81 mg aspirin tablet while the patient was being transported to the ED. On arrival to the unit, the patient exhibits increased chest pain 8/10, and a repeat 12-lead ECG shows sinus bradycardia HR 58,

with new, inverted T waves and ST elevation in V1. ED labs show positive troponins. Which of the following drugs should be used cautiously in the initial treatment of this patient?

    A) morphine sulfate

    B) oxygen

    C) lactated Ringer's IV solution

    D) heparin bolus and continuous drip

36. A patient presenting with polyuria, nausea and vomiting, Kussmaul respirations, and a fruity odor to their breath is diagnosed with DKA. Which of the following signs would indicate that DKA is worsening?

    A) fluid volume overload

    B) oliguria

    C) metabolic alkalosis

    D) decreased blood glucose level

37. What symptoms may be seen with fulminate hepatitis?

    A) jaundice, decreased bilirubin levels, elevated NH_3

    B) asterixis, epistaxis, decreased glomerular filtration rate

    C) decreased glomerular filtration rate, hyperkalemia, hypoglycemia

    D) hypertension, ascites, bradykinesia

38. The following labs return on a patient being treated for congestive heart failure secondary to chronic kidney disease:
WBC 12,000/μL
HgB 6.8 g/dL
potassium 6.2
phosphate 2.8 mEq/L
The patient will be receiving dialysis today. What treatment would the nurse expect to be administered after dialysis?

    A) PRBCs

    B) potassium supplement

    C) epoetin alfa (Epogen)

    D) heparin

39. The nurse is assessing for compartment syndrome in a patient recovering from a femur fracture. Which of the following is NOT a sign of this condition?

A) poikilothermia

B) pain that is unresponsive to analgesics

C) decreased serum CK

D) reduced pedal pulse

40. A patient has been diagnosed as brain dead after a drowning accident. When the family has arrived for their first visit since the patient was admitted, a nurse and an aide are providing range-of-motion exercises with the patient. The family is confused about why their loved one is being treated as though they are going to get better. What is the nurse's best response?

A) Discontinue providing care to avoid offending the family.

B) Explain that the nurse and the aide are following the facility's protocols.

C) Ask if the family would like to participate in the care being provided.

D) Ask the family to leave until care is complete.

41. A patient with suspected sepsis is directly admitted to the ICU. The patient describes having a sinus infection attributed to a virus last week. Which of the following are appropriate actions to implement as part of the sepsis bundle?

A) Begin IV fluid resuscitation with crystalloids.

B) Hold antibiotics because initial infection was viral.

C) Start norepinephrine drip if MAP is 70.

D) Draw blood cultures after antibiotics are started.

42. The nursing staff in an ICU forms a self-governed, unit-based council. After discussion, they vote on the goal of decreasing catheter-associated UTI rates in patients with indwelling catheters. A volunteer is delegated to reach out to infectious disease for guidance on this initiative. What competency does this action uphold?

A) collaboration

B) response to diversity

C) systems thinking

D) clinical inquiry

43. The nurse is assisting the neurologist in completing a brain function test on a 24-year-old patient who had a seizure a week ago and who has been sustained on mechanical ventilation. The apneic test is conducted, and there is no respiratory drive noted and the test is aborted after the O_2 sat declines to 75% and remains so for 35 seconds. What should the nurse prepare to do next?

A) Notify the family that the brain death test was positive.

B) Repeat apnea test in 2 hours.

C) Extubate the patient.

D) Obtain an ABG.

44. The code team is resuscitating a patient who went into ventricular fibrillation. ACLS has been started, and the patient has been defibrillated 1 time with a biphasic defibrillator. A rhythm check finds that the patient continues to be in ventricular fibrillation. What intervention would be expected next?

A) amiodarone 150 mg

B) defibrillate at 360 J

C) adenosine 6 mg

D) defibrillate at 300 J

45. The CCRN candidate notes a decrease in the documentation of hourly blood glucose levels and therapeutic adjustments for patients on IV insulin therapy in the ICU. The candidate asks the clinical nurse specialist for assistance in creating a study on the issue. The candidate's interest and initiative are an example of

A) advocacy.

B) caring practices.

C) clinical inquiry.

D) clinical judgment.

46. A patient has been extubated after being mechanically vented for 6 days because of acute respiratory distress syndrome. The patient is no longer sedated and is sitting up and talking with family members. The patient's spouse asks when the patient may have something to eat. What should the nurse verify before the patient begins eating or drinking?

   A) that a diet order has been entered by the physician

   B) that a swallow assessment has been completed

   C) that the patient can tolerate ice chips

   D) any cultural or personal nutritional preferences

47. A 72-year-old patient is admitted with a diagnosis of bilateral pneumonia and sepsis. An ABG drawn 4 hours post-extubation is as follows: pH 7.35, PaO_2 64 mm Hg, $PaCO_2$ 59 mm Hg, HCO_3 32 mEq/L. How should the nurse interpret these findings?

   A) compensated metabolic acidosis

   B) compensated respiratory acidosis

   C) uncompensated respiratory alkalosis

   D) uncompensated respiratory acidosis

48. A patient is admitted for a hypotensive episode with syncope. The nurse notes that the patient had bariatric surgery within the past 6 months. What medication in the patient's history may indicate that the patient has experienced dumping syndrome?

   A) octreotide acetate

   B) metoprolol

   C) vancomycin

   D) insulin

49. A patient arrives to the ED after an attempted suicide by a self-inflicted gunshot wound. The patient is determined to be brain dead, but life can be sustained for organ procurement. The patient is identified as an organ donor. Which of the following is the next step for the ED nurse?

   A) Notify the local organ procurement organization.

   B) Remove all life-supporting interventions.

   C) Perform postmortem care on the patient.

   D) Complete the death certificate.

50. A 40-year-old female, 3 days postpartum, is in the ICU when the patient required mechanical ventilation after a cardiac arrest and subsequent respiratory failure occurred several hours after giving birth. The patient is now profusely bleeding from the C-section site, and the lab notifies the nurse of a critical PLT level of 30,000/μL. What is likely occurring with this patient?

   A) postpartum hemorrhage

   B) phase 1 amniotic fluid embolism

   C) phase 2 amniotic fluid embolism

   D) placenta accreta

51. A patient who was being treated with buprenorphine is admitted with a complex femur fracture. The patient is transferred from the medical-surgical floor 2 days after surgery to the ICU after having symptoms of severe withdrawal. What treatment plan would be expected?

   A) Restart buprenorphine and cease further opioid use.

   B) Increase amount of opioids to treat pain.

   C) Refuse patient requests of pain control, as they are a drug seeker.

   D) Immediately cease using any opioids.

52. A patient with amyotrophic lateral sclerosis is admitted for new-onset weakness and difficulty walking. The nurse reviews the home medications and sees that the patient takes 75 mg of clopidogrel daily after receiving a peripheral stent 3 months ago. What should the nurse verify before administering this medication?

   A) PLT values

   B) swallowing ability

C) PT/INR values

D) diet order

53. Which of the following complications can occur if more than 1000 – 1500 mL is removed from the pleural space by a thoracentesis?

A) pneumothorax

B) empyema

C) reexpansion pulmonary edema

D) opposite lung collapse

54. Which of the following are typical signs of opioid withdrawal?

A) piloerection, diaphoresis, and tremors

B) tachycardia, tachypnea, and hypotension

C) nausea, vomiting, and abdominal cramping

D) insomnia and headache

55. A patient returns to their ICU room after having a fistulagram with sedation. The nurse gets a report that the patient was given 3 mg of midazolam. The patient is hard to arouse during assessment. Vital signs are HR 62, BP 105/75, RR 4, and O_2 sat 86% on 3 L. The nurse puts a nonrebreathing mask on the patient and increases the O_2. The sats do not increase, and the patient is no longer responding to their name. What intervention would be appropriate?

A) Administer naloxone 1 mg via IV push.

B) Increase fluids to help kidneys clear the medication.

C) Call a code blue.

D) Administer flumazenil 0.2 mg via IV push.

56. A patient requires an ICU bed after surgery to repair an abdominal aortic aneurysm. The family is notified that the patient will be going to a unit that is closed to visitors because of COVID-19. How can the nurse best help the family visit with the patient?

A) Notify them of the policy that does not allow visitors.

B) Give them the phone number of the unit.

C) Provide a web link to a teleconference app that is used by the facility to allow virtual visits.

D) Tell the family that the primary nurse will call with updates.

57. A 90-year-old female who is a member of the Orthodox Jewish faith has been diagnosed with metastasized liver cancer. How can the care team ensure that the patient's end-of-life care options are supported?

A) Ask the patient if she would like her rabbi to attend a patient care conference.

B) Involve only the patient in care decisions.

C) Recognize that the Jewish law mandates that all measures be taken to extend a dying person's life, and do not bring up hospice or palliative care.

D) Limit family visiting to three people.

58. A patient is a direct admit from a physician's office to the CCU to be evaluated for intermittent, severe chest pain that is relieved with rest and positional changes and for tachycardia and hypotension. The initial ECG revealed a bundle branch block, and troponin levels were negative. The nurse assesses the patient and auscultates a pericardial rub. What diagnostic test would the nurse anticipate to be ordered?

A) cardiac catheterization

B) repeat ECG

C) repeat troponin levels

D) chest X-ray

59. A patient with a history of hypertension has a serum glucose of 62 mg/dL but presents with no symptoms of hypoglycemia. What medication should the nurse suspect is masking the patient's symptoms?

A) ACE inhibitors

B) opioids

C) antihistamines

D) beta blockers

60. A 28-year-old male patient is admitted to the ICU with a diagnosis of gastric ulcer bleed, hypovolemia, and dehydration. Vital signs are temp 37.1°C, HR 128, and BP 96/58. Labs show HgB 9 g/dL and Hct 34%. The patient was admitted to the ICU with transfusion orders for 2 units of PRBCs based on ED labs, and NG tube placement for gastric decompression. Which of the following measures would be contraindicated?

A) NPO, elevate head of bed

B) pain relief with NSAIDs

C) fluid resuscitation

D) administration of proton pump inhibitors

61. A patient is started on a loop diuretic for fluid volume overload. What electrolyte must be monitored for depletion?

A) magnesium

B) calcium

C) phosphate

D) potassium

62. A charge nurse is notifying the oncoming shift that a patient suspected of having viral meningitis is expected to be transferred in the next hour. What safety precautions related to this diagnosis are required?

A) contact precautions

B) droplet precautions

C) neutropenic precautions

D) seizure precautions

63. A nurse is closely monitoring ICP in an unresponsive patient with TBI and severe cerebral edema. Which of the following should the nurse use as the first-line intervention to maintain cerebral perfusion pressure in this patient?

A) fluid management

B) vasodilators

C) mannitol

D) sedation to prevent increased stimulation

64. A patient with a witnessed ventricular fibrillation is resuscitated in the field. The patient is subsequently admitted to the CCU for initiation of therapeutic hypothermia and is cooled via endovascular catheter with a target of 32 – 36°C. The nurse knows that this cooling is aimed at preventing what?

A) cardiac ischemia

B) vascular thrombus

C) neurological damage

D) multisystem organ failure

65. A nurse arrives at the start of his shift, and he is approached by the house supervisor. The neuro-stepdown unit needs extra assistance. Despite being unfamiliar with this unit, the nurse is agreeable to help. What is the expectation of standards of care on that unit?

A) telling the neuro-stepdown charge nurse that because the assisting nurse is not familiar with the unit, he will assist in a nursing assistant role

B) following the care expectations of his home unit

C) following this unit's policies and procedures

D) simply getting through the night and providing what care he has time for

66. A patient in the ICU has been transitioned to palliative care per their wishes. The patient is requesting for family to be at the bedside. They arrive at 7:30 p.m., and visiting hours end at 8 p.m. What should the nurse tell the patient's family?

A) Family is welcome to stay at the patient's bedside until they get caught and are asked to leave.

B) Visiting hours will be over in half an hour, so the visit must be short.

C) It would be better for the family to come in the morning.

D) She will check with the nursing supervisor for permission for the family to stay late.

67. A 49-year-old transgender woman is nonresponsive after a near-drowning boating accident. The patient's sister is upset that the health care team has been referring to the patient using male pronouns. What is the most appropriate action for the nurse to take?

A) Listen attentively to the sister, and communicate the pronoun preference request to the charge nurse.

B) Respectfully inform the family member that legal pronouns are used when discussing HIPAA-sensitive treatment and care options.

C) Acknowledge the sister's concern, and communicate the information with the entire health care team.

D) Consult an ethics committee on the legality of the family request for use of gender pronouns of choice.

68. After an end-of-life discussion with the physician, the patient asks the nurse to clarify the meaning of the terms "do not resuscitate" and "allow natural death." Which of the following would be an appropriate response from the nurse?

A) I cannot discuss end-of-life care, but I will let the physician know you have questions.

B) "Do not resuscitate" means that resuscitative efforts are withheld.

C) "Allow natural death" withholds all care.

D) You should choose to keep full code.

69. What lab marker is used to determine adequate tissue perfusion during sepsis?

A) ALT

B) creatinine

C) lactate

D) WBC

70. An external ventricular drain is ordered for a patient with a GCS of 4 and cerebral edema. What is the purpose of this procedure?

A) noninvasive monitoring of ICP

B) determines the neurological pupil index

C) prevents infection related to retention of CSF

D) provides monitoring of ICP and CSF drainage

71. A 36-year-old male patient who presented to the ED in respiratory arrest after an overdose of fentanyl is being treated for alcohol and drug dependence. CIWA protocol has been initiated, and for the past day, the patient's symptoms are being managed with lorazepam, per protocol. On the next assessment, the nurse finds the patient lethargic and unable to hold up a cup of water on his own. Labs are drawn with the following results: potassium 6 mmol/L, calcium 14 mmol/L, creatinine 2.6 mg/dL, and CK 4900 U/L. What order would the nurse expect?

A) hemodialysis

B) fluids and sodium polystyrene sulfonate

C) discontinue CIWA protocol

D) calcium gluconate

72. A patient with chronic kidney disease is being cared for in the ICU after an ischemic stroke. Routine lab work reveals the patient's potassium level is 7.4 mEq/L. Which priority intervention should the nurse prepare for?

A) an IV bolus of NS

B) oral administration of sodium polystyrene sulfonate

C) emergent dialysis

D) administration of IV dextrose followed by IV insulin

73. A patient is recovering from myocardial revascularization and has started treatment on an ARB, a beta blocker, and an anticoagulant. Labs are drawn and show an increasing trend in creatinine and BUN. The urine output totals for the day have increased from 250 mL/day to 2500 mL/day. What intrarenal disease phase is the patient in?

   A) diuretic phase

   B) oliguric phase

   C) onset phase

   D) recovery phase

74. A patient has been admitted for acute pancreatitis. The nurse completes a head-to-toe assessment, reviews medications, and addresses pain. What other assessment should occur with this patient population?

   A) behavioral

   B) CIWA

   C) sepsis

   D) STOP-Bang

75. Laboratory results for a patient with fluid overload caused by congestive heart failure are most likely to reveal

   A) increased BNP.

   B) increased Hct.

   C) increased sodium levels.

   D) increased serum osmolality.

76. A patient presents to the ED with chest pain, dyspnea, and diaphoresis. The nurse finds a narrow complex tachycardia with an HR of 210, a BP of 122/72, and an RR of 18. The nurse should first prepare to

   A) administer adenosine 6 mg IV.

   B) perform synchronized cardioversion at 100 J.

   C) perform defibrillation at 300 J.

   D) perform vagal maneuvers.

77. A 64-year-old patient with a recent diagnosis of stage 3 cancer is admitted to CCU with chest pain 2/10. An ECG on admission indicates mild ST elevation with low-voltage QRS segments. On examination, the nurse notes jugular vein distension, muffled heart sounds, hypotension with a narrow pulse pressure, and weakly palpable peripheral pulses. A nurse should suspect

   A) chronic aortic regurgitation.

   B) cardiac tamponade.

   C) aortic stenosis.

   D) thyrotoxicosis.

78. The nurse is caring for a patient post-hypophysectomy. Over the last shift, the patient's urine output has been 25 mL/hr. What measures should the nurse anticipate for this patient?

   A) neuro precautions, Foley insertion, and vasopressin

   B) telemonitoring, seizure precautions, and fluid resuscitation

   C) seizure precautions, fluid restriction, and sodium replacement

   D) telemonitoring and hypotonic fluid administration

79. The practice council decides to put together care packages for patients who are at end-of-life care. The package includes aromatherapy, a journal to leave messages to loved ones, and a soft blanket. How does this practice support clinical practice?

   A) works on behalf of community

   B) bases clinical judgment on immediate grasp of situation

   C) has global outlook

   D) compassionately stands with patient and family through the end-of-life process

80. A 19-year-old male who is suicidal is brought into the ED after consuming a bottle of extra-strength acetaminophen. He was found unconscious by his roommate 2 hours ago. After the patient is admitted to the ICU, the nurse notes in the orders that the patient is to be assessed using the Rumack-Matthew nomogram. What is this assessment used for?

A) to assess for kidney damage

B) to guide dosage of N-acetylcysteine

C) to verify if activated charcoal was effective

D) to predict the risk of hepatoxicity

81. A nurse is planning to complete a capstone project to fulfill the BSN degree requirement. The project aims to look at long-term outcomes for patients who require resuscitative efforts while hospitalized. What should the first step of the project be?

A) Ask if there have been any recent codes, and look that patient up in the EMR.

B) Consult the facility librarian for evidence-based practice and articles related to the subject.

C) Form a PICOT question.

D) Consult the Code Blue committee to guide the project.

82. What action best demonstrates being involved and working on behalf of patient, family, and community?

A) participation in education health fair at local event center to promote gun safety

B) enrollment in class working toward a BSN degree

C) development of a care plan for a patient and family member while patient is admitted to hospital

D) recruiting an RN associate to work in same facility

83. A patient's cardiac monitor shows the rhythm in the figure. The patient is awake and alert but is pale and confused. BP is 64/40. What is the priority nursing intervention for this patient?

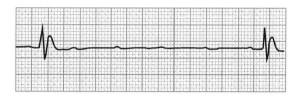

A) Defibrillate at 200 J.

B) Prepare for transcutaneous pacing.

C) Administer epinephrine 1 mg.

D) Begin CPR.

84. A patient is admitted for an acute exacerbation of COPD. The patient says that he was prescribed ProAir HFA. However, it was too expensive, so he has been using the fluticasone inhaler prescribed for his spouse, who has asthma. What important education should the nurse provide to the patient to prevent another exacerbation?

A) The importance of continuing chest physiotherapy if he cannot afford his medications

B) A list of medications that may be substituted for ProAir HFA

C) The proper use of a fluticasone inhaler

D) The difference between corticosteroid and bronchodilator medications

85. A patient has been diagnosed with pulmonary fibrosis and is currently on ventilatory and hemodynamic support. The patient's family asks the nurse if there is any chance that the disease can be cured. What does the nurse know about the treatment trajectory of this disease?

A) Life expectancy is unchanged with treatment.

B) Hospice should be discussed and recommended.

C) With treatment, a patient's life may be extended for 3 – 5 years.

D) Lung transplants are not an option to treat this disease.

86. Which of the following ECG changes is not associated with a PE?

A) transient right bundle branch block

B) tall, peaked T waves in leads II, III, and aVF

C) negative QRS in lead I

D) ST elevation in lead I and aVL

87. A family member calls for help from the patient's room and says the patient is no longer responding to her. A rapid response is called, and the primary nurse assesses the patient. The patient's rhythm on telemetry is sinus bradycardia, and a pulse is not found. What should be the initial intervention?

A) Begin defibrillation.

B) Administer 1 mg of epinephrine.

C) Initiate chest compressions.

D) Continue to monitor.

88. The nurse is caring for a patient with delirium who tells the nurse, "There are snakes crawling up on my bed." How should the nurse respond?

A) "That's just the wrinkles in your blanket."

B) "I will see if I can move you to another room."

C) "I will call maintenance to come and remove them."

D) "I know you're scared, but I don't see any snakes on your bed."

89. A 19-year-old is brought into the ED for a closed-head injury after a fall while skateboarding. The patient was not wearing a helmet when they fell. What assessment would indicate increasing ICP?

A) A&O × 3

B) pupils bilaterally dilated and fixed

C) GCS 13

D) Kussmaul respirations

90. A nurse is caring for a patient who is not expected to survive the night. The patient's family has stated they are on their way but have not arrived. The patient is tearful and continues to ask when family will arrive. What is the best action for the nurse to take?

A) Stay with patient until family arrives.

B) Remind patient that family stated they are on the way, and check on the other patients.

C) Avoid the room until family arrives.

D) Administer PRN midazolam so that the patient takes a nap until family arrives.

91. A nurse begins an initiative to improve a policy in an effort to prevent falls among patients who use mobility devices. What core nursing competency does this align with?

A) Advocacy/moral agency

B) Clinical inquiry

C) Facilitation of learning

D) Caring practices

92. A patient is in shock because of postpartum hemorrhage. How would this shock be classified?

A) hypovolemic

B) cardiogenic

C) obstructive

D) distributive

93. Occlusion of the right coronary artery may cause ischemia in all the following parts of the heart EXCEPT this one:

A) anterior wall

B) right atrium

C) inferior-posterior wall of the left ventricle

D) atrioventricular node

94. A patient with dilated congestive cardiomyopathy is admitted to the ICU for acute kidney failure. The patient's dilated congestive cardiomyopathy is managed with beta blockers and ACE inhibitors. What lab value should be closely monitored?

A) HgB

B) calcium

C) potassium

D) blood glucose

95. The nurse is caring for a patient receiving PRBCs. Vital signs at the start of the transfusion are as follows:
BP 99/70
HR 92
RR 16
temp 37.2°C
After the transfusion has been running on a pump for 1 hour and 30 minutes, the patient's vital signs are as follows:
BP 103/72
HR 85
RR 25
temp 38.3°C
What action would NOT be warranted by the nurse?

A) Administer acetaminophen.

B) Stop transfusion, and administer NS.

C) Administer antihistamine.

D) Notify physician and blood bank.

96. Prone position for ventilation is used in patients with which of the following disorders?

A) acute respiratory distress syndrome

B) pneumothorax

C) sepsis

D) hydrocephalus

97. A 95-year-old male is admitted to observation overnight after an emergent cardiac catheterization with angioplasty and stenting. The patient's wife accompanied him and is still in the room after visiting hours are over. When the nurse asks if she has a way home tonight, she answers that her husband does all the driving and they have no family in the state. The patient reveals that his wife becomes confused at night. What should the nurse do?

A) Attempt to find accommodations for the patient's wife at a nearby hotel.

B) Tell the patient and wife that they should have planned better and that she cannot stay.

C) Provide the patient with a reclining chair to stay in overnight in the patient's room.

D) Call a family member, and tell them that they need to figure something out.

98. A patient in the ICU has coded for a second time after return of spontaneous circulation is achieved. Family members are at the bedside visiting. The code team arrives, and the family is asked to step out of the room to allow the team to resuscitate the patient. The family members are requesting to stay at the bedside. What option would best empower the family to make an informed choice?

A) Identify the durable power of attorney, and allow this person to observe from outside the room.

B) Escort them to a waiting room, and leave.

C) Allow all of them to stay if they want.

D) Allow them to stay outside the room, and close the curtains.

99. A fluid bolus is given to a patient being treated for sepsis. What is the best method to determine if tissue perfusion is responding to the fluid boluses?

A) improved capillary refill

B) dry, pink skin

C) 10% decrease in lactate level

D) cardiac output 6 L/min

100. A patient has an organized rhythm with a HR of 45 and tall, peaked T waves. The nurse should suspect

- **A)** hypokalemia.
- **B)** hyperkalemia.
- **C)** hyponatremia.
- **D)** hypernatremia.

101. A 38-year-old morbidly obese patient is admitted for a stabbing wound resulting in retroperitoneal hemorrhage. The patient has received 2 L 0.9% NS and 2 units of PRBC. He is currently on BiPAP for fluid overload and acute congestive heart failure. Which action is a priority for this patient?

- **A)** insertion of Foley catheter
- **B)** increase positive end-expiratory pressure on noninvasive ventilation
- **C)** placing patient in high Fowler's position
- **D)** placing NG tube for enteral nutrition

102. The nurse is caring for an 82-year-old patient who presented to the ED with poor appetite, confusion, and weakness. Which of the following lab findings is most concerning?

- **A)** chloride 99 mEq/L
- **B)** calcium 9.4 mg/dL
- **C)** sodium 118 mEq/L
- **D)** potassium 4.2 mEq/L

103. Which patient is most at risk for hyperosmolar hyperglycemic state?

- **A)** 43-year-old male with diet-controlled diabetes and BMI 32
- **B)** 86-year-old female with type 2 diabetes, congestive heart failure, and BMI 38
- **C)** 18-year-old female with type 1 diabetes managed with an insulin pump and BMI 22
- **D)** 52-year-old male with COPD managed with corticosteroids and BMI 42

104. Which of the following assessment results is consistent with a diagnosis of acute left-sided systolic heart failure?

- **A)** BNP lab result < 70 pg/mL
- **B)** ejection fraction > 70%
- **C)** transient, intermittent auscultated pericardial friction rub
- **D)** bilateral pleural effusions

105. A nurse is basing a school project on promoting competency in caring practices on her own unit. Which of the following would be an expert action in implementing the unit change into practice?

- **A)** Anticipate resistance from staff, and work to gain buy-in before making the change.
- **B)** Announce the changes at the beginning of shift huddle.
- **C)** Have the manager tell all staff about the change in practice.
- **D)** Only implement the change with her own patients.

106. A nurse is teaching a patient with new-onset diabetes the importance of caring for their skin. Which of the following indicates that the patient needs additional instruction?

- **A)** The patient says that they are going to incorporate healthy eating habits provided by the dietician.
- **B)** The client intends to seek a referral to a foot care clinic.
- **C)** The patient can teach back the steps of insulin administration with minimal assistance.
- **D)** The patient says that they are glad that they will still be able to wear sandals in the summer.

107. A patient displays a narrow complex supraventricular tachycardia on the cardiac monitor. Assessment shows mild dyspnea, chest pain 2/10, mild diaphoresis, and anxiety. Vital signs are HR 168, BP 82/50, and RR 23. Which of the following drugs should NOT be used as a first-line treatment for this patient?

A) adenosine

B) digoxin

C) amiodarone

D) verapamil

108. Which of the following drugs is administered to decrease myocardial workload and prevent dysrhythmias after an acute MI?

A) amiodarone

B) clopidogrel

C) beta blockers

D) morphine sulfate

109. A 23-year-old patient with a history of status asthmaticus is a direct admit to the ICU with severe dyspnea despite the patient's use of a rescue inhaler. Stat ABGs are as follows:
PaO_2 52 mm Hg
$PaCO_2$ 65 mm Hg
pH 7.08
SpO_2 82%
Repeat ABGs after 60 minutes show the following:
PaO_2 76 mm Hg
$PaCO_2$ 60 mm Hg
pH 7.10
SpO_2 93%
How can the repeat ABGs be interpreted?

A) respiratory acidosis and resolved hypoxemia

B) respiratory alkalosis and resolved hypoxemia

C) respiratory acidosis and hypoxemia

D) respiratory alkalosis and hypoxemia

110. Hyperosmolar hyperglycemic state is most often caused by

A) inadequate glucose monitoring.

B) dehydration.

C) noncompliance with insulin therapy.

D) a breakdown of ketones.

111. A patient with an upper GI bleed has had a mass transfusion protocol with fluid resuscitation because of severe hemorrhage. The following day, the nurse reviews the labs and finds that the creatinine is increased. What medical exam should be conducted with caution?

A) X-ray

B) CT scan without contrast

C) angiogram

D) HIDA scan

112. The nurse is assessing the skull fracture of a patient being cared for after the patient was hit in the head with a baseball bat during an altercation. The fracture is depressed 7 mm. What should the nurse's next action be?

A) Continue to monitor, and report if depression increases.

B) Notify physician, and prepare patient for immediate surgery.

C) Redress the wound, and document findings.

D) Administer ordered antibiotics.

113. The nurse is obtaining history and home medications during the admission process. The patient identifies as a transgender woman. What should the nurse find out when communicating with this patient?

A) allergies

B) preferred pronouns

C) social support system

D) risk of suicide

114. Four hours after femoral-access interventional cardiac angioplasty, a patient shows the following symptoms: Grey Turner's sign, back pain, bradycardia, hypotension, sinus rhythm with new-onset unifocal premature ventricular contractions, and a right lower extremity that is cool to touch with reduced pedal pulses. The nurse should suspect

A) respiratory embolism.

B) retro-peritoneal bleeding.

C) papillary muscle rupture.

D) myocardial Infarction.

115. A patient with an insulin-secreting tumor is awaiting surgery and is treated for a blood glucose level of 35 mg/dL. The following are the blood glucose levels every 15 minutes over 1 hour: 85, 120, 135, and 72 mg/dL. What action would be anticipated next?

A) Administer 12.5 g of D50.

B) Give 4 oz of juice and recheck blood glucose in 15 minutes.

C) Continue to monitor.

D) Start continuous infusion of D10.

116. After a myocardial infarction, how soon will the initial troponin elevation occur?

A) immediately

B) 2 – 4 hours

C) 12 – 24 hours

D) > 24 hours

117. A 63-year-old patient is admitted to the ICU after being hit by a car while riding a bicycle. Chest X-ray on admit showed several rib fractures. The patient suddenly becomes hypotensive, with BP noted at 84/34. Rhonchi are auscultated on the right side, and breath sounds on the left side are dim to absent. What intervention should the nurse anticipate?

A) immediate chest tube insertion

B) chest X-ray

C) CT scan

D) intubation

118. Which of the following is NOT a cause of acute kidney injury?

A) MAP < 65 for > 30 minutes

B) dopamine IV at 16 mg/kg/min

C) vancomycin trough of 22.3

D) acetaminophen toxicity

119. The physician requests that the nurse prepare a patient who has left upper extremity cellulitis and an open wound for a dressing change along with wound debridement. The patient describes their pain level as currently 4/10. Family is at the bedside. What is the priority with this patient?

A) Provide analgesia prior to changing dressing.

B) Set up a sterile tray for debridement.

C) Ask family to leave room before changing dressing.

D) Swab exudate of dressing to send for culture.

120. A 65-year-old patient sustained a head injury from a fall on the bathroom floor at home after showering. Two days after admission, the nurse notes bruising behind both ears, raccoon eyes, and clear rhinorrhea that produces a "halo" sign when captured on a paper strip. Which type of skull fracture would the nurse suspect?

A) frontal

B) parietal

C) basilar

D) temporal

121. A physician is discussing with a patient's family a procedure that would be lifesaving but that would also require extensive therapies and medications for the rest of the patient's life. The physician does not elaborate on the extent of these therapies and that the patient would require around-the-clock care. What ethical principle violation could the nurse consult the ethics team on?

A) beneficence

B) confidentiality

C) utilitarianism

D) autonomy

122. After a hernia removal, a patient is repeatedly asking for increasing doses of hydromorphone before the time scheduled for the next dose. The nurse assesses the patient and finds that all vitals are within normal levels and that the patient has no distension or pain around the incision site. The patient says that the pain is in the lower back and is at 8/10. The nurse reviews the list of home medications and sees that the patient is on hydrocodone for chronic back pain. What should the nurse do to establish limits on appropriate pain control with this patient?

A) Tell the patient that they are exhibiting drug-seeking behavior.

B) Call the physician to increase the dosage and frequency of IV pain medications.

C) Establish a functional pain goal with the patient.

D) Notify the physician that the patient's hydrocodone needs to be ordered, and continue to give both oral and IV push medications.

123. After a fall from a cliff, a patient is being observed in the ICU for a spinal cord injury. The patient is A&O×3 and is being kept stable with a C-collar in place. The patient is describing a reduction of feeling in the lower extremities and has been incontinent several times today. A grasp reflex is documented at 1+, down from 3+ yesterday. What syndrome is the patient likely experiencing?

A) anterior spinal cord syndrome

B) cauda equina syndrome

C) central cord syndrome

D) neurogenic shock

124. A 38-year-old patient is admitted to the CCU with vague pressure-like chest discomfort that developed after social cocaine and alcohol usage. The responding paramedics report that the patient's chest pain was unresponsive to nitroglycerin. The ECG shows coved-type ST segment elevation with T-wave inversion in leads V1 and V2. CBC is unremarkable, and serial troponin levels are below the 99th percentile range. What pathology should the nurse suspect?

A) posterior wall MI

B) vasospastic angina

C) Brugada pattern

D) papillary muscle rupture

125. Which of the following symptoms is characteristic of a nondominant right hemisphere stroke?

A) right hemiparesis

B) emotional lability

C) difficulty in problem solving

D) sensory loss in all 4 limbs

126. A patient has been transferred to the ICU preoperatively for surgical repair of a bowel obstruction. The patient calls the nurse to the room and reports feeling chest tightness, dizziness, and dyspnea. The patient says they have had anxiety in the past and feels that this is similar. How should the nurse proceed?

A) Administer benzodiazepine, and continue to monitor.

B) Obtain a 12-lead ECG.

C) Tell the patient that anxiety is common but not a medical emergency.

D) Give the patient a paper bag to breathe into.

127. A nurse working in the open-heart preop unit is responsible for educating patients and their families when patients are scheduled to undergo coronary artery bypass grafts surgery. A considerable number of patients are from the nearby Native American community and are dissatisfied with the limit on the number of family members allowed to attend the educational sessions. What action by the nurse would be at the highest level of competency within clinical inquiry?

A) Allow an additional two family members to attend if patient is Native American.

B) Approach the department director with the observations, and inquire about changing this policy.

C) Make sure the receptionist stresses the permitted number of family when confirming appointments.

D) If additional family comes, tell them that they will have to wait outside.

128. The nurse is reviewing the chart of a patient who will be transferred from surgical step-down for respiratory depression and lethargy after a glioblastoma debulking. The chart notes that the patient has diplopia. How can the nurse best facilitate the patient's comfort during assessments?

A) Thoroughly explain each part of the assessment before touching patient.

B) Perform the assessment quickly to avoid overstimulating patient.

C) Delay assessment until the patient is more alert.

D) Copy and paste the previous nurse's assessment since it was completed recently.

129. A 28-year-old female is admitted to the ICU after an ATV accident where the patient hit the handlebars with her chest. Assessing the patient, the nurse notes jugular vein distention and muffled heart sounds on auscultation. The patient gasps and says that she is having severe pain in the mid chest. The arterial line in the right wrist suddenly reads 95/63. What assessment finding may indicate aortic dissection?

A) manual BP measurement in left arm 130/52

B) pulsus paradoxus

C) bradycardia

D) manual BP measurement in right lower extremity 170/62

130. A MICU patient is intubated with a diagnosis of status asthmaticus. A morning ABG was obtained with the following results: pH 7.54, PaO_2 88 mm Hg, $PaCO_2$ 24 mm Hg, and HCO_3 24 mEq/L. How should the nurse interpret these findings?

A) compensated respiratory alkalosis

B) uncompensated metabolic alkalosis

C) compensated metabolic alkalosis

D) uncompensated respiratory alkalosis

131. A patient with status asthmaticus shows a significant left upper lobe pneumothorax on chest X-ray. What is the nursing priority?

A) Set up for an immediate thoracentesis.

B) Call for a stat paracentesis tray.

C) Set up for an immediate chest tube insertion.

D) Draw a stat ABG, and notify the respiratory intensivist.

132. Which of the following would be a contraindication for noninvasive positive pressure ventilation?

A) atrial fibrillation

B) RASS of −5

C) hypercapnic failure

D) flail chest

133. Which of the following patients is at the highest risk for developing diabetes insipidus?

A) 32-year-old female with bilateral pneumonia

B) 47-year-old male with bleeding esophageal varices being treated by vasopressin therapy

C) 26-year-old male who sustained a basilar skull fracture sustained in a motor vehicle crash

D) 86-year-old female with an acute exacerbation of chronic heart failure

134. A patient with hepatic failure has a peritoneal drain on the left outer quadrant to drain ascites. The nurse notes that drainage has decreased from 25 mL/hr to no output. The insertion site appears reddened and has a purulent exudate around the tube. What intervention would be most likely?

A) Flush catheter with a 3 mL syringe to encourage drainage.

B) Remove catheter at bedside, and notify physician.

C) Use IR to check the drainage tube for possible replacement.

D) Redress, and continue to monitor.

135. A MICU patient is intubated with a diagnosis of status asthmaticus. The nurse auscultates this patient's lung fields and finds bilateral wheezes present, with markedly diminished breath sounds in all areas. This finding indicates

A) the presence of bilateral pneumothorax.

B) that the patient is not moving air and that respiratory collapse is imminent.

C) consolidated pneumonia in all lung fields.

D) that the endotracheal tube is dislodged.

136. A patient with COPD required increasing levels of O_2 decompensated and was placed on a vent. The vent settings were at FiO_2 55% with a positive end-expiratory pressure of 8 cm for the past 24 hours. What condition is this patient at risk for?

A) ARDS

B) CO_2 retention

C) sepsis

D) pneumothorax

137. Which of the following IV solutions should be administered to a patient with DKA who is placed on an insulin drip?

A) lactated Ringer's

B) NS

C) NS with potassium

D) NS with dextrose

138. What learning tool is the gold standard for ensuring that the patient understands learning objectives?

A) The patient can teach the knowledge back to the nurse.

B) The patient's family member actively listens and has health care experience.

C) The patient nods when listening to instructions.

D) The patient states that they will rely on home care to take care of needs on discharge.

139. The nurse is calculating the initial dose of N-acetylcysteine for a 93 kg patient who overdosed on acetaminophen. What is the correct loading dose for this patient?

A) 1.5 g

B) 5 g

C) 13 g

D) 28.6 mg

140. The ED nurse is waiting for a bed for a 72-year-old patient with Alzheimer's disease who has episodes of confusion. Which of the following will be included in the plan of care for this patient?

A) Prescribe haloperidol to prevent agitation.

B) Provide toileting every 2 hours.

C) Use restraints at night to prevent wandering.

D) Allow choices when possible to promote feelings of respect.

141. A patient with delirium has scored high on a fall risk assessment tool. Standard precautions have been initiated, but the patient continues to try to get up without using the call light. What nursing intervention would be best for this patient?

A) Move this patient closer to the nurse's station.

B) Place the patient on a bed or chair alarm.

C) Restrain the patient.

D) Utilize a patient safety companion.

142. Which of the following electrolyte abnormalities is positive Chvostek sign associated with?

A) hyponatremia

B) hypomagnesemia

C) hyperphosphatemia

D) hypocalcemia

143. A 63-year-old female with thyroid cancer had a tracheostomy tube placed 1 week ago. The patient has been utilizing a 1-way valve to enhance communication. What must the nurse ensure when placing the 1-way valve?

A) that the cuff is deflated

B) that multiple sizes of tracheostomy tubes are available at the bedside

C) that the cuff is inflated to 10 mm

D) that there is an extra nurse at the bedside

144. A patient with cardiogenic shock is expected to have

A) hypertension; dyspnea.

B) decreased urine output; warm, pink skin.

C) increased urine output; cool, clammy skin.

D) hypotension; weak pulse; cool, clammy skin.

145. A patient with V/Q mismatch should be placed

A) in a non-recumbent position with the head of the bed raised 45 – 90 degrees.

B) with the left lung down.

C) in the reverse Trendelenburg position.

D) with the least affected area of the lung in the most dependent position.

146. Which of the following clinical presentations is consistent with a diagnosis of SIADH?

A) hyperosmolar state with systemic edema

B) reduced urine output with dilutional hyponatremia

C) hypotensive state with hyperkalemia

D) neurogenic shock with urinary output > 10 L/24 hr

147. Which of the following is a barrier to incorporating systems thinking into patient care?

A) using available resources

B) negotiating on behalf of patient and family

C) solving issues by relying only on personal experience

D) initiating change to improve patient care

148. A nurse receives a report from EMS of a 40-year-old patient who is unresponsive after a motor vehicle crash. EMS states that they suspect the patient has a spinal injury at C2. The patient will be admitted directly to the ICU. What should the nurse do first to prepare for the patient's arrival?

A) Call respiratory to set up a ventilator in the room.

B) Notify the charge nurse that this patient does not require ICU care.

C) Request a portable telemetry unit to maximize patient mobility.

D) Prepare a vial of methylprednisolone for immediate injection.

149. A 24-year-old patient with idiopathic pulmonary fibrosis is receiving fluids, O_2 supplementation, and supportive care in the ICU after being admitted for dyspnea and pleuritic chest pain. Labs are drawn in the morning and are as follows: WBC 22,000/ μL, HgB 13.5 g/dL, PLT 223,000/μL, and fasting blood glucose 215 mg/dL. What is the most likely cause of the elevated blood glucose?

A) underlying undiagnosed diabetes

B) nebulizer albuterol treatments

C) broad-spectrum antibiotic

D) IV hydrocortisone

150. Which of the following increases a patient's risk for a PE?

A) long-term ticagrelor use after percutaneous coronary intervention

B) factor V Leiden

C) asthma

D) BMI of 19

PRACTICE TEST TWO ANSWER KEY

1. **D)** Compensated pulmonary hypertension is marked by a return to adequate cardiac output, and right atrial pressures will have normalized. The heart compensates by increasing the size of the right ventricle. Increased right atrial pressure, decreased cardiac output, and increased right ventricular hypertrophy are all seen in decompensating pulmonary hypertension. Decompensated pulmonary hypertension is marked by decreased pulmonary artery pressure and right-sided heart failure.

   Objective: Respiratory

   Subobjective: Pulmonary hypertension

2. **A)** Fluid boluses of 1 – 2 L normal saline (NS) should be used to treat hypotension. The patient is dehydrated at the cellular level and needs fluid resuscitation. Furosemide is used as a diuretic and would further dehydrate the patient, exacerbating the issue. Inotropes such as dopamine are used to promote cardiac contractility and will not hydrate the patient. D5W is not indicated, because it is not an isotonic solution that will add to the systemic fluid volume.

   Objective: Cardiovascular

   Subobjective: Acute coronary syndrome

3. **D)** The signs and symptoms of HELLP include hypertension, tachycardia, dyspnea, jaundice, fatigue, dehydration, and right upper quadrant pain. Bradycardia, left upper quadrant pain, fluid volume overload, and hypotension are not typically associated with this condition.

   Objective: Multisystem

   Subobjective: Life-threatening maternal/fetal complications

4. **A)** An intra-aortic balloon pump (IABP) is used to augment diastolic aortic pressure, thereby decreasing afterload and increasing cardiac output. The statement that it decreases cardiac output is incorrect. Blood flow is increased to the coronary arteries during inflation, which occurs during diastole and therefore directs blood flow toward the coronary arteries. Heparin therapy should be initiated during IABP insertion to prevent thrombus formation. Aortic regurgitation is a contraindication to IABP because leakage would make counterpulsation ineffective.

   Objective: Cardiovascular

   Subobjective: Manage patients requiring IABP

5. **D)** Type 2 respiratory failure causes marked hypercapnia of > 45 mm Hg due to failure of CO_2 exchange. ($PETCO_2$ reflects $PaCO_2$ values.) A PaO_2 of 48 mm Hg or an O_2 sat of 88% would be a type 1 respiratory failure due to hypoxemia. A $PaCO_2$ of 35 mmHg is within normal limits.

   Objective: Respiratory

   Subobjective: Acute respiratory failure

6. **C)** Clopidogrel is an alternative blood-thinning medication for before and after cardiac interventions when aspirin is contraindicated. The patient should be educated on the importance of adhering to a blood-thinner regimen for 6 months after TAVR placement. Prasugrel is used in conjunction with aspirin to prevent restenosis of stents. Tirofiban hydrochloride is an IV medication used during cardiac catheterization and given via bolus, then by continuous infusion for ≤ 18 hours after percutaneous coronary intervention. Enoxaparin is a blood thinner used prophylactically for the prevention of DVT.

   Objective: Cardiovascular

   Subobjective: Structural heart defects

7. **D)** Heparin should be held, and the physician notified immediately, as this patient has had recent surgery, may have been placed on an anticoagulant protocol postsurgery, and has an extremely low platelet count.

   Objective: Hematology and immunology

   Subobjective: Thrombocytopenia

8. **C)** Because of the caustic nature of the infusing medication, the nurse should suspect infiltration and should immediately stop the infusion and follow hospital protocol for extravasation.

   Objective: Integumentary

   Subobjective: IV infiltration

9. **A)** Asterixis is a reflex tested by having the patient hold out their arms and spread fingers. In patients with asterixis, this position of the hands elicits a flapping response. Because a patient with a GCS of 7 could not follow directions to perform this test, this charting should be questioned for accuracy. PERRLA is the evaluation of pupil size, shape, and reaction to light. Decorticate positioning is an involuntary posturing that involves rigid flexion of the arms with clenched fists and extended legs. Tremors may be noted on comatose patients.

   Objective: Neurological

   Subobjective: Encephalopathy

10. **C)** The patient is not tolerating liquid or soft food intake. This is a sign of a kink in the surgical sleeve and would require surgical intervention. The patient should be prepared for surgery and placed on NPO status until evaluated by the physician. If there is a kink in the surgical sleeve, the other options would not correct the issue, and progressing to a full diet may cause more harm.

    Objective: Multisystem

    Subobjective: Bariatric complications

11. **C)** Early mobility has been proven to improve patient outcomes, and the patient should be walking as soon as possible. The patient should be educated on safe pain relief options, and by including the patient in a plan they find acceptable, the nurse will increase likelihood that the patient will participate. The patient's pain should not be ignored, and forcing the patient to walk does not promote autonomy or learning. Ibuprofen is contraindicated with mitral valve replacement as the patient will be on anticoagulants.

    Objective: Multisystem

    Subobjective: Pain

12. **A)** To facilitate discharge planning for a patient diagnosed with a terminal illness and with no immediate social support network, the nurse should recommend a hospice consult. The goal of hospice care is to help the patient have the best quality of life for as long as possible. It would not be appropriate for the nurse to request a second opinion unless the patient specifically requested one. With no home care treatments mentioned in the scenario, hospice care is appropriate, given the patient's diagnosis. The patient is progressing through stages of grief, and tearfulness and depression are expected responses; a psychiatric evaluation for these responses is not warranted.

    Objective: Professional caring and ethical practice

    Subobjective: Caring practices

13. **B)** Even though the nurse is no longer in orientation, reaching out to mentor others is an advanced level of collaboration. Answer B provides support while still allowing the newer nurse to work through the problem. Leaving the nurse to fend for themselves or printing out instructions may lead to a delay in patient care.

    Objective: Professional caring and ethical practice

    Subobjective: Collaboration

14. **C)** Patients starting mood stabilizers and antidepressants often feel better very quickly. The risk is that they will assume they are better and discontinue treatment without a physician's supervision. Before discharge, a patient who has attempted suicide should be evaluated by a psychiatrist. A patient should never be restrained if they are not actively attempting to hurt themselves or others.

    Objective: Behavioral and psychosocial

    Subobjective: Suicidal ideation and/or behaviors

15. **D)** Residuals > 250 mL indicate a high gastric residual volume, and this patient has had increasing residuals. The patient is experiencing poor motility, and metoclopramide would improve motility. Omeprazole is a proton pump inhibitor; sodium polystyrene sulfonate is used to excrete potassium; and metolazone is a diuretic.

    Objective: Gastrointestinal

    Subobjective: Intervene to address barriers to nutritional /fluid adequacy

16. **B)** Before starting the infusion, the potassium value must be evaluated and corrected if < 3.3 mEq/L. WBC, sodium, and INR have no clinical significance in this scenario.

    Objective: Endocrine

    Subobjective: Diabetic ketoacidosis

17. **B)** As the patient's vital signs are stable, the patient's pain is a priority. Once pain is controlled, the assessment can continue. It is likely that breath sounds would be more easily identified when the patient can comfortably take a deeper breath. Documentation should never take precedence over treating a patient or their comfort level.

    Objective: Respiratory

    Subobjective: Thoracic trauma

18. **A)** A patient with an acute heart failure exacerbation requires positive airway pressure to improve oxygenation and decrease right ventricular afterload. The patient should be placed in Fowler's or semi-Fowler's position. Calcium channel blockers are contraindicated in patients with heart failure. The patient does not need a chest tube.

    Objective: Cardiovascular

    Subobjective: Heart failure

19. **B)** ST depression in the precordial leads should be considered a STEMI of the posterior wall. Anxiety disorder and mitral valve prolapse would not cause significant ECG changes. The ECG changes caused by a PE include tall, peaked T waves in II, III, and aVF, right bundle branch block, and right axis deviation.

    Objective: Cardiovascular

    Subobjective: Acute coronary syndrome

20. D) Patient dignity is important, as is respecting individuals' preferences. The nurse must be sure to put aside any biases based on age, sex, religion, or gender. The name and date of the patient should be verified for safety purposes, but the patient's preference for how they should be addressed must be acknowledged. As long as the hairpiece is not interfering with any patient care and is not a potential danger to the patient, the request to remove it is not appropriate. Patients should always be addressed by the name they prefer; a gender-nonconforming name is no different from a nickname.

Objective: Professional caring and ethical practice

Subobjective: Caring practices

21. C) The priority action is to remove the medications securely to prevent any accidental double dosing. It is imperative that the care team be aware of and control the medications that the patient is receiving while under the care of the hospital to prevent sentinel events. After medications are secure, the physician and pharmacy may be consulted on the possibility that the patient may continue to receive their own supplements. The patient should not be encouraged to take any medication that is not given by nursing staff.

Objective: Professional caring and ethical practice

Subobjective: Systems thinking

22. D) Benzodiazepines are typically used to treat recurrent seizure activity due to eclampsia. Labetalol and hydralazine hydrochloride are used to treat refractory hypertension. Phenytoin may be ordered, but it is diluted and infused slowly with a filter to prevent precipitation.

Objective: Multisystem

Subobjective: Life-threatening maternal/fetal complications

23. B) Weakness that is progressing from the feet upward after a recent infection is indicative of myasthenia gravis. Further evidence comes from the vitals, including classic signs of autonomic dysfunction. Neither cerebral palsy nor muscular dystrophy would be new onset for a patient in their late 50s. Tachycardia, not bradycardia, would be expected in untreated Guillain-Barré syndrome.

Objective: Neurological

Subobjective: Neuromuscular disorders

24. A) HHH therapy (induced hypertension, hypervolemia, and hemodilution) aims to prevent and treat cerebral vasospasms after the onset of subarachnoid hemorrhage. Hyponatremia is an electrolyte imbalance that may occur because of HHH therapy. The nurse should monitor for this condition, which may cause seizures and coma.

Objective: Neurological

Subobjective: Stroke (hemorrhage)

25. C) While all these responses are correct, the first actions should be to notify the physician and, because the fall was unwitnessed and the patient is on anticoagulant therapy, to complete a CT scan to rule out a cranial hemorrhage.

Objective: Musculoskeletal

Subobjective: Functional issues

26. D) Fecal management devices should not be used in patients who have had a bowel surgery within the past year. A fecal management device would cause significant discomfort to a patient with hemorrhoids. Anticoagulant therapy is not a contraindication but does bear close observation. A urinary tract infection is not a contraindication for use of a fecal management device.

Objective: Integumentary

Subobjective: Wounds (infectious)

27. C) A pneumothorax, a complication of total parenteral nutrition, is caused by improper central catheter placement or by a catheter that has migrated. Air embolism, fluid overload, and refeeding syndrome do not present with absent breath sounds.

Objective: Gastrointestinal

Subobjective: Manage patients requiring enteral and parenteral nutrition

28. D) The patient has a suspected UTI with markers of possible sepsis. This patient should be screened for sepsis, and protocol followed. A lactate test and blood cultures would be ordered before the nurse would initiate a fluid bolus and antibiotics.

Objective: Renal and Genitourinary

Subobjective: Infections

29. D) The patient who is diagnosed with disseminated intravascular coagulation (DIC) has both a clotting and a bleeding problem. Increased prothrombin time and partial thromboplastin time (PT/PTT), elevated D-dimer levels, decreased platelets, decreased hemoglobin, and a decreased fibrinogen level are all expected lab values for this patient.

Objective: Hematology and immunology

Subobjective: Coagulopathies

30. **C)** Threats cannot be tolerated within a health care facility, and the most appropriate response would be to call security for support. It is best if security is present to assist with deescalating the situation or to escort her out. Neither the nurse nor the other family members should attempt to remove the daughter from the room. The physician should be notified of the situation once safety concerns have been addressed.

Objective: Professional caring and ethical practice

Subobjective: Collaboration

31. **B)** The compensatory respiratory response of respiratory alkalosis through hyperventilation reduces the severity of metabolic acidosis, which can lead to cardiac arrest and death. As pCO_2 increases, there is a rapid increase in the flow of salicylates crossing the blood-brain barrier. Therefore, intubation and mechanical ventilation should be avoided unless absolutely necessary. Mechanical ventilation cannot keep the respiratory drive to flush CO_2 from the system. Correcting electrolyte imbalances, fluid resuscitation, and preventing hypoglycemia are all expected treatments for salicylate toxicity.

Objective: Multisystem

Subobjective: Toxic ingestion/exposure

32. **B)** Positioning the patient on the right side, not left, may help with lung expansion and perfusion. A thoracentesis to drain fluid evidenced by the white opacities seen on the X-ray and culture could ensure that antibiotic therapy is directed at the identified bacteria and would be reasonable to expect in this situation. Diuretics and an infusion of albumin are appropriate when the effusion is caused by congestive heart failure or low blood protein levels.

Objective: Respiratory

Subobjective: Acute respiratory infection

33. **C)** Although the vital signs are showing improvement, the patient's condition is not stable, especially with the syncope. The patient should be immediately transcutaneously paced. Because phenylephrine is a vasopressor that may induce bradycardia, this medication is contraindicated for this patient's situation. The patient has already received the maximum recommended dosage of atropine. Because the patient's HR is palpable, the ACLS dosage of epinephrine would not be indicated. A titratable IV infusion of dopamine or epinephrine would be more appropriate.

Objective: Cardiovascular

Subobjective: Dysrhythmias

34. **C)** PT (prothrombin time) and PTT (partial thromboplastin time) are blood tests that monitor the effectiveness of anticoagulant therapy. Hematocrit measures PRBCs, not necessarily anticoagulant effectiveness. HDL and LDL are components of cholesterol measurement. Troponin levels measure myocardial muscle injury.

Objective: Respiratory

Subobjective: Acute pulmonary embolus

35. **A)** Nitrates cause reduction in left ventricle and right ventricle preload by peripheral arterial and venous dilation. Patients with an inferior wall MI and RV infarction are highly dependent on RV filling pressures to maintain BP and cardiac output. In suspected RV infarct, morphine sulfate (a vasodilator) is contraindicated.

Objective: Cardiovascular

Subobjective: Acute coronary syndrome

36. **B)** Initially, a patient will present with rapid onset of polyuria and Kussmaul respirations with fruity breath odor, and they may have nausea and vomiting. As the symptoms progress, fluid deficit is common, resulting in oliguria. DKA causes metabolic acidosis. Blood glucose levels would typically increase as DKA progresses.

Objective: Endocrine

Subobjective: Diabetic ketoacidosis

37. **B)** Because of high ammonia levels, patients often develop asterixis. Coagulopathies may present as a bleeding nose. There is a high correlation between acute kidney injury and liver failure. Bilirubin levels will be increased, potassium will be decreased, and hypotension is common.

Objective: Gastrointestinal

Subobjective: Hepatic failure/coma

38. **C)** Although the patient is anemic, the baseline of renal patients is often lower than normal. The patient is having symptoms of congestive heart failure and might not tolerate the extra fluid of PRBCs. The potassium is already elevated, and dialysis will correct this imbalance. Heparin is used during dialysis to prevent thrombolysis and is not typically administered after. In chronic kidney disease, the kidneys cannot produce enough erythropoietin. Administering epoetin alfa (Epogen) stimulates bone marrow to increase RBC production.

Objective: Renal and genitourinary

Subobjective: Chronic kidney disease

39. B) In patients with compartment syndrome of the extremities, serum CK (creatine kinase) levels will increase as muscle breaks down. Patients developing compartment syndrome often experience increasing pain that is not expected for their injury and does not respond to analgesics. Poikilothermia and reduced pulses should be recognized as signs of compartment syndrome.

Objective: Musculoskeletal

Subobjective: Compartment syndrome

40. C) It is important to give family the opportunity to participate in the care of the patient and to work through the grieving process. An explanation that the nurse and aide are following protocols is insufficient. The nurse should explain the dying process and explain that although the brain is dead, the body continues to have normal functional processes. The family should not be made to leave for asking questions.

Objective: Multisystem

Subobjective: End-of-life care

41. A) A sepsis bundle should include IV fluid resuscitation, antibiotics, and vasopressors after fluid resuscitation if MAP is < 65. Antibiotics are used to treat sepsis regardless of the suspected initiating infection. If blood cultures are ordered, they should be drawn before the administration of antibiotics.

Objective: Multisystem

Subobjective: Septic shock

42. A) Collaboration includes working with health care colleagues to promote individual contributions to advance patient care. Professionals may collaborate through group meetings, like councils, that allow team members to contribute ideas focused on improving care delivery. Reaching out to an expert department further demonstrates a group's willingness to learn new strategies; such openness is key for higher-level collaboration.

Objective: Professional caring and ethical practice

Subobjective: Collaboration

43. D) The neurologist, not the nurse, should notify the family of results. Repeating the apnea test would be called for if there was spontaneous respiratory effort. The patient would not be extubated until the physician received further results and the family was notified. ABG results should be drawn after 8 minutes, and results would be included in the evidence for a clinical diagnosis of brain death.

Objective: Neurological

Subobjective: Brain death

44. D) In ventricular fibrillation, it is appropriate to attempt defibrillation 2 times before administering medications. As this would be the second attempt at defibrillation, the joules should be set to 300. A setting of 360 J would be appropriate for the third attempt at defibrillation. Epinephrine would be administered before amiodarone. The initial dose for amiodarone utilizing ACLS protocol would be 300 mg, not 150 mg.

Objective: Cardiovascular

Subobjective: Dysrhythmias

45. C) In identifying a patient safety issue and collaborating with an advanced practice expert, the nurse is using evidence-based practice, research, and experiential knowledge to advance nursing care.

Objective: Professional caring and ethical practice

Subobjective: Clinical inquiry

46. B) A diet order will be required before the nurse can order any food or drink for the patient, but such an order is not the top safety priority. Aspiration leading to nosocomial pneumonia and longer patient stays are associated with post-extubation dysphagia. To reduce the risk of aspiration, a swallow assessment should take place within 24 hours of extubation and passed before the patient can take anything by mouth (including ice chips). Cultural and personal nutritional preferences should be updated in documentation and referred to when ordering sustenance.

Objective: Respiratory

Subobjective: Aspiration

47. B) This was a compensated blood gas because the pH is normal, but other values are not normal. A pH of 7.35 – 7.39 would fall on the compensated acidosis side of the continuum, whereas a pH of 7.41 – 7.45 would fall on the compensated alkalosis side. Normal $PaCO_2$ is 35 – 45 mm Hg, so in this case, the elevated $PaCO_2$ indicates a primary respiratory acidosis. Normal HCO_3 is 22 – 26 mEq/L, so the body has worked hard to compensate for the identified respiratory acidosis, as seen by an HCO_3 of 32 mEq/L. Therefore, the answer is a compensated (normal) respiratory (elevated $PaCO_2$) acidosis (pH on the acidotic side).

Objective: Respiratory

Subobjective: Interpret blood gas results

48. A) Octreotide acetate, an antidiarrheal medication administered via subcutaneous injection, is used in the treatment of dumping syndrome. Metoprolol may be the cause of the hypotensive episode, but it is not used to treat this condition. Insulin is a contraindication because late dumping syndrome may be caused by a hypersecretion of insulin. Vancomycin is a broad-spectrum antibiotic and is not used in the treatment of this condition.

Objective: Multisystem

Subobjective: Bariatric complications

49. **A)** When an organ donor patient dies in the ED, the nurse should first contact the organ procurement organization because of time sensitivity. Life-supporting interventions such as ventilators and medications should be continued until the organ procurement agency arrives. Postmortem care can be provided and the death certificate completed after organ procurement has taken place.

Objective: Professional issues

Subobjective: Patient (end-of-life issues)

50. **C)** Phase 2 amniotic fluid embolism presents as profuse hemorrhage and DIC. This phase progresses from cardiac arrest, acute respiratory distress syndrome, and multisystem organ failure that is seen in phase 1 amniotic fluid embolism. Postpartum hemorrhage is a symptom of this condition and is not the overall diagnosis for these sequelae. Placenta accreta presents as hemorrhage but without the other signs and symptoms noted.

Objective: Multisystem

Subobjective: Life-threatening maternal/fetal complications

51. **A)** The patient should be restarted on buprenorphine by an authorized provider, and treatment should avoid further use of opioids. The nurse should expect to use alternative and adjuvant treatments to control pain. Increasing opioid use or immediately ceasing use of any opioids is detrimental to the patient's recovery from addiction.

Objective: Behavioral and psychosocial

Subobjective: Substance use disorders

52. **B)** While a bleed risk does accompany this medication, clopidogrel is not evaluated via PLT or PT/INR values. This medication should not be held unless there is a specific order to not administer medication. Amyotrophic lateral sclerosis exacerbation often involves swallowing difficulty. Because clopidogrel is a large tablet that may pose a choking risk for someone with dysphagia, a swallow evaluation should be completed as soon as possible. The patient may require an NG tube to ensure that the medication is administered.

Objective: Neurological

Subobjective: Neuromuscular disorders

53. **C)** The major sequela to too-aggressive removal of fluid accumulation by thoracentesis is the emergent condition of reexpansion pulmonary edema. A pneumothorax, or collapsed lung, may occur spontaneously or be induced through a puncture to the pleural wall. Empyema is purulent fluid within the pleural space and may be drained via pleurocentesis. An opposite lung collapse would not be a risk associated with thoracentesis.

Objective: Respiratory

Subobjective: Thoracentesis

54. **C)** Nausea, vomiting, and abdominal cramping typically accompany opioid withdrawal. Tremors and insomnia are more typical with alcohol withdrawal. Tachycardia, tachypnea, and hypertension, not hypotension, would be more accurate signs of opioid withdrawal as well.

Objective: Behavioral and psychosocial

Subobjective: Substance use disorders

55. **D)** The patient is in respiratory distress because of oversedation. Because a benzodiazepine was administered, a dose of flumazenil should be administered with monitoring for improvement in O_2 sats and alertness. Naloxone would be given if the oversedation was caused by opioid administration. If the medication is not effective, the nurse should call a rapid response. Increasing fluids would not be effective in treating the oversedation and may put the patient into fluid volume overload.

Objective: Multisystem

Subobjective: Toxic ingestion/exposure

56. **C)** All possible measures should be used to allow for patient visitation, even during the pandemic crisis. The family and patient should be notified of the patient visitor policy but also given alternatives that are available. By sharing the teleconference app with the family members, the nurse gives them a way to visit with the patient virtually. Answers B and D help the family contact the facility and primary nurse, but these options ignore the virtual visit option.

Objective: Professional caring and ethical practice

Subobjective: Caring practices

57. **A)** Followers of the Jewish faith may consult their rabbi when making decisions. Care conference should be made to accommodate for a large number of individuals if the patient requests it. Jewish law does generally mandate extension of life. However, easing the patient's suffering may take priority, depending on interpretation of the religious law.

Objective: Professional caring and ethical practice

Subobjective: Response to diversity

58. D) A cardiac catheterization may be completed after less invasive diagnostic testing is completed. As the patient has a bundle branch block, an ECG will not rule out ST elevation. Troponin levels should be repeated 6 hours from the initial draw, but this test is not the priority. A pericardial rub, tachycardia, hypotension, and severe chest pain that is reduced by rest and changing positions are signs of cardiac tamponade. A chest X-ray should be ordered to rule out cardiac tamponade. Alternatively, an echocardiogram would also be an appropriate diagnostic test for these symptoms.

Objective: Cardiovascular

Subobjective: Cardiac tamponade

59. D) Beta blockers may mask cardiovascular symptoms of hypoglycemia such as tachycardia, diaphoresis, irritability, restlessness, and cool skin.

Objective: Endocrine

Subobjective: Hypoglycemia (acute)

60. B) NSAIDs, including aspirin, are inappropriate as they can cause further bleeding. The patient is kept NPO because of gastric bleeding, and the head of bed is elevated to prevent aspiration. Fluid resuscitation will restore hemodynamic stability. Proton pump inhibitors can help relieve pain and prevent further gastric damage.

Objective: Gastrointestinal

Subobjective: Acute GI hemorrhage

61. D) Loop diuretics waste potassium. Supplements are usually initiated when treatment is started.

Objective: Renal and genitourinary

Subobjective: Life-threatening electrolyte imbalances

62. D) Patients with suspected viral meningitis should be placed under seizure precautions. Bacterial meningitis requires droplet precautions until 24 hours have passed since antibiotics have been started. Neutropenic precautions are to protect immunocompromised patients undergoing chemotherapy. Contact precautions are not indicated.

Objective: Neurological

Subobjective: Neurological infectious disease

63. A) Patients with severe cerebral edema lose autoregulation control, and the result is hypotension that is difficult to control. Fluid management to maintain a cerebral perfusion pressure > 70 mm Hg

and MAP > 60 mm Hg has the greatest effect on outcomes. Vasopressors, not vasodilators, would be used to maintain pressures. Mannitol may further induce hypotension. Sedatives can cause vasodilation and should be used cautiously when needed to maintain patient comfort. Because this patient is nonresponsive, they should not be receiving sedatives, which may mask neurological responsiveness.

Objective: Neurological

Subobjective: Traumatic brain injury

64. C) Targeted temperature management is used to prevent neurological damage in post-cardiac-arrest patients. The lowered temperature decreases cerebral metabolism, and the brain requires less oxygen. The inflammatory response is also reduced, as is the amount of reperfusion injury. This therapy is not aimed at preventing damage to any other organ system.

Objective: Cardiovascular

Subobjective: Manage patients requiring defibrillation

65. C) The nurse should review the care expectations of this unit because he is responsible for providing care at that level. Policies may differ from his home unit, and vital sign frequency and documentation should be clarified with the charge nurse. The nurse would be expected to work at the level of his license; demanding to work as an assistant would not be appropriate. Answer D may jeopardize patient safety if the standard of care for this patient population is unmet.

Objective: Professional caring and ethical practice

Subobjective: Clinical judgment

66. D) Visitation during end-of-life care should be as allowable and accommodating to the patient as possible. Gaining permission from the nursing supervisor before notifying the patient's family is the best option so that it has been approved. The family should not feel as if they are breaking rules and may be caught. Requiring the patient and family to wait until morning may cause undue stress for both parties. Rushing the visit to fit within the stated times in this case is insensitive to the patient's needs.

Objective: Multisystem

Subobjective: End-of-life care

67. C) A transgender woman is clinically identified as someone who was assigned as male at birth but who has chosen to be identified as a woman. The sister is advocating for the patient's preferences, and the health care team must be made aware of the appropriate pronouns to address the patient.

Communicating this preference only to the charge nurse does not ensure that other health care team members are using the correct pronouns. Patients should be addressed by preferred, not legal, pronouns. There is no reason to escalate this simple request to an ethics committee.

Objective: Professional caring and ethical practice

Subobjective: Response to diversity

68. **B)** "Do not resuscitate" allows for medications and non-resuscitative action, while "allow natural death" gives all care aside from interventions that would prevent a natural progression to death. Neither action withholds appropriate and nonemergent care. Nurses can and should have discussions with patients and family to clarify end-of-life and lifesaving options. Option D projects the nurse's bias onto the family.

Objective: Professional caring and ethical practice

Subobjective: Collaboration

69. **C)** Lactate levels are drawn at the initial identification of sepsis and after 6 hours to evaluate for tissue ischemia. An elevated level that is sustained for > 6 hours is associated with an increase in mortality rates. Alanine aminotransferase (ALT) is a liver enzyme, while creatinine evaluates kidney function. Both these lab values are important in monitoring for progression to multiple organ dysfunction syndrome. WBC is used in the initial diagnosis of sepsis.

Objective: Multisystem

Subobjective: Septic shock

70. **D)** An external ventricular drain is an invasive procedure that places a drain in the ventricle of the nondominant hemisphere to enable ICP monitoring and to drain CSF. Neurological pupil index is read via a handheld infrared pupillometer. Because the drain is placed transcutaneously, infection is a risk.

Objective: Neurological

Subobjective: Increased intracranial pressure

71. **B)** The muscle weakness, electrolyte imbalances, and severely elevated creatine kinase (CK) indicate that the patient has developed rhabdomyolysis secondary to alcoholism. Fluid support and sodium polystyrene sulfonate to correct the elevated potassium would be the appropriate treatment for this condition. Discontinuing CIWA protocol places the patient at risk for developing delirium tremens. Because the patient's calcium levels are elevated, calcium gluconate would put him at risk for coma and dysrhythmias.

Objective: Musculoskeletal

Subobjective: Rhabdomyolysis

72. **D)** The patient's potassium levels are critically high. Administering IV dextrose and insulin is the priority intervention, as this will shift potassium to intercellular spaces. Sodium polystyrene sulfonate is used to lower potassium levels but will not work fast enough. IV fluids should be administered cautiously in patients with chronic renal failure and will not lower potassium levels. The patient will need dialysis, but this is not the priority intervention.

Objective: Renal and genitourinary

Subobjective: Chronic kidney disease

73. **A)** The patient has transitioned from the oliguric phase, which is characterized by urine output of < 400 mL/day, to the diuretic phase, which may have output of up to 3 L per day.

Objective: Renal and genitourinary

Subobjective: Acute kidney injury

74. **B)** One of the most common causes of pancreatitis is alcohol abuse. This patient should be screened for alcohol history and be monitored for development of alcohol withdrawal while hospitalized. The other assessments, including the STOP-Bang test for severe sleep apnea, are important but are not specific to this patient population.

Objective: Gastrointestinal

Subobjective: Pancreatitis

75. **A)** B-type natriuretic peptide (BNP) levels are used to assess cardiac function and can help diagnose fluid overload. In fluid overload, sodium levels would be decreased through hemodilution. Hct and serum osmolality would also be decreased because of extra fluid volume.

Objective: Cardiovascular

Subobjective: Heart failure

76. **D)** The patient is stable in supraventricular tachycardia (SVT), so the most noninvasive treatment (vagal maneuvers) should be performed first. Adenosine is the first drug of choice if vagal maneuvers are unsuccessful. Defibrillation is not used in conscious patients with organized heart rhythms. Synchronized cardioversion is not indicated for a stable patient in SVT.

Objective: Cardiovascular emergencies

Subobjective: Dysrhythmias

77. **B)** The classic signs of cardiac tamponade, an emergency situation, include Beck's triad: jugular vein distension due to the impaired venous blood flow returning to the right side of the heart, muffled

heart sounds as the pericardial effusion builds, and hypotension as the mechanical pressure from fluid in the pericardial sac reduces stroke volume and therefore cardiac output. Widening pulse pressure is reflective of aortic stenosis, thyrotoxicosis, and chronic aortic regurgitation, among other systemic disease processes.

Objective: Cardiovascular

Subobjective: Cardiac tamponade

78. **C)** The patient may be retaining fluid because of syndrome of inappropriate antidiuretic hormone secretion (SIADH). Because of the high risk for seizures due to decreased sodium levels, seizure precautions would be appropriate. Fluid restriction and sodium replacement are also appropriate treatments. The other options would be appropriate treatment for central diabetes insipidus.

Objective: Endocrine

Subobjective: SIADH

79. **D)** Choice D best exemplifies patient-centered care and caring practices. The other responses are in line with advocacy/moral agency and clinical judgment.

Objective: Professional caring and ethical practice

Subobjective: Caring practices

80. **D)** The Rumack-Matthew nomogram is used to predict the risk of hepatoxicity by comparing serum acetaminophen concentrations with the estimated time since ingestion occurred. This chart does not evaluate for any damage that may have occurred; it just predicts risk. N-acetylcysteine is administered as an initial loading dosage followed by a weight-based dose. The Rumack-Matthew nomogram does not predict the efficacy of activated charcoal in treatment.

Objective: Multisystem

Subobjective: Toxic ingestion/exposure

81. **C)** The first step of implementing an evidence-based practice project is to define the scope of the project. The scope is best defined with a PICOT question (patient, intervention, comparison, outcome, time). The nurse should not look up patients in the electronic medical record (EMR) without permission or without being involved in patient care; doing so violates HIPAA. The librarian will be better able to locate resources with the direction of the PICOT. The Code Blue team is an excellent resource, but the nurse should maintain responsibility for project management.

Objective: Professional caring and ethical practice

Subobjective: Clinical inquiry

82. **A)** The participation in the community health event on a topic that the ED nurse would see in patients in the clinical setting demonstrates advocacy for the patient, family, and community. Developing an inpatient care plan that includes family advocates for the patient and family but fails to meet community involvement. Working toward a BSN or recruiting an RN may benefit patient care but does not directly advocate for the community.

Objective: Professional caring and ethical practice

Subobjective: Advocacy/moral agency

83. **B)** The patient is unstable in a third-degree or complete heart block, so transcutaneous pacing is indicated.

Objective: Cardiovascular emergencies

Subobjective: Dysrhythmias

84. **D)** The patient should be educated on the difference between his prescribed medication (a bronchodilator) and his spouse's medication (a corticosteroid). Inhaled corticosteroids are minimally effective at relieving symptoms of COPD, and if he continues to rely on his spouse's inhaler he will likely experience another acute exacerbation. Some form of chest physiotherapy may be ordered for the patient, but it should not replace his prescribed medications. While the nurse may suggest the patient inquire about other medication options, only the pharmacist or prescribing provider may suggest specific medications. The patient should be discouraged from using another person's medication and should not be taught to use the fluticasone inhaler.

Objective: Respiratory

Subobjective: Chronic conditions

85. **C)** Without lung transplant, pulmonary fibrosis progresses and death typically occurs within 3 – 5 years of initial diagnosis. Hospice should not be recommended without a thorough consultation from the physician.

Objective: Respiratory

Subobjective: Pulmonary fibrosis

86. **D)** Transient right bundle branch block and peaked T waves in leads II, II, and aVF are typical ECG changes in the presence of a PE. Right axis deviation, also commonly seen, causes a deflection of the QRS in lead I. ST elevation is not an expected sign of PE and should always be ruled out as a possible cardiac infarction.

Objective: Respiratory

Subobjective: Acute pulmonary embolism

87. C) Since the patient has no palpable pulse, the first intervention should be immediate initiation of CPR. Since there is a rhythm being detected, the patient is in pulseless electrical activity (PEA). This is not a shockable rhythm, so defibrillation is not indicated. A 1 mg dose of IV push epinephrine would be administered as soon as possible, but chest compressions are the priority. D is not appropriate; PEA is a medical emergency and requires intervention.

Objective: Cardiovascular

Subobjective: Dysrhythmias

88. D) When a patient is experiencing hallucinations, the nurse should acknowledge the patient's fear but reinforce reality. Telling the patient that it is the wrinkles in the blanket dismisses the patient's fear and does not reorient the patient. Offering to move the patient to another room suggests that the snakes are real and does not help the patient with reality. Offering to call maintenance reinforces the patient's belief that the snakes are real.

Objective: Neurological

Subobjective: Delirium

89. B) Bilateral dilation and fixation of the pupils are signs of a midbrain injury that could be caused by increased ICP. Answers A and C are within normal limits. Kussmaul respirations are seen with diabetes or metabolic acidosis; rather, Cheyne-Stokes breathing pattern would indicate increasing ICP.

Objective: Neurological

Subobjective: Traumatic brain injury

90. A) The patient is distressed that family has not arrived. The nurse should recognize that the patient wants companionship through the dying process and should fulfill that surrogate role. Avoidance is ignoring this patient's needs. Administering an anxiolytic to cause sedation and compliance may be considered a chemical restraint.

Objective: Multisystem

Subobjective: End-of-life care

91. D) The nurse's identification of a need to improve patient care on the basis of policy, procedure, and standards falls under the core competency of *caring practices*.

Objective: Professional caring and ethical practice

Subobjective: Caring practices

92. A) The patient's shock would be categorized as hypovolemic because the hemorrhage has caused a reduction in intravascular volume. Cardiogenic and obstructive shock are due to reduced cardiac output. Cardiogenic shock originates from cardiac tissue damage, whereas obstructive shock is unrelated to cardiac tissue damage. Distributive shock is caused by massive vasodilation.

Objective: Multisystem

Subobjective: Shock states

93. A) The anterior wall of the heart is supplied by the left anterior descending artery, a major branch of the left coronary artery. The right coronary artery supplies the right atrium, the right ventricle, and the inferior-posterior wall of the left ventricle. For 90% of people, the right coronary artery supplies blood to the atrioventricular node.

Objective: Cardiovascular

Subobjective: Acute coronary syndrome

94. C) The patient is taking an ACE inhibitor, which increases the risk for hyperkalemia. Potassium is wasted by the kidneys, and the patient is at risk for retaining further potassium. Lab values and ECG changes should be closely monitored for signs of hyperkalemia. Anemia would be a concern with chronic kidney failure as the kidneys produce erythropoietin, which stimulates RBC production. Calcium and blood glucose changes are not of significant concern with ACE inhibitor usage.

Objective: Cardiovascular

Subobjective: Cardiomyopathies

95. C) The patient has developed dyspnea and increased temperature from baseline. Although the symptoms may be a febrile nonhemolytic reaction, the transfusion should be stopped until acute hemolytic reaction and sepsis are ruled out. Administering an antipyretic to address the fever is appropriate. Since these are not symptoms of an allergic reaction, administering an antihistamine would not be appropriate.

Objective: Hematology and immunology

Subobjective: Transfusion reactions

96. A) Prone positioning is an effective therapy for the patient with acute respiratory distress syndrome (ARDS) on a ventilator. Prone positioning reduces compression of the heart and abdominal muscles (compared with supine position), redistributes blood and air flow more evenly in the lungs, reduces ventilator-induced lung injury, and decreases aspiration risk.

Objective: Respiratory

Subobjective: ARDS

97. C) Keeping the wife with the husband would be the best solution for this night. It is not reasonable to expect that the wife could care for herself should a room at a nearby hotel be available. Calling a family member to let them know the situation would be appropriate, but to demand that they do something is not the best solution. Chastising the patient and wife will not change or help the situation. The social worker should be consulted to assist with their living situation and offer further resources.

Objective: Professional caring and ethical practice

Subobjective: Advocacy/moral agency

98. A) All accommodations should be made to allow family members their request if it is not impeding the efforts of the code team and is not a risk to patient care. It is best practice to allow family to witness code situations in a safe manner. Allowing the durable power of attorney to observe from outside the room is the best compromise in this situation. Leaving the family in the waiting room alone does not advocate for the patient or family. Allowing all the family to stay in the room is likely to distract the response team and may interfere with patient care. Closing the curtains prevents the family from witnessing the resuscitative efforts on the patient and would not help the family members make informed choices.

Objective: Professional caring and ethical practice

Subobjective: Advocacy/moral agency

99. C) With each fluid bolus, the elevated lactate level should decrease by 10%. The first 2 responses are interpretive and do not ensure that tissue perfusion is adequate. A cardiac output of 6 L/min is within normal limits but will not determine adequate tissue perfusion if the patient has severe vasodilation or systemic vascular resistance.

Objective: Multisystem

Subobjective: Septic shock

100. B) Hyperkalemia will cause bradycardia and tall, peaked T waves. Patients with hypokalemia will have ventricular dysrhythmias like premature ventricular contractions, ventricular tachycardia, ventricular fibrillation, or the presence of U waves. Hyponatremia can cause such neurologic effects as a decreased level of consciousness or seizure activity.

Objective: Cardiovascular

Subobjective: Dysrhythmias

101. A) Being morbidly obese and having a retroperitoneal bleed, this patient is at a very high risk for developing abdominal compartment syndrome. A Foley catheter that measures intravesical pressure may be used to monitor intra-abdominal pressures. Excessive positive end-expiratory pressure is contraindicated as it may decrease cardiac output. A supine position should be maintained; raising the head of bed increases intra-abdominal pressure. Although an NG tube may be placed for nasogastric decompression, enteral nutrition delivery is not a priority at this time and the patient should remain NPO in anticipation of the possible need for surgery.

Objective: Gastrointestinal

Subobjective: Abdominal compartment syndrome

102. C) The normal sodium range is 135 to 145 mEq/L. Levels < 120 mEq/L are critical and may lead to death if left untreated. The values given for chloride, calcium, and potassium are within the normal range and do not require treatment.

Objective: Renal and genitourinary

Subobjective: Life-threatening electrolyte imbalances

103. B) Hyperosmolar hyperglycemic state most often affects adults > 65 with cardiovascular disease. The 86-year-old has those 2 conditions plus obesity. Patients A and D have 2 risk factors, while C may be at risk for DKA.

Objective: Endocrine

Subobjective: Hyperosmolar hyperglycemic state (HHS)

104. D) Cardiac silhouette enlargement and bilateral pleural effusion is a classic sign of heart failure. An elevated BNP (> 100 pg/mL) is a strong diagnostic sign for heart failure, so BNP < 70 pg/mL is not of concern. Acute left-sided systolic heart failure would result in a reduced ejection fraction (< 40%). Pericarditis may add to or cause acute heart failure, but is not a common sign in heart failure.

Objective: Cardiovascular

Subobjective: Heart failure

105. A) Expertise requires insightful anticipation of potential obstacles and recognition and intervention when these obstacles are encountered. The nurse needs staff acceptance and support to make a change that will affect the whole unit. Changes should be discussed over a longer period of time than a single shift huddle to ensure all staff understand and will be compliant. The nurse should take responsibility for the practice change rather than relying on the manager to introduce the project. Implementing the change only with the nurse's own patients creates a deviation in practice and does not allow for a unit change.

Objective: Professional caring and ethical practice

Subobjective: Caring practices

106. D) Patients with diabetes are instructed to protect their feet because neuropathies can diminish feeling and lead to injury and infection. The patient's statement is contradictory to best practice and indicates that further teaching is required. The comment about healthy eating habits demonstrates that the patient is open to change and willing to follow the advice of a health care expert. Seeking a referral to a foot care clinic shows that the patient understands the importance of follow-up care. The ability to teach back with minimal assistance shows that the patient is progressing with this skill.

Objective: Professional caring and ethical practice

Subobjective: Facilitation of learning

107. C) The American Heart Association suggests that amiodarone should be used only if chemical or electrical cardioversion is not successful in correcting unstable supraventricular tachycardia. Short-term management of the condition can be initiated with vagal maneuvers and the administration of adenosine 6 mg (an antidysrhythmic), verapamil (a calcium channel blocker that causes vasodilation and reduces the pumping work of the heart), or digoxin (a glycoside that controls rate and rhythm of the heart as well as strengthening the pumping action of the heart).

Objective: Cardiovascular

Subobjective: Dysrhythmias

108. C) Beta blockers work by inhibiting the action of epinephrine (adrenaline). This results in decreased preload and afterload, thereby lessening workload. Amiodarone is an antiarrhythmic that treats certain ventricular tachycardias and other dysrhythmias. Clopidogrel is an anticoagulant. Morphine sulfate is an opioid analgesic that also causes vasodilation and is used in the acute MI stage to reduce myocardial workload.

Objective: Cardiovascular

Subobjective: Acute coronary syndrome

109. A) The patient continues with severe hypercapnia and respiratory acidosis, both of which are now showing some improvement, and the SpO_2 is markedly improved and indicates the hypoxemia is resolved. This ABG does NOT indicate a compensated

hypercapnia ($PaCO_2$ 35 – 45 mm Hg is normal). Hypoxemia is resolved (> 90% SpO_2 as indicated on pulse oximeter), and there is nothing alkalotic on these postintubation ABG measurements (normal pH range is 7.35 – 7.45).

Objective: Respiratory

Subobjective: Interpret blood gas results

110. B) Hyperosmolar hyperglycemic state (HHS) is often caused by dehydration, especially in patients > 65. Inadequate glucose monitoring and medication noncompliance are not the most common causes of HHS. A breakdown of ketones causing ketoacidosis would be found in DKA.

Objective: Endocrine

Subobjective: Hyperosmolar hyperglycemic state (HHS)

111. C) An angiogram uses dye that is nephrotoxic. The performing physician should be notified to ensure that a minimal amount of dye is used or that an alternative medium, such as CO_2, is used. An X-ray and CT scan without contrast would be safe for this patient. A hepatobiliary iminodiacetic acid (HIDA) scan uses a radioactive tracer that does not affect kidney function.

Objective: Gastrointestinal

Subobjective: Acute GI hemorrhage

112. B) The patient's skull fracture depression is greater than 6 mm and requires immediate attention; it will likely need to be treated via surgical depression. Antibiotics are standard treatment for all skull fractures, but their administration is not the nurse's priority in this scenario.

Objective: Neurological

Subobjective: Traumatic brain injury

113. B) Before moving forward in the admission process, the nurse should verify what pronouns the patient would prefer to be addressed with. The other responses should be obtained regardless of a patient's gender identity.

Objective: Professional caring and ethical practice

Subobjective: Response to diversity

114. B) Grey Turner's sign is ecchymosis on the flank, a clear indication of a retro-peritoneal bleed from the angioplasty. The accumulation of blood leads to the assessed back pain. Hypotension, bradycardia, rhythm changes are additional indications of an unstable cardiovascular condition. Reduction in pedal pulses, especially on the operative side, and coolness to touch indicate impairment to circulation.

Objective: Cardiovascular

Subobjective: Cardiac/vascular catheterization

115. D) The patient's blood glucose level does not indicate a need for D50. The patient is going to surgery and would be NPO; juice would be contraindicated. This is refractory hypoglycemia and should be treated. Starting continuous infusion of D10 via peripheral IV or D20 via central line is the appropriate action to treat refractory hypoglycemia.

Objective: Endocrine

Subobjective: Hypoglycemia (acute)

116. B) After a myocardial infarction, elevation in troponin levels may be detected within 2 – 4 hours of symptom onset.

Objective: Cardiovascular

Subobjective: Acute coronary syndrome

117. A) Although another chest X-ray may be obtained, the nurse should prepare the patient and set up the room for an immediate chest tube insertion. Because of the blunt-force trauma to the chest with rib fractures, the patient is probably experiencing either a hemothorax or a pneumothorax. Even though the initial chest X-ray did not detect either condition, hemothorax and pneumothorax can present quickly and must be treated emergently. In light of the patient's symptoms, it would be inappropriate to transport them and await a CT scan. Intubation would not alleviate the symptoms.

Objective: Respiratory

Subobjective: Thoracic trauma

118. D) Acetaminophen is cleared by liver metabolism, not kidney, and would not be implicated as a causative agent of acute renal failure. An MAP < 65 for > 30 minutes can create acute renal failure due to vasoconstriction of renal profusion and cellular hypoxia. Dopamine at 16 mg/kg/min also causes vasoconstriction of renal blood flow and cellular ischemia, resulting in acute renal failure. A vancomycin trough of 22.3 is nephrotoxic, a causative agent of acute renal failure.

Objective: Renal and genitourinary

Subobjective: Acute kidney injury

119. A) The patient should be provided analgesia preemptively to allow it enough time to take effect before the procedure. A sterile tray will need to be set up, but controlling the patient's pain and maintaining comfort throughout the procedure is the priority. Including a family member in the dressing change provides an educational opportunity because the patient will be sent home requiring further changes. Cultures should always be obtained from the bed of the wound.

Objective: Integumentary

Subobjective: Cellulitis

120. C) A blunt injury to the back of the head can produce a basilar fracture that affects the middle fossa. Battle sign is an accumulation of blood that pools behind the ears in the mastoid area, but it is not typically present during the initial evaluation. On day 2 onward, evidence of bruising will appear and is strongly indicative of a basilar fracture. Periorbital ecchymosis (raccoon eyes) is blood pooling around the eyes. When bilateral, this sign is highly predictive of a middle cranial, rather than anterior cranial, fossa basilar fracture. Rhinorrhea (CSF fluid leaking from the nose) may be delayed days after the initial head trauma.

Objective: Neurological

Subobjective: Traumatic brain injury

121. D) Because the physician is withholding the full long-term consequences of this procedure, the principle of autonomy is being violated. Response B is incorrect; the physician is not discussing the case outside the care team and patient's family. The physician's personal bias may be that extending the person's life is the highest achievable good for the patient and attempting to promote life for the patient (utilitarianism and beneficence).

Objective: Professional caring and ethical practice

Subobjective: Collaboration

122. C) A pain goal should be set with the patient as the IV medications were initially ordered for postsurgical pain, and the pain is now consistent with what the patient chronically experiences. Setting a goal will allow the nurse and the patient to agree on an established pathway to treat the pain more effectively. Accusations of drug-seeking behavior negate the patient's subjective pain experience and compromise a trusting relationship. Options B and C are not appropriate for the treatment of chronic pain and are likely to lead to complications of oversedation.

Objective: Multisystem

Subobjective: Pain

123. B) Cauda equina syndrome includes symptoms of sensory loss in the lower extremities, loss of reflexes in the upper extremities, and bowel and bladder dysfunction. Anterior spinal cord syndrome results in complete loss of motor and sensory function below the lesion. With central cord syndrome, there is greater motor function and paresthesia in the upper extremities than in the lower extremities, without urinary or bowel dysfunction. Neurogenic shock results in marked hypotension caused by the automatic nervous system's inducing system-wide vasodilation.

Objective: Neurological

Subobjective: Acute spinal cord injuries

124. **C)** The distinctive Brugada morphology on an ECG can be caused by sodium channel blockade (such as cocaine), hyperkalemia, beta blockers, anti-angina medications, psychotropic drugs, or alcohol. While the ST elevation strain pattern may look like a STEMI, it is not and will resolve in 3 – 4 hours as active cocaine is metabolized. The presence of troponin elevation below the 99th percentile reference range indicates no myocardial infarction. The patient's unresponsiveness to nitroglycerin rules out angina. Papillary muscle rupture usually occurs 2 – 7 days post-MI.

Objective: Cardiovascular

Subobjective: Myocardial conduction system defects

125. **C)** A nondominant right hemisphere stroke will have signs such as rambling speech, left-sided vision changes and sensory loss, spatial disorientation, and difficulty with problem solving. Right hemiparesis and emotional lability are associated with ischemia of the dominant left hemisphere. Sensory loss in all 4 limbs is noted with involvement of the posterior hemisphere, cerebellum, or brainstem.

Objective: Neurological

Subobjective: Stroke (ischemic)

126. **B)** Although the patient has had anxiety in the past and feels that the symptoms are similar, a cardiac origin for the symptoms should first be ruled out. Option A would be reasonable if a full assessment shows no cardiac or respiratory sources for the symptoms. Options C and D are not appropriate.

Objective: Behavioral and psychosocial

Subobjective: Anxiety

127. **B)** Recognizing a recurrent source of patient dissatisfaction, the nurse approaches the director about a policy change that would take into account different patient populations. The policy should be adjusted to accommodate any patient, not just Native Americans. Reminding family of the limit does not fix the issue or improve patient relations. An expert nurse would individualize the policy to accommodate the family that is already there and not send them away.

Objective: Professional caring and ethical practice

Subobjective: Clinical inquiry

128. **A)** The nurse should verbally notify the patient with each step of the assessment or procedure, because a patient with diplopia (double vision) may not be able to clearly see what is about to happen. The nurse should also avoid quick movements to avoid startling or causing the patient to become dizzy. The patient is being transferred because of a need for a higher level of care, and the primary nurse must perform an assessment as soon as the patient arrives to the ICU.

Objective: Professional caring and ethical practice

Subobjective: Clinical inquiry

129. **A)** Blunt aortic injuries may cause a pressure gradient between upper extremities. Since the BP in the left arm is > 30 mm Hg systolically, it can be considered clinically significant and should be reported to the physician. Pulsus paradoxus is a BP change during inspiration and is seen with cardiac tamponade; tachycardia would be expected. Aortic disruption may also cause a difference in upper and lower extremities, but typically, the hypertension would occur in the upper extremity, and hypotension in the lower.

Objective: Cardiovascular

Subobjective: Cardiac trauma

130. **D)** As the ABG shows that the pH is > 7.45 (normal range 7.35 – 7.45), the CCRN candidate knows that this patient is alkalotic. The $PaCO_2$ is low (normal range 35 – 45 mm Hg), indicating respiratory alkalosis. Since the HCO_3 is normal at 24 mEq/L (normal range 22 – 26 mEq/L), this is not a metabolic problem, and therefore, the patient has an uncompensated respiratory alkalosis.

Objective: Respiratory

Subobjective: Interpret blood gas results

131. **C)** Re-expansion of the left lung by the insertion of a chest tube is indicated for a 40% or larger pneumothorax. A small pneumothorax could heal on its own but is a high risk factor when mechanical ventilation is in place. A thoracentesis is used to remove a pleural effusion, which is not what occurs with a pneumothorax event. A paracentesis procedure is done to remove ascites to relieve symptoms and analyze the fluid collected to identify underlying disease. Drawing a stat ABG is inappropriate, as lung re-expansion is necessary to correct any ventilation/perfusion mismatch.

Objective: Respiratory

Subobjective: Status asthmaticus

132. B) Noninvasive positive pressure ventilation should never be utilized in a patient who is not conscious. A RASS (Richmond Agitation-Sedation Scale) rating of −5 indicates that the patient is not arousable. Atrial fibrillation is not an arrythmia contraindicated with noninvasive ventilation. Nor are hypercapnic failure and flail chest contraindicated with this sort of noninvasive ventilation.

Objective: Respiratory

Subobjective: Manage patients requiring noninvasive positive pressure ventilation

133. C) Basilar skull fractures from head trauma are the second most common cause of diabetes insipidus. Diabetes insipidus may also be seen in neurosurgical patients and patients with meningitis, Hodgkin's disease, tumors, sarcoidosis, and syphilis. Pneumonia and a high level of vasopressin administration would predispose a patient to develop SIADH. Heart failure is not generally seen as a cause of diabetes insipidus.

Objective: Endocrine

Subobjective: Diabetes insipidus

134. C) The physician should be notified of the reduced output and irritation at site. Interventional radiology (IR) can be used to check tube placement and to reveal whether a new tube needs to be placed. The tube may be cultured for potential microbials. When flushing, the nurse should use a syringe ≥ 10 mL to prevent excessive pressure. These catheters are sutured in and must be removed surgically. The findings are concerning and require follow-up.

Objective: Gastrointestinal

Subobjective: Manage patients requiring GI drains

135. B) Decreased breath sounds is a clinical sign of grave concern. It indicates that the patient is not moving air, and both ventilation and perfusion will be profoundly affected, leading to respiratory collapse. If the patient was showing evidence of bilateral pneumothorax, the breath sounds would be diminished (or absent) in the lower lobes but clearly audible to auscultation in the upper lobes. Pneumonia is heard as bronchial breath sounds: continuous loud breath sounds heard on exhalation. A dislodged endotracheal tube will cause unilateral breath sounds.

Objective: Respiratory

Subobjective: Status asthmaticus

136. A) Patients maintained at > 50% FiO_2 have a higher chance of developing acute respiratory distress syndrome (ARDS). The patient is being ventilated, so CO_2 clearance is optimized. There is no indication

that this patient has an infection that would escalate to sepsis. Vented patients are at an increased risk for pneumothorax at high positive end-expiratory pressures of > 10 cm.

Objective: Respiratory

Subobjective: ARDS

137. C) Insulin administration shifts potassium into the cells and causes hypokalemia, so fluids with potassium are indicated for this patient. The other fluids are not indicated for this patient.

Objective: Endocrine

Subobjective: Diabetic ketoacidosis

138. A) Having patients teach the health education material or skills back to the nurse ensures that the patient can competently address their own health care needs. Although family may assist the patient at home, the patient, when capable, should be fully engaged in their own care. Nodding does not indicate understanding. Relying on home care for the patient's needs leaves them vulnerable and may produce a poor outcome if the care is not provided as intended.

Objective: Professional caring and ethical practice

Subobjective: Facilitation of learning

139. C) The loading dose of N-acetylcysteine to treat acetaminophen overdose is 140 mg/kg. So, 93 kg × 140 mg/kg = 13,020 mg. The correct dosage is 13 g.

Objective: Multisystem

Subobjective: Toxic ingestion/exposure

140. B) As Alzheimer's disease progresses, confusion increases. Providing regular toileting can prevent possible falls that result when a patient is hurrying to the bathroom to maintain continence. Haloperidol should be used with extreme caution in geriatric patients with Alzheimer's. Restraints can increase confusion in these patients and should be used only per facility guidelines. Offering too many choices can overwhelm the patient and lead to increased confusion and frustration.

Objective: Neurological

Subobjective: Dementia

141. D) Options A and B would be reasonable if the patient did not have a high fall risk. The patient should only be restrained as a last option. This patient would benefit most from having a safety companion at the bedside.

Objective: Musculoskeletal

Subobjective: Functional issues

142. D) Chvostek sign (an abnormal spasm of the facial muscles when the lower jaw is lightly tapped) is an early sign of low calcium, although it may occur in 20 – 25% of non-calcium-depleted patients. The sign is considered a strong indicator for treatment to prevent tetany. Chvostek sign will not be apparent if patient has clinical tetany, because the involuntary response to stimuli cannot overcome strong facial muscle contractures inherent in advanced hypocalcemia.

Objective: Renal and genitourinary

Subobjective: Life-threatening electrolyte imbalances

143. A) Placing a 1-way valve while the cuff is inflated will block the patient's airway. The cuff must always be deflated before placement. An extra tracheostomy tube should be at the bedside of every patient with a tracheostomy, but multiple sizes are not needed. An extra nurse is required during tracheostomy tube changes, but not when placing a 1-way valve.

Objective: Respiratory

Subobjective: Tracheostomy

144. D) Classic signs of cardiogenic shock include a rapid pulse that weakens; cool, clammy skin; and decreased urine output. Hypotension is another classic sign.

Objective: Cardiovascular

Subobjective: Cardiogenic shock

145. D) Reducing anatomical pressure exerted by the abdominal organs on the heart and lungs will help the lung fields more fully expand during ventilation and improve perfusion. The reverse Trendelenburg position will also increase the flow of more oxygen-saturated blood throughout the system. Positioning with the least affected area of the lung in the most dependent position reflects this rationale. Prone positioning for the intubated, mechanically ventilated patient has been shown to improve ventilation/perfusion (V/Q) mismatch issues, when done with careful management. The other options will increase the amount of abdominal pressure.

Objective: Respiratory

Subobjective: Chronic conditions

146. B) Syndrome of inappropriate antidiuretic hormone secretion (SIADH), the result of increased ADH levels, reduces urine output. The cardinal sign of SIADH is hyponatremia because the body's "holding on to water" dilutes serum sodium levels. A hyperosmolar state is typically caused by dehydration and may result in cerebral edema. Hyperkalemia increases the risk of cardiac dysrhythmias, which can induce

hypotension and shock. Neurogenic shock is related to spinal injuries, while SIADH is a hormonal imbalance that stimulates the kidneys to retain water.

Objective: Endocrine

Subobjective: SIADH

147. C) When approaching an issue, the CCRN candidate should view the problem from numerous perspectives and consider how it could best be solved with the available resources pertinent to the situation. The other responses are all ways that systems thinking can be used and upheld.

Objective: Professional caring and ethical practice

Subobjective: Systems thinking

148. A) C1 and C2 injuries require mechanical ventilation and are completely ventilatory dependent; a ventilator should be prepared before the patient arrives. This patient would require critical care nursing. Because the patient will not be mobile and will likely remain in spinal precautions and traction indefinitely, promoting mobility would not be a priority at this time. Methylprednisolone is not an emergent, resuscitative medication and would not be administered without an order.

Objective: Neurological

Subobjective: Acute spinal cord injury

149. D) IV steroids, such as hydrocortisone, have the side effect of elevating both WBC and blood glucose. As these patient populations are closely monitored, it is unlikely that the patient has new-onset undiagnosed diabetes. Albuterol treatments and antibiotics have not been found to cause a significant change in blood glucose levels of people with diabetes or those who are not diabetic.

Objective: Respiratory

Subobjective: Pulmonary fibrosis

150. B) Factor V Leiden, a mutation of one of the blood clotting factors, can increase a person's chance of developing thrombus in the lower extremities and lungs. Ticagrelor is an anticoagulant and would decrease the risk for blood clot formation. Asthma may be exacerbated by a PE because of the increased risk for bronchoconstriction but does not increase a patient's risk of PE. A BMI > 26 puts patients at a greater risk for blood clots.

Objective: Respiratory

Subobjective: Acute pulmonary embolism

15 APPENDIX A: ABBREVIATIONS

A

A&O×3: awake and oriented to person, place, and time

A-a gradient: alveolar-arterial gradient

AAA: abdominal aortic aneurysm

ABC: A1c (hemoglobin), blood pressure, and cholesterol

ABCs: airway, breathing, circulation (emergency treatment)

ABG: arterial blood gas

ABPI: ankle-brachial pressure index

AC ventilation: assist-control ventilation

ACA: anterior cerebral artery

ACE inhibitors: angiotensin-converting enzyme inhibitors

ACLS: advanced cardiovascular life support

ACPE: acute cardiogenic pulmonary edema

ACS: acute coronary syndrome *or* abdominal compartment syndrome

ACTH: adrenocorticotropic hormone stimulation test

ADH: antidiuretic hormone

AFE: amniotic fluid embolism

A-fib: atrial fibrillation

AHRQ: US Agency for Healthcare Research and Quality

AIDS: acquired immunodeficiency syndrome

AIS: acute ischemic stroke

AKI: acute kidney injury (formerly called acute renal failure, ARF)

ALI: acute lung injury (no longer used; instead use mild, moderate, or severe ARDS)

ALL: acute lymphocytic leukemia

ALP: alkaline phosphatase

ALS: amyotrophic lateral sclerosis

ALT: alanine aminotransferase or alanine transaminase

AMA: against medical advice or American Medical Association

AML: acute myeloid leukemia

AND: allow natural death

AOM: acute otitis media

APP: abdominal perfusion pressure

aPTT: activated partial thromboplastin time

AR: aortic regurgitation

ARBs: angiotensin II receptor blockers

ARDS: acute respiratory distress syndrome

ARF: acute respiratory failure (sometimes acute renal failure, which is now called acute kidney injury [AKI])

AS: aortic stenosis

ASCVD: atherosclerotic cardiovascular disease

ASIA: American Spinal Injury Association

AST: aspartate aminotransferase or aspartate transaminase

ATN: acute tubular necrosis

AUB: abnormal uterine bleeding

aVF: augmented vector foot (ECG lead)

aVL: augmented vector left (ECG lead)

AVM: arteriovenous malformation

aVR: augmented vector right (ECG lead)

B

BAI: blunt aortic injury

BBB: bundle branch block

BCI: blunt cardiac injury

BiPAP or BPAP: bilevel positive airway pressure

BNP: B-type natriuretic peptide

BP: blood pressure

BPH: benign prostatic hyperplasia

bpm: beats per minute (in all caps [BPM], breaths per minute)

BPS: Behavioral Pain Scale

BRAT: banana, rice, applesauce, toast (e.g., BRAT diet)

BSA: body surface area

BUN: blood urea nitrogen

BZK: benzalkonium chloride (e.g., BZK wipes)

C

CA-MRSA: community-acquired methicillin-resistant *Staphylococcus aureus*

CABG: coronary artery bypass graft

CAD: coronary artery disease

CAM-ICU: Confusion Assessment Method for the ICU

CaO₂: arterial oxygen content

CAOD: carotid artery occlusive disease (stenosis)

CAP: community-acquired pneumonia

CAUTI: catheter-associated urinary tract infection

CBC: complete blood count

CBF: cerebral blood flow

CCB: calcium channel blocker

CDC: Centers for Disease Control and Prevention

CHF: congestive heart failure

CI: cardiac index

CISD: critical incident stress debriefing

CISM: critical incident stress management

CIWA-Ar: Clinical Institute Withdrawal Assessment for Alcohol

CK: creatine kinase

CK-MB: creatine kinase–muscle/brain

CKD: chronic kidney disease

CLABSI: central line associated bloodstream infection

CLL: chronic lymphocytic leukemia

CML: chronic myelogenous leukemia

CMP: comprehensive metabolic panel

CN: cranial nerve

CNS: central nervous system

CO: cardiac output

COBRA: Consolidated Omnibus Budget Reconciliation Act

COCA: color, odor, clarity, amount (urinary assessment)

COPD: chronic obstructive pulmonary disease

COWS: Clinical Opiate Withdrawal Scale

CP: cerebral palsy

CPAP: continuous positive airway pressure

CPG: clinical practice guideline

CPP: cerebral perfusion pressure

CPR: cardiopulmonary resuscitation

CrCl: creatinine clearance

CRF: chronic renal failure

CRI: cutaneous radiation injury

CRP: C-reactive protein

CRRT: continuous renal replacement therapy

CRT: capillary refill time

CS: culture and sensitivity

CSF: cerebrospinal fluid

CSM: circulation, sensation, and movement

CT scan: computed tomography scan

cTnI: troponin I

cTnT: troponin T

CTPA: computed tomography pulmonary angiography

CVA: cerebrovascular accident

CVP: central venous pressure

CVVH: continuous venovenous hemofiltration

CXR: chest X-ray

D

D&C: dilation and curettage

D50: dextrose 50% solution

D5W: dextrose 5% in water

DAI: diffuse axonal injury

DBP: diastolic blood pressure

DCCM: dilated congestive cardiomyopathy

DDS: dialysis disequilibrium syndrome

DI: diabetes insipidus

DIC: disseminated intravascular coagulation (or coagulopathy)

DKA: diabetic ketoacidosis

DM: diabetes mellitus

DMARDs: disease-modifying antirheumatic drugs

DNA: deoxyribonucleic acid

DNI: do not intubate

DNR: do not resuscitate

DO$_2$: oxygen delivery

DPL: diagnostic peritoneal lavage

DPOA: durable power of attorney

DSRS: distal splenorenal shunt

DT: diphtheria and tetanus (vaccine)

DTs: delirium tremens

DTaP: diphtheria, tetanus, and pertussis (vaccine)

DTI: deep tissue injury

DTPA: diethylenetriamine pentaacetate

DTs: delirium tremens

DUBB: dangerous underwater breath-holding behaviors

DVT: deep vein thrombosis

E

EAPs: Employee Assistance Programs

EBP: evidence-based practice

ECF: extracellular fluid

ECG: electrocardiogram

ECMO: extracorporeal membrane oxygenation

ECR: extracorporeal core rewarming

ED: emergency department

EDH: epidural hematoma

EEG: electroencephalogram

EF: ejection fraction

EGD: esophagogastroduodenoscopy

EIA: enzyme immunoassay

ELISA: enzyme-linked immunosorbent assay

EMB: ethambutol

EMTALA: Emergency Medical Treatment and Active Labor Act

EN: enteral nutrition

EPAP: expiratory positive airway pressure

ERCP: endoscopic retrograde cholangiopancreatography

ESI: Emergency Severity Index

ESR: erythrocyte sedimentation rate

ESRD: end-stage renal disease

ESWL: extracorporeal shock wave lithotripsy

ETCO$_2$: end-tidal CO_2 measurement (capnography)

ETT or **ET tube**: endotracheal tube

EVD: external ventricular drain

EVL: endoscopic variceal band ligation

F

FAST ultrasound (or exam): focused assessment with sonography for trauma

FDP: fibrin degradation products

FES: fat embolism syndrome

FFP: fresh frozen plasma

FiO$_2$: fraction of inspired oxygen

FLT3: fms-related tyrosine kinase 3

FRC: functional residual capacity

FSH: follicle-stimulating hormone

FSP: fibrin split products

G

G-tube: gastrostomy tube

GABA: gamma-aminobutyric acid

GCS: Glasgow Coma Scale

GER: gastroesophageal reflux

GERD: gastroesophageal reflux disease

GFR: glomerular filtration rate

GGT: gamma-glutamyl transferase

GI: gastrointestinal

GRV: gastric residual volume

GSW: gunshot wound

GU: genitourinary

H

H/H: hemoglobin and hematocrit

HA-MRSA: hospital-acquired methicillin-resistant *Staphylococcus aureus*

HAP: hospital-acquired pneumonia

HBO: hyperbaric oxygen therapy

HBSS: Hanks' Balanced Salt Solution

HCAHPS: Hospital Consumer Assessment of Healthcare Providers and Systems

hCG: human chorionic gonadotropin

HCM: hypertrophic cardiomyopathy

HCS: Hazard Communication Standard

Hct: hematocrit

HELLP syndrome: hemolysis, elevated liver enzymes, low platelet count

HF: heart failure

HFpEF: heart failure with preserved ejection fraction (diastolic heart failure)

HFrEF: heart failure with reduced ejection fraction (systolic heart failure)

HgB: hemoglobin

HHH: hypertensive, hypervolemic, hemodilution therapy

HHNK: hyperglycemic hyperosmolar nonketotic syndrome

HHS: hyperosmolar hyperglycemic state

HIET: hyperinsulinemia euglycemia therapy

HIPAA: Health Insurance Portability and Accountability Act

HIT: heparin-induced thrombocytopenia

HIV: human immunodeficiency virus

HOB: head of bed

HR: heart rate

HSV: herpes simplex virus

I

I:E ratio: inspiratory-expiratory ratio

I/O or **I&O**: intake and output

IABP: intra-aortic balloon pump

IAP: intra-abdominal pressure

IBD: inflammatory bowel disease

IBS: irritable bowel syndrome

IC: inspiratory capacity

ICD: implantable cardioverter defibrillator

ICDSC: Intensive Care Delirium Screening Checklist

ICF: intracellular fluid

ICH: intracerebral hemorrhage

ICP: intracranial pressure

ICS: incident command system

ICU: intensive care unit

IgM: immunoglobulin M

IM: intramuscular

INH: isoniazid

INR: international normalized ratio

IO: intraosseous (infusion)

IPAP: inspiratory positive airway pressure

ITP: idiopathic thrombocytopenic purpura

IUD: intrauterine device

IV: intravenous

IVAC: infection-related ventilator-associated conditions

IVH: intraventricular hemorrhage

IVIG: intravenous immunoglobulin

IVP: intravenous pyelography

J

JVD: jugular vein distention

K

KUB: kidney, ureter, bladder

L

LAD: left anterior descending

LBBB: left bundle branch block

LD or **LDH:** L-lactate dehydrogenase

LET: liquid emulsion therapy

LFT: liver function test

LLQ: left lower quadrant

LMA: laryngeal mask airway

LOC: level of consciousness

LPN: licensed practical nurse

LPV: lung-protective ventilation

LUQ: left upper quadrant

LV: left ventricle

LVAD: left ventricular assist device

LVEDP: left ventricular end-diastolic pressure

LVN: licensed vocational nurse

LVO: large-vessel occlusion

M

MAP: mean arterial pressure

MAR: medication administration record

MCA: middle cerebral artery

MCH: mean corpuscular hemoglobin

MCHC: mean corpuscular hemoglobin concentration

MCI: mass casualty incident

MCV: mean corpuscular volume

MD: muscular dystrophy

mEq: milliequivalent

MG: myasthenia gravis

MI: myocardial infarction

MICU: mobile ICU

MMI: methimazole

MMSE: mini-mental state exam

MODS: multiple organ dysfunction syndrome

MPAP: mean pulmonary artery pressure

MR: mitral regurgitation

MRI: magnetic resonance imaging

MRSA: methicillin-resistant *Staphylococcus aureus*

MS: multiple sclerosis *or* mitral stenosis

MSDS: material safety data sheets

MVC: motor vehicle crash/motorized vehicle crash

N

NAAT: nucleic acid amplification test

NG tube: nasogastric tube

NIF: negative inspiratory force

NIH: National Institutes of Health

NIHSS: National Institutes of Health Stroke Scale

NIV: noninvasive ventilation

NMB: neuromuscular blockade

NO: nitric oxide

NPE: noncardiogenic pulmonary edema

NPi: neurological pupil index

NPO: *nil per os* (Latin for "nothing by mouth"; patient should consume no food or fluids)

NPWT: negative pressure wound therapy

NSAID: nonsteroidal anti-inflammatory drug

NSTEMI: non-ST-elevation myocardial infarction

NSTIs: necrotizing soft-tissue infections

O

OG tube: orogastric tube

OME: otitis media with effusion

P

PA: pulmonary arterial

PAC: pulmonary artery catheter

PaCO$_2$: partial pressure of carbon dioxide

PACU: post-anesthesia care unit

PAD: peripheral arterial disease

PALM-COEIN: polyp, adenomyosis, leiomyoma, malignancy, coagulopathy, ovulatory disorder, endometrial, iatrogenic, not otherwise classified (risk factors for abdominal uterine bleeding)

PAP: pulmonary artery pressure

PaO$_2$: partial pressure of oxygen

PAOP: pulmonary artery occlusion pressure

PCA: posterior cerebral artery

PCC: prothrombin complex concentrate

PCI: percutaneous coronary intervention

PCR: polymerase chain reaction

PCWP: pulmonary capillary wedge pressure

PE: pulmonary embolism *or* pulmonary embolus

PEA: pulseless electrical activity

PEEP: positive end-expiratory pressure

PEFR: peak expiratory flow rate

PETCO$_2$: patient end-tidal CO$_2$ measurement (capnography, also called ETCO$_2$)

P/F ratio: PaO$_2$ divided by patient's FiO$_2$

PH: pulmonary hypertension

PHH: postprandial hyperinsulinemic hypoglycemia

PHI: protected health information

PICC: peripherally inserted central catheter

PICS: post-intensive-care syndrome

PID: pelvic inflammatory disease

PLT: platelet count

PO: *per os* (by mouth)

PPE: personal protective equipment

PPI: proton pump inhibitor

PPN: peripheral parenteral nutrition

PRBCs: packed red blood cells

PRN: *pro re nata* (as needed)

PSP: primary spontaneous pneumothorax

PSV: pressure support ventilation

PT: prothrombin time

PTA: percutaneous transluminal angioplasty

PTH: post-traumatic headaches

PTSD: post-traumatic stress disorder

PTT: partial thromboplastin time

PTU: propylthiouracil

PVC: premature ventricular contraction

PVD: peripheral vascular disease

PVR: pulmonary vascular resistance

PZA: pyrazinamide

R

RAAS: renin-angiotensin-aldosterone system

RAP: right atrial pressure

RASS: Richmond Agitation-Sedation Scale

RAWS: refractory alcohol withdrawal syndrome

RBBB: right bundle branch block

RBC: red blood cell

RCA: right coronary artery

RCM: restrictive cardiomyopathy

RhoGAM: Rho(D) immune globulin

RIF: rifampin

RIG: rabies immune globulin

RLL: right lower lobe (e.g., lung)

RLQ: right lower quadrant

ROM: range of motion

ROSC: return of spontaneous circulation

RPR: rapid plasma reagin

RR: respiratory rate

RSBI: rapid shallow breathing index

RSI: rapid sequence intubation

RSV: respiratory syncytial virus

RT–PCR: real-time polymerase chain reaction

RUQ: right upper quadrant

RVEDP: right ventricular end-diastolic pressure

RYGB: Roux-en-Y gastric bypass

S

SA: sinoatrial

SAH: subarachnoid hemorrhage

SANE: sexual assault nurse examiner

SaO$_2$: arterial oxygen saturation

SARS: severe acute respiratory syndrome

SAT: spontaneous awakening trials

SBP: systolic blood pressure

SBT: spontaneous breathing trials

SCCM: Society of Critical Care Medicine

SCI: spinal cord injury

ScvO$_2$: central venous oxygen saturation

SDH: subdural hematoma

SDS: safety data sheets

SG: vertical sleeve gastrectomy

SGOT: serum glutamic-oxaloacetic transaminase

SIADH: syndrome of inappropriate antidiuretic hormone secretion

SICU: surgical intensive care unit

SIMV: synchronized intermittent mandatory ventilation

SIRS: systemic inflammatory response syndrome

SND: sinus node dysfunction

SpO$_2$: peripheral capillary oxygen saturation or pulse oximetry

SSEP: somatosensory evoked potential

SSP: secondary spontaneous pneumothorax

SSS: sick sinus syndrome

START: simple triage and rapid treatment

STEMI: ST-segment elevation myocardial infarction

STI: sexually transmitted infection

SV: stroke volume

SvO$_2$: mixed venous saturation

SVR: systemic vascular resistance

SVT: supraventricular tachycardia

T

T&C: blood type and crossmatch

T&S: blood type and screen

TACO: transfusion-associated circulatory overload

TAVR: transcatheter aortic valve repair

TBI: traumatic brain injury

TBSA: total body surface area

TCCS: transcranial color-coded duplex sonography

TCD: transcranial Doppler study

TCP: transcutaneous pacing

Td: tetanus and diphtheria (vaccine)

Tdap: tetanus, diphtheria, and pertussis (booster DTaP vaccine)

TEE: transesophageal echocardiogram

TEN: total enteral nutrition

TF: tissue factor

TIA: transient ischemic attack

TIPS: transjugular intrahepatic portosystemic shunt

TLC: total lung capacity

TMJ: temporomandibular joint

tPA: tissue plasminogen activator

TPN: total parenteral nutrition

TRALI: transfusion-related acute lung injury

TSH: thyroid stimulating hormone

TTM: targeted temperature management

U

U/L: units per liter

ULQ: upper left quadrant

URQ: upper right quadrant

UTI: urinary tract infection

V

VAC: ventilator-associated conditions or vacuum-assisted wound closure

VAD: ventricular assist device

VAE: ventilator-associated events

VAP: ventilator-associated pneumonia

VATS: video-assisted thoracoscopic surgery

VBG: vertical band gastroplasty

VC: vital capacity

VDLR: venereal disease research laboratories

V-fib: ventricular fibrillation

VO$_2$: oxygen consumption

V/Q ratio: ventilation/perfusion ratio

VRE: vancomycin-resistant enterococci

V$_T$: tidal volume

V-tach: ventricular tachycardia

vW: von Willebrand factor

W

WBC: white blood cell

WHO: World Health Organization

16 APPENDIX B: SIGNS AND SYMPTOMS GLOSSARY

asterixis: bilateral tremor or "flapping" of the wrist or fingers

ataxia: abnormal, uncoordinated movements

bradycardia: slow heart rate

bradypnea: slow respiration rate

crepitus: abnormal cracking sounds heard in fractures, joints, or the lungs or in subcutaneous emphysema

diaphoresis: excessive sweating

dyspnea: difficulty breathing

ecchymosis: bruising

epistaxis: bleeding from the nose

erythema: redness of the skin

guarding: voluntary contraction of abdominal muscles to avoid pain

hematemesis: blood in vomit

hematochezia: bright red blood in stool

hemoptysis: blood in expectorate from respiratory tract

hepatomegaly: enlargement of liver

hyperpigmentation: darkening of the skin

hyperpyrexia: body temperature > 106.7°F (41.5°C)

hyperreflexia: overreactive reflexes

jaundice: yellowing of the skin or sclera

jugular vein distention: bulging of the superior vena cava due to increased pressure

lacrimation: excessive secretion of tears

lymphadenopathy: swollen lymph nodes

melena: dark, sticky digested blood in the stool

myalgia: muscle pain

mydriasis: pupil dilation

myoclonus: twitches or jerks of muscles

myoglobinuria: urine that is brown due to presence of myoglobin

nocturia: excessive urination at night

nuchal rigidity: inability to place the chin on the chest (neck flexion) due to muscle stiffness (indicator of meningitis)

nystagmus: repetitive, uncontrolled movement of the eyes

oliguria: low urine output

orthopnea: dyspnea that occurs while lying flat

otorrhea: drainage from the ear

pallor: pale appearance

paresthesia: abnormal dermal sensation such as burning or "pins and needles"

pericardial rub: characteristic heart sound caused by inflammation of the pericardium

petechiae: tiny red or brown spots on the skin caused by subcutaneous bleeding

photophobia: sensitivity to light

piloerection: erection of the hair

poikilothermia: inability to regulate body temperature

polydipsia: excessive thirst

polyphagia: excessive hunger

polyuria: abnormally high urine output

pruritus: severely itchy skin

pulsus alternans: alternating strong and weak pulse

pulsus paradoxus: abnormally large drop in blood pressure during inspiration

purpura: purple coloring on the skin caused by blood pooling around damaged blood vessels

rhinorrhea: drainage from the nose

S3 (ventricular gallop): an extra heart sound heard after S2, caused by a rush of blood into a ventricle; a normal finding in children and young adults

S4 (atrial gallop): an extra heart sound heard before S1, caused by the atrial contraction of blood into a noncompliant ventricle; can be a normal finding in older adults

spider angiomas: red skin lesions caused by dilated blood vessels

splinting: voluntary shallow breathing done to avoid pain caused by inspiration

steatorrhea: excretion of excess fat in the stool

syncope: temporary loss of consciousness

tachycardia: fast heart rate

tachypnea: fast respiratory rate

APPENDIX C: MEDICAL SIGNS

Battle sign: bruising behind the ears caused by a basilar skull fracture

Brudzinski's sign (indicator of meningitis): passive flexion of the neck elicits automatic flexion at the hips and knees

Chvostek sign: contraction of facial muscles in response to tapping over the facial nerve (CNVII)

Cullen sign: a bluish discoloration to the umbilical area

Grey Turner sign: ecchymosis in the flank area

Homans' sign: pain in the calf following dorsiflexion of the foot

Kehr sign: referred left shoulder pain caused when the diaphragm irritates the phrenic nerve

Kernig's sign (indicator of meningitis): patient in supine position with the hips and knees flexed, unable to straighten leg due to hamstring pain

Levine's sign: a clenched fist held over the chest in response to ischemic chest pain

Markle test (heel drop): pain caused when patient stands on tiptoes and drops heels down quickly or when patient hops on one leg

McBurney's point: RLQ pain at point halfway between umbilicus and iliac spine

Murphy sign: pain and cessation of inspiration when RUQ is palpated

Psoas sign: abdominal pain when right hip is hyperextended

Rovsing sign: pain in the RLQ with palpation of LLQ (indicates peritoneal irritation)

Trousseau sign: contraction of the hand and wrist following compression of the upper arm

Made in the USA
Monee, IL
13 October 2023

44565575R00199